TIME ZONES

Slipping Away....

by Wayne Glenn Terry

Cover photo by Mary Z. Smith.

The author, Wayne Glenn Terry, can be contacted at:

retcwo@yahoo.com

First printing, January 2009
© Nov, 2008 Wayne Glenn Terry
Printed in the United States. All rights reserved.

ISBN: 978-0-9795394-7-3

Father's Press, LLC
Lee's Summit, MO
(816) 600-6288
www.fatherspress.com
E-Mail: fatherspress@yahoo.com

Publisher's Comments

It's not often that an author asks his/her publisher to make a comment about their work, in their work, but Wayne put his head on the chopping block and asked me to give my thoughts on this piece. I know what you may be thinking. What risk is there from a publisher who has already decided to publish the book? But keep in mind that in many publishing houses projects are sometimes selected based on their marketing potential and the publisher may not share the sentiments of the author, especially if the author strays from the popular views of secular humanism and espouses Christian values. I guess Wayne's bravery comes from a lifetime of risk-taking in the service of our country and the realization that no matter what happens in this life, ultimately we all (believers) serve a higher power and will spend eternity in paradise.

It's impossible to predict where a book will land when you hurl it into the public sphere. When it comes to the invisible movement of God's hand, our finite minds cannot comprehend the ways that He uses unworthy vessels like Wayne, and me. But in His infinite wisdom, grace and perfect planning, He sometimes finds ways to use the most inept and afflicted of us to do His greatest works.

As you read this book, you will note that Wayne jumps around a lot. He spills his thoughts on a myriad of issues, most related to Alzheimer's, then takes you into prayer and Scriptural quotes. As you read you will, as I have, deeply admire Wayne's courage and unshakable faith in God. But this is not a book about Wayne. It is not even a book about Alzheimer's Disease. That is merely the vehicle through which Wayne illustrates God's grace and love for us.

Don't get me wrong. This book is a wonderful resource for anyone who is or may someday be afflicted with Alzheimer's, or is or may have to interact or care for someone with Alzheimer's. But the broader, overarching theme is that no matter what your affliction or condition, we believers are wrapped in the greatest strength and comfort in the universe to see us through.

So! Learn about Alzheimer's and benefit from Wayne's experience with this horrible disease. But keep in mind that life here is so temporary, and none of us are going to get off this planet alive. Ultimately, someday, sooner for some than others, we will all be on our knees before Jesus Christ as He judges us. You can be on your knees weeping with joy at the realization of what an eternity in Heaven really means, or you can be on your knees crying hysterically and trembling in stark fear as you realize the horror of the eternity that you will face in the lake of fire. But don't deceive yourself, on your knees you will be.

Therefore, friend, as you read, I urge you to open your mind and heart. Take an introspective look inward and identify your own affliction, whether it be physical, emotional, mental, or the many other conditions that can afflict us to the point that we are unable to connect with God, such as pride, self-absorbed humanism, materialism or procrastination and the lack of courage to face the tough questions. Then examine Wayne's analysis of God's grace, mercy and benevolence, and apply it to your own life.

Take a hard look and figure out for yourself what it is that is stopping you from facing the truth. What is it that you don't want to change or give up? Examine your motives. Let me assure you that no matter where you look, whether in your bank account, your resume, your toy-chest or your mirror, you will find nothing that entitles you to one ounce of pride or arrogance. By God's standards, we are all miserably unworthy, until we humble ourselves and accept His salvation.

As for your work, Wayne, well done. Your words will impact peoples' lives for generations to come. Thanks for setting aside your own pain and fear and spending your final days helping God expand His Kingdom. It's been one of the great honors of my life to have been a small part of this project. Hang tough, Brother.

Mike Smitley,
Publisher - Father's Press

FOREWORD

Alzheimer's disease is the quintessential adversary, the enemy at the gate, and the pervasive disease of mankind. By whatever label or measuring stick you use, the disease does get and deserve our constant attention.

It strips the individual of their uniqueness, those hard earned attributes we prize as memory, awareness, judgment, and indeed personality among others. Soon we have to rely on others to remind us and piece together our journey here on Earth. With the cruelest of intentions, it is no respecter of race, religion, economic status, or philosophy, but its strong suit is its ability to ravage the aged of the population and occasionally the younger.

There is hope that medical research will define a reliable biomarker, its pathophysiology, and a disease-modifying treatment worthy of consideration.

Winston Churchill once said, "Never, never, never quit!". No doubt, this statement encouraged his embattled countrymen of World War II. That phrase is appropriate for the task at hand, if only we can all remember never to lose that resolve.

John J. Hennessey, IV, MD.
Diplomat in Neurology
Associated Neurologist, P.C.
Richmond, VA

Wayne G. TERRY

This retired Naval officer; author and world traveler really does not have a bio sketch filled with much loftiness or anything that is considered greatness (writes Wayne Terry). *In fact, when I first sat down to scrawl it down, the only person I could think of was my earthly father, Glenn G.*

Dad was the one who had written to me not long before his death, asking what the sands and heat of North Africa felt like, and with questions about the view from the crow's nest of what would later be my Guided Missile Destroyer in the seventies. He always seemed to know where I was headed before I did. Sorta reminds you of another Father.

Should anything worthy at all be mentioned, it would be that this writer, now in the harvest years, has had lots of great breaks, seen lots of great places, and known lots of neat folks over the years. Another thing seemingly important to him: raising a family or two and knowing that Someone has been and *is* greater than anything else we might meet along the way; greater than any circumstance or misfortune or what we might even call success.

Wayne continues to worship and sometimes serve (as possible) in his beloved New Hope Fellowship in Powhatan, Virginia, not far outside of Richmond, Virginia. He attends Alzheimer's Association meetings, and is a co-facilitator with the gracious program director, Mary Ann Johnson. He has, as you might note, also returned to one of his greatest labors of love: that of writing. He calls it that *bit in the mouth* that causes the sound of the galloping hooves and the wind in his hair, something he continues to chase after. Yet what he really chases after is how he might assist others who are coping with disabling and often disastrous experiences. He is hopeful that his words will reach far and wide, so that others, both caregivers and patients as well as family members, might find hope and solace in what he has and is unveiling.

Wayne was first published in book format in the nineties by Royal Fireworks Press. His children's work, *GIRLS CAN DO ANYTHING!* is a self-esteem read that can be found in many libraries across this nation, especially in schools. His rich and full life, which has been anything and everything betwixt and between scrubbing floors and serving with the U.S. State Department; those broad and varied experiences have helped to yield him some logical placement of ideas that he hopes will be of use to those suffering with, and/or living with Alzheimer's disease. His latest effort, *TIME ZONES (Slipping away...)* began germinating in what remains of his lobes (frontal, occipital and so on), as he through the years ministered to persons in various stages of health and/or attitude.

The author and his wife were fortunate not long ago to begin and close a media services documentary, published by one Dr. Roberta Fountain of Henrico County, Virginia entitled *NO WAY BACK: Coping with Alzheimer's.* He again congratulates her, Roberta, as well as her co-worker, Bruce Berryhill, for their Emmy-winning media services documentary.

Although not divinely steeped in education, the author has had enviable careers in the military, and without, and was one of a few who was granted a commission by the President, with the advice and consent of the Senate, without having obtained a sheepskin. Indeed, however, there has been lots of hard, dedicated, meticulous work and often long hours behind the obtaining of such a commission. But once again, the Relationship that he speaks of throughout this work is what remains his consistent theme, as he strives to reach the mark, and strives to *Never Give Up!*

His work through the years as a *Stephen Minister*, under the instruction of Dr. Kenneth Haugk, the founder of the *Stephen Ministry Series,* has been of invaluable assistance as Wayne learned the importance of listening to and going to where the care receiver is; of being empathetic and then later perhaps praying and even studying Scripture with a care receiver.

Word about Wayne's forthcoming work has appeared in several newspapers, on television and in documentaries. He was also chosen to tell his story in a *StoryCorps* format which is held on CD in the Library of Congress. Wayne and Donna have also appeared in *Virginia Sheriff* magazine, as well as when they make trips here and there to places such as Washington, D.C. or wherever the Alzheimer's team happens to travel (when possible). Their appearance in the Sheriff's Magazine was upon the occasion of receiving his GPS bracelet that allows law enforcement personnel to locate him more quickly, should he wander. Six out of ten Alzheimer's patients do wander.

Mr. Terry currently resides with his loving wife, Donna, their dogs and cats and gardens, and an occasional visiting grandson or granddaughter or other loving family members and friends. Although their friends are their most important assets, Wayne often speaks of his favorite subject: 'crossing the river' where he longs to continue praising, singing, praying and dancing before a benevolent and loving Father. The One Who offered His all, so all could be saved unto Him.

Acknowledgements

There is no writing of a dedication. Yet herein is elucidated much the same. Hopefully. I believe you will come to know to Whom this work is solely dedicated by the reading of it.

Unfortunately, not everyone is attune to *spirituality*, many seem to call it nowadays. And because of my deep friendships and relationships, forged especially with God, it may well be more difficult to get this work into print. That is rather a shame to have to say, but it seems that too many have today forgotten who is in charge: the One with the hugest shoulders and longest loving and awaiting arms. Indeed the One who knocks upon your very heart's door; the unforeseen One. I will not forget. It is something not negotiable for me. So I may search for quite a while until God leads me to the proper house. (But I'll come clean now: it did not take too long to find a *home*, a *launch pad* if you will, and in that way the past has become present.) Or at least today has finally caught up with yesterday. It is the tomorrow and tomorrow that I sometimes concern myself with, at least if I allow myself to.

It is a prayer this does not sound too outward-bound, but rather that I have announced an awakening if you will. Or at the very least, that parts of me have become more acutely awakened to what and Who has been with us all along.

Setting out to concentrate upon ones who have influenced my life and who have become friends prior to and during this process became a challenge in itself. Again, my *Acknowledgements* section is somewhat different than/from many others. I owe a lot of what I have become in this life to organizations of comradeship, such the *Military Officers Association of America,* the *Veterans of Foreign Wars,* the *Ruritan Club* and *Kiwanis International*, and you might note that I am familiar with many other fraternal and non-fraternal outfits who have as their goal 'good deeds' for those around them. Then there is the *Stephen Ministry Program*, as well as various church bodies that I have been affiliated with throughout my lifetime. All this (mostly past) socialization and my traveling around the globe have meant a lot to me in becoming who I am.

Our environment certainly helps to mold us in many ways. At least, as much as we allow it to. Of course, once again, it is not about who I am, but who God is.

One of the first possibilities I considered when swishing this story around inside my head, swirling it around my soul's palate, was: *What happens when one forgets or merely leaves out a person's name?* For that reason, especially since I live with a form of dementia, I have grouped family and friends into an all-encompassing enclave so *every one who has ever known me has been included, whether your name appears or not, I love you. Not only do I love you, and have not overlooked you, be it known that I diligently pray for each of you and yours, whether you are a caregiver or one suffering, or simply a friend I met somewhere along the way.* And as is written in Galatians 6:14-15: **'I have striven to boast in Him alone.'** That is my first and most hearty acknowledgement. I encourage you to always place God first. I suspect it may be an encouragement of **'Thou shalt have no any other Gods before Me.'** I *believe* those warning words and daily strive to achieve them.

Without our loving Lord, not one word of this could have come into being, or ever been shared, for He led me all the way. He so humbled me during this process, for I never had to ask. He indeed answered before I could ask! *He was here, is here, and shall always be! Do not fool yourself otherwise.*

My *Lucy,* Donna, and her being able to put up with my shenanigans throughout this endeavor have helped make the whole work possible as well. She supported me all the way. Sometimes even quietly, (Yes, a joke at my risk.)

(And Donna: I do not regret this not being that heart-felt romance novel that you always wanted me to write.) You're my soul mate, and without you, dear wife, there would be no book, and a life that would seem much less filled with love and purpose! Indeed we are a team, even though marriage counselors bet against our odds.

That said, there are others included as family and friends. Some are listed separately, no particular reason. Much of this work came along as it came into my noggin, such as it was and is. I am prayerful that I have not become too clouded to cause you not to understand parts of this, but that is one of the great reasons for finding editors and publishers. They can be quite helpful, if you allow them to be.

Not only will you read names herein, but sometimes within the work itself. Let me simply add at this point, if something not quite so heart-felt has been issued throughout this work, it is not meant in any manner that it should pull anyone down, for it is my intention that this be a work of edification and perhaps education as well.

Often a name is so very much more than a simple mentioning or reflection. One such person is Joan, who has worked for Congressman J. Randy Forbes (Virginia) for more years than she desires to let on. She has been diligent concerning my particular situation, *Thank you, so much, Joan!* You are the epitome of what our Republic today needs in my opinion in the governmental sector. You are unique, tireless, and have been nothing short of a *vein of hope* for my wife and me. You are not only a caring soul, but a prayer warrior as well. And so is the congressman. Those are praise items! (I simply wish we could get all the leadership to drop the *R* and *D* next to their respective names, and have folks center-in on the job at hand instead of so much partisan gamesmanship.) I am thankful that I found you and the congressman to be straight shooters at all times. It has been my honor and privilege. One I shall attempt not to forget or ever take for granted. Good listeners (and leaders) are difficult to cultivate today.

Sue Ash, of Powhatan, Virginia, has a great *Frame Shop* in town. Sue accomplished the graphic art for my model of *Ezekiel's Wheel Vision* illustrated in Chapter 12. *Thanks for the beautiful and professional job. Well done, Sue.* By the way, Sue is one of Powhatan's quiet rays of hope, here, in this somewhat bucolic section of the world. Yet it, too, Powhatan, is an area that is also growing much too rapidly. I just hate the thought of driving another thirty or forty miles outside town again and probably will not.

Doctors D. Annette Reid and John J. Hennessey IV, are not only good friends and mainstays in my life; they have always gone above and beyond for my family and me. Never were they too busy or unable to assist, both have been blessings to my rather confused (at times) state of mind. *Thanks, Dr. John, for the marvelous Foreword. You were one of the first doctors to recognize that I have two invasions set upon me at similar times. Kudos! Thanks, too, Dr. Reid, for your quality care and love and prayers for Donna and myself. And might I add for others, as well. There is also you, Dr. Michael Fielding. You have shown more insight than any doctor I believe I have ever met.* And these doctors, folks similar to Joan, mentioned earlier, are angels of His, sent to walk and work the face of this sphere. Dr. Isaac Wornom, III (or three-sticks as I sometimes call him), is my plastic surgeon, that tenderly removes suspicious portions of me before they become troublesome. *You, too, Isaac, are much appreciated… you and yours.* (Now if I could just convince the government that sunburn turns to cancer sometimes, and that *they* sent me to all those sun-drenched locations, but that, too, is an unfortunate game with many of them not wishing to understand or hear it.) *See no evil, I think they call it.*

There are so many others who have either provided direct support and/or were not only supportive during my more active working years, and many have just plain stuck by my side and pushed me to continue on. How I love the upward-looking folks, especially now, some are, or were associates, and closer. Among them: Bill and Debbie Moran, Senator John McCain, Commander Myron Young, (VFW Post 9571), Reverend/Dr. Steve Brown of Keylife Network fame, and a friend to me whenever I got in over my head which has been often. You, too, Reverend Pete, my dear friend. I'm not using your complete name, for Father knows it well, then again, it may appear on the jacket cover. Another old favorite of mine is Reverend Alan Hutchison as well as Reverend Reese Wills. (Reese is now retired, along with many others. I am not even certain where you are hiding out, but I miss you, Reese).

Some of these folks mentioned are from long ago and far away: Skip and Barb Fischer, Pete and Mary Peterson, Ralph and Grace

Taylor (Ralph is an old NSA buddy). Then there's Mr. Herman Figueroa of Panama, (formerly of New York), as were: John C. Lacy, Bernard McLaughlin, Ross Driver, Bob Curd, and several NISO (Naval Investigative Service Office), agents I can recall: Dave Planton, Joe Mulvehill, Ralph, you still have New York's finest bar and grill? Then there was an old Marine friend: Agent Cabellis; "Andy" Anderson, John Gentile, just a few associates that I can recall and miss from the old Naval Investigative Service outfit. It was a workplace filled with fond memories that made the falling of the WTC another personal tragedy in my life, along with too many others. I yet cannot believe it happened; cannot believe that we are so often looked at jealously, or have just happened upon some who seem incapable of humane-reasoning and/or are unwilling to *flex* and/or to act less than a savage or a coward might. (God seems to be nudging me somewhat about the fact that we are not always the most docile, loving folks either. But then again, at least we have used our ideas to form a grand union that has worked this far along. Right?)

Colonel and Mrs. Bruce Deakin, USAF (ret), will never be far from my heart. That good man drove me around in a country so densely populated and so far down the culture chain at the time, you had to go and find medicine for your sick kids, otherwise they would surely have died on the spot. Fortunately, I have been richly blessed to know many men and women such as these two. I keep you in prayer.

Then there's Gunnery Sergeant David Leonard, USMC (retired), my *Promise Keeper's* and lifelong friend, him and his sweetie, St. Barb. *There's a real woman.* Any woman who could put up with 'Lenny' as long as she has! Okay, he's about as pleasant to live with as I sometimes am. Something about warriors I suppose. Next, there's Connie and Bill Howard (another Marine family). Bill's finally back from his African hiatus. These two have adopted Donna and me. *We love you both, as we do the couples mentioned afore!* There's another couple that we prefer greatly who are getting married only days after these words are tapped out: Danny and Ruthie. *All the best; we love you so. Might God continue to shower you both as you are led.*

I also miss a long-ago friend, James Elroy Brown of Baton Rouge.

Morocco, wasn't it? How's life treating you? Did you marry? Start a family? I did catch it one year that you were commissioned. Congrats! (I knew you had the 'stuff' before you did. Miss ya.)

There was a dear friend and attorney, Mark Myers, who so loved Psalm 119 and often talked of God's *Book of Life,* Mark and his lovely family. These guys and gals and Christian families are also held in God's powerful hand: Rusty George and Paul Ortz, of Ohio, a new friend, Bob Schaeffer (locally). God bless you, Bob. *What you have had to endure with your sweetheart and her Alzheimer's! (And naturally, there are mates, ladies whose names I have not left out on purpose, I guess I have opted to feel too much the part of the male gender at this particular sitting.)*

And yes, you, too, Carolyn (of *Four Seasons* fame, here in Powhatan). I must thank you for your friendship, and that we share such a strong bond especially since your mother's passing. *You called it: that this work would become published. And now you get to see it in print. I love you and yours.*

And while I am addressing those who have lost loved ones to AD, let me just ask: *You know how you feel when you really miss someone?* This book not only acknowledges those who are daily getting closer to the veil, it is a memorial to the thousands upon thousands of other grand folks who have already marched on. There is nothing sadder in this life than losing someone you hold so dear.

Yet, as we standing, *live,* we will one day, just as the notes of music strike lobes on both sides of the brain, join those who have enjoyed life's strains and joys thanks only to the One who led me to write these words, the One who first loved you, and me. The One we are to glorify and enjoy forever. *Sound familiar?*

I have found it a great and awesome privilege to realize, thanks to good folks around me, and to a wonderfully written Guidebook, I have no doubt whatsoever that Holy God knows every little situation that will take place in our lifetime, even before we are conceived. And that is such a grand comfort to any Christian. You would think it would shake the foundation of those who'd rather talk all the time.

Captain Kim Novak, RN: *I listened to you (on CSPAN) for only two minutes, and you became indelibly etched upon my mind and soul. I can identify.* (Kim was one of the restless cast-aside military folks who got to say a few words at the Walter Reed committee hearings, whatever they called the aftermath of that covered-up mess.) And yes, I have first-hand reports of it as well, not simply what we heard in the media.

You were 'right on' Captain, I wish you only the best from hereon. I've read about changes since... time will tell. Check with me in five years, okay?

Those good folks remind me of Richard 'Dick' and Ann Nelson, surely two of God's, as is Reverend David Dennis and Reverend Charles Warren (the forty-plus years servant-sent-to-India-giant-for-God). Maude and Drewer Johns are two more grand missionaries I so adore. I've always admired a fairly new acquaintance: Mr. John W. Jones and his lovely spouse, as well as the retired Sheriff Lynn Woodcock and his bride. (Lynn shares my Grandma Reba's maiden name.) I didn't realize it until I'd learned of it: Lynn's wife's mom had also been an Alzheimer's person. (They are projecting a million new AD cases annually by 2050, should it reign that long.) Amazing.

Then there's Mr. Paul Hook, now of Port Royal, (formerly a British Army dude). We'd get started talking in the library and I often wanted to ditch whatever project I was working, just to hear his grand stories. Hook reminds me of me, that is, he's been lots of places, seen lots of things, and done as many. *Really have enjoyed our companionship, man. You always brightened my day. Thanks.*

There's Mary Ann Johnson and others associated with our local Alzheimer's Association in Richmond, Virginia; Nancy Lentz, Bridget Soyars (a volunteer coordinator), Bob Schaefer (again), and Janina Bognar, Sherry Peterson (CEO), Alyssa McBride and Melisa, to name a few. All are counted as friends, friends and a new family thrown together by this albatross I call one of my thorns. Forgive me for any omissions. The 'association' has been a very real and rich blessing to Lucy and me. *Thanks so much; so very much. You have all so touched our hearts; so given us a reason to hope* (as our purple armbands remind us).

I look forward to another trip to D.C. this coming year (to get the word out).

I cannot forget Carter Harrison, Kevin Northrop and Paul Miller as well as Paul Izzo and Michael Larkin (although some meetings were very brief, yet so very insightful). *I love each of you working for this grand cause that you pray and work for/with, this malaise that may yet be unraveled by stem-cell research, or another of God's wondrous miracles. The gift will come. God never fails!* Most of us are far more blessed than we deserve to be, and fearful for some reason to admit that He never fails.

I can never say enough about Congressman J. Randy Forbes, 4th District, Virginia. He has done so much for so many (especially warriors). *Kudos! And many thanks. You are folks who don't simply give lip service.* There are also other loving friends: Reverend Mike Lamm and his sweet Linda, and the New Hope Fellowship of Powhatan, Virginia. They have prayed and shared and loved my wife and me beyond description. It is a love-filled congregation extraordinaire! There are so many friends that have made us feel at home in God's amazing house of praise. One of those with a very big heart is a recent friend, Harold Watson. What a great guy and loving family, so many wonderful, loving, caring, praying people. *I'll attempt to never forget one of you. Continue about God's work. He loves you, too.*

Then there's lovely Danielle Wheelis, yes, one who lives in Arizona. She has aided me in keeping my 'saneness' during times of near insanity or what I considered near to it. She has fought and won so many battles for a family striving to endure certain trauma. *Thank you, so much.* I must also acknowledge a name from long ago, that of Attorney Ginger Paad. *You cannot be forgotten my little marathon girl. I always keep you and yours in prayer, and always will. How is San Diego and how are your girls? They'd be young ladies by now.*

There are many others who I've thought of during this endeavor, some I served with, others, just names from the past and/or folks or family who I simply admire and/or love: Bubba and Ann, Betty and her professorial daughter, SSG Luis Melendez: sacrificed in uniform in East Africa, December 2005. *We miss ya, Luis!* Colonel William P. King, USA (ret), Colonel Robert A. Mountel, USA (ret), YNCM Vicky Carroll, USN (ret), as well as ENCM Rick Stucky, another retired Navy pal. CWO Charles Barber, USCG (probably either retired or near flag rank by now). He had such a neat 'collective' family. They were in the child custody (loving) business, as my sweet sister, Gale and her husband were for so many years. It has been a blessing for them to watch over and love literally hundreds of children with their heart-felt love and security in their loving, God-filled homes. *How proud of you all I am.*

While I'm addressing many formerly uniformed folks, modern-day fighters who happen to remain first-rate citizens, it is here when I request your deepest, noblest and most sincere prayers for our warriors, both men and women. And don't forget the thousands missing and even greater number of veterans who have been forgotten and live on the streets of our sometimes wave-tossed and at times rather cold, apathetic Republic. I love this land, but sometimes we lost sight of the ball at kickoff time, one seemingly not to be recovered again for quite some time. We need to go the extra innings for these folks! Especially for the ones who went 'all the way' for you and me, we *owe* them that! They *earned* it.

There was Chaplain Joe Howland, Chaplain Robert Moser (and a lady I always called Mom #2). Both chaplains are retired Navy fellows, as are many of my chums, such as Chaplain "P" "J" McNabb (one of the only shipmates to visit me when I had declared 'Stop the world, I wanna get off'). PTSD, way back, and yet…

I'll not forget Reverend Jan Douglass and the great guy I introduced her to: Gene. There's Reverend Robert Allman of Georgia, and Rev/Dr. Steven Booth, Rev/Dr. Frank Reding, and James Pardue (who officiated for Lucy and me), all are of Virginia (with the exception of Douglass and the Allman's), at least, when I knew everyone more actively. Reverend Richard E. Fruit of Ohio: *I miss YOU and yours.*

Hey! Chuck Moffett. *Miss you and yours and keep you in prayer, always.*

I could go on and on. And incidentally, I could name many more great and God-fearing chaplain types and/or reverends that it has been my special privilege to know and serve with, whom I yet keep in prayer. (You would not believe the stations (assignment locations) that I am purposefully skipping.) Yet all these folks are such grand samplings of a loving God, and so many other grand workers such as my sweet Aunt June Ann.

And of late, there's a new name to be added to this list of God-fearing folks; that of Mike Smitley. *Thanks, Mike, for your tireless, devoted, dedicated and constructively conscientious work to this book. I have sensed God's Presence when talking/sharing with you. Love ya, Mike.* I am honored by your selection of my work and especially enamored with the name of your house: *FATHER'S PRESS.*

There was an older (long ago) friend, LCDR C.D. Older, a Great Lakes unit commander and working dynamo that I am proud to mention having served with. He took care of his troops! There's ENCM Osteen Mishoe, USN (ret); Colonel Charlie Beckwith, USA (ret); VADM Mike Kalleres, USN (ret). RADM Robert R. Fountain, USN (ret). More on him later, as well as the surreal meeting that I had with his cousin who did a media documentary that began with Lucy and me. She along with Bruce Berryhill: *you were there with your associate, many thanks! Congrats to your outfit for the Emmy award, Roberta. You deserve it!*

Thanks as well to the folks at *The Richmond Times-Dispatch,* the *Virginia Sheriffs* magazine and the Institute, Genworth Financial and others, following herein. Thanks to Jennifer, my favorite Ohio reporter, TV channel 33, who caught Lucy and me at the great Canfield County fair (up in snowbird country) not so very long ago. *I recall your Alzheimer's-ridden loved one, too. Yes, I keep you in prayer. Thanks for the lovely letter to my daughters and son, and your great compassionate reporting.*

While I am thanking and congratulating folks, I have to say *thanks so much* to Deputy John Mattox. He's the deputy that normally stops by our place and places a new battery in my GPS bracelet. It is a life-saving device, you probably know. It enables law enforcement officials to be able to locate me by satellite in a short period of time. I believe the sheriffs call it a transmitter. (It is part and parcel of Project Lifesaver.) I said 'places' (concerning the battery) back there, but it should have been 'placed' as John has been transferred closer to his wife's folks. Thanks also to Chris, one of his sidekicks! And I'd be remiss if I didn't once again mention Sheriff Lynn Woodcock, who was responsible for getting the program off the ground. *Thanks to all,* that includes Deputy Brad who has taken John's place at our place, and others as well. Most law enforcement types really do care.

A special thanks to so many folks in the loving community of Powhatan, for donations, prayers and special caring and service; service and love and money not only for Alzheimer's folks, but those suffering with Autism as well. (That of course includes folks of my local church and the Christian Motorcyclists, Wings of Hope and others, some who come from far and wide to do great philanthropic acts of kindness.) *God does NOT forget your acts of kindness and they are the true measure of a society and people who really care one for another. I am thankful for the folks who offer more than lip service.* Yet I do recall how we are also called to pray, and that is good as well. Pray always. It's in our Book.

While I am speaking of *acts,* one of the most important revelations of this book (to me) (not to be confused with God's Book), has been that you and I need to continue to be contemplative, keep working what we have; realize that new neuron pads can be created by working your noggin daily. I am living proof the 'experts' are on to something here. This is especially important for those of us with early on-set of the disease. And one more important piece of all of this, as you will read over and again within the work: *Never give up!*

Captain Joseph Bailey, USMC (at the time I knew him): Joe presented me, a Navy guy, with an honorary *Semper Fi* plaque, upon retirement. One of the greatest days of my life! *Thanks, Joe. Don't forget you are Department of the Navy, too!*

I miss Captain Gerald Egan, USN (ret), my last skipper and by far the best. *(You were right, about retiring; I should have listened.)*

I have met and served with folks of all branches of our beloved Armed Forces. (I even had an uncle who served in the National Guard.) It has been a rare privilege and an honor to be part of the professionalism, pride and dedication of these warriors (present, and now some missing or gone). I was elated to hear of our nation's approval rating of our military back in June, 2007. The military topped the list! It is overwhelming as well as heart-warming to me. You cannot fool Americans. Not for long at least. I only wish we had not been allowed to be drawn-down so much. I hope the ol' SecDef, Rumsfeld, did not make a drastic mistake by cutting back on numbers of personnel. Were it up to me, I'd restart the draft, especially when I spot some of these young guys running around with their pants down way too low. If it's a secret message, they're not doing so hot with it. Kids wondering why they can't grow up, I suspect. Some of it caused by non-parenting parents, unsure of where their own compass is pointed. Then again, we all have choices.

I find myself instead, fondly reflecting upon the heroic survivors of Hill 488, probably the most highly decorated small unit in American military history (according to a VFW article in their April, 2007 magazine). And man, again, do not forget today's (Army) National Guard, what a great bang up job they've been doing for our nation; being toured and double-toured, as others have before. What a mess (for Army and Marines, Airmen and the Naval services as well). And let's not forget our Coast Guard folks. So many have been pitching-in since 9/11. *Thank you all!*

I later got to thinking that perhaps I should have attempted to recall all the names from the 19 locations (and more) where I'd been stationed (temporarily or permanently), but when your brain is running on not-quite-full any longer, it would've been an almost futile task, so please forgive me one and all. *I love you and think of you each, as I am able. Yes, I pray for you and yours!* It just now hit me: ENS Eugene Babich (submarines) was another guy I so admired and figured if he had remained in uniform, he'd be a four-star Admiral by now, but I suspect that he is long out of uniform. *Hello, Vince and kids. Best to all. Miss you, too. I know, the kids are no longer kids.*

I must mention an old yeoman-type friend, Ronald Thomas Jones (who passed suddenly and much too early in life). What a grand relationship we had. Also Tony Jones of Mississippi, Dennis Mudger (formerly of SC), David Grubaugh (probably still in Ohio), Chuck Orr, Jerry Mugerditchian (an Air Force fighter pilot and close friend); another Jerry, Jerry Milan of Orange Park, FL. Gerald relieved me onboard a coffee-ground-locked sub-tender and allowed me to gain some weight. So many co-workers and friends I dearly miss. (Names, which may be *ho-hum* to readers yet *vital* and *dear* to me.) My kind of people: God, country and family.

Then there's my extended as well as immediate family: Mickey and Lori, Levi and Jessica, Chuck and Debbie, Jim and Amy and always my Angie. Anjuli is more than family, though: she's my shining star! Then there's Jenna Cetto and the rest of the family, living in this 'spiritual battle' today. Michele and boys; other nephews and nieces, grandsons and granddaughters, what blessings God presents, cares for, provides for! (J&J)…

This listing could be much more voluminous. The memory of most of these folks and loved ones inspired me to be as good a writer as I could, especially when thinking of each of you. Aunt June, Lorraine and Jody, Linda and all. Forgive my shortcomings, absences, and lapses of memory. Any selfishness.

There's sweet Norma Jean, as well as my remaining uncles: Jack and Bob: *I keep you and yours in prayer. Really.* If not already mentioned, I so miss and revere Autumn and T.J. (and 'Rhett'), Jeff, Brandy and sweet Emma. Timigeon, Michelle and her boys; Amber and Greg (still newly-weds to me). Ronen and sweet Holly and the baby, as well as Adi. What a sweetheart. (I'll want to crawl under a rock for the ones I've left out.) Chris and Betty and girls.

Miss ya, man! (Lots of kids and grandkids from my sweet siblings. Each so special.)

So once again your faces are here even if your names are somehow missing. Honestly, it would make me crazy reliving and trying to recall all my grand years in and out of uniform and all the wonderful people I've met and served with. What a team! What a dream; what a sweet life! (I could have died in uniform, I so loved it.)

I'd be more than remiss if I failed to mention brother/citizens from 'back home', who *gave their all* during the Vietnam War: Bill Berry, Ralph Crytzer, Ray Holman, Thomas Webster and Howard Vaughn, to name a few from my old alma mater, Jackson-Milton. May God continue to bless their families and the sweet memory of each one of these special departed hero/warriors. Forgive me for any omissions; I was not present to compile that complete listing, and there are others I know of and yet picture in my heart, mind and very soul, all of them heroes. And there are many I yet miss and recall from the three rivers city. For me long ago.

Thanks Samuel Dewey for your devoted service for our beloved extended family and our beloved country. The same words apply to so many of you in my immediate family, Gale and Glenn and Dave, all uniformed folks; Barry, Richard Cetto and ones even before us: Glenn G., (Dad), Robert and Thomas, all served this country well! And again, Luis and Michelle.

One thing that burdens my heart to the core right now, is not simply the dastardly things that we are facing at present in this beacon of hope called America, my heart is hurting for the approximately 29,000 children who are daily dying around the globe due to hunger and the lack of medicines necessary to sustain them. I hope and pray that somehow we might one day be able to pull together with other outward-looking nations of this world and look after the children of this growing world; as iron sharpens iron, so must one man sharpen another. Certainly we have all heard it. The secret is learning how to live it! How to once again gain possession of the ball. And I'm sorry, we cannot only look within, there's a big world out there. And it is God's tenderness that can show us the way to move ahead together.

For a brief moment I seem to at the same time realize that I am feeling a knot in my throat, for as I think of brothers, Dave and Glenn, (and then step dads), Tom and Bob, another Navy brother, Barry, that we all shared in a grand love for the Navy, it is because I right now picture the boat in <u>Crimson Tide</u>, as they are taking her down, (for me about the 200th time). I visualize that beautifully powerful SSBN 731 and her smooth, titanium skin silently slipping beneath the waters as I hear in the background a wonderfully melodic hymn that I'll always remember (God willing): *Eternal Father, Strong To Save*. It is a hymn I long to have played at my final earthly celebration, although I will have by then been long-gone in spirit; and with that departure perhaps the end of thoughts of carriers and destroyers and missile cruisers and submarine tenders and PCFs (Swift Boats) and boomers and so on; memories of comradeship, albeit some of them haunting memories as well. Then again, there's the sweet other side, the sweet by-and-by. (Don't look for them to all be of your ancestry and/or background either, when we get there.) I think our *special conversations* in our own little places are quite often silly, don't you?

What guy could forget three great dads? Glenn G., Thomas and Bob, all princes in their own right. Wish I could have been more like any one of them! Each was unique, devoted and faithful; all were better spiritual men than I'll ever be. I'm one that strives, but may never quite reach the goal. Let it suffice for me to say that I'd be content to stand by *The Door*. Just let me peek in now and again to check on all of you.

I must repeat, as I do within the forthcoming pages: *family is everything, and that includes you, Momma! Especially you. So touched and loved I've felt throughout my lifetime, what I've lived thus far; so fortunate was I to be surrounded by your special love, and the love of many others.* And what great siblings! All of 'em top notch: Again, Gale and Mary, Glenn and David, your sweet mates. How proud I am of each and every one of you, and the families you have raised and blessed, and will be blessed by. *Keep looking up! You all made my life more wonderful.*

Mucho thanks to the kind assistance often rendered to me by the great staff at the Powhatan Public Library, Kim and the gang. And it is a must to thank all the endorsers of this effort: Pete, Steve, Ken, and Mary Ann. I look forward to many more gatherings for those who suffer the strains and often sprains of a world clouded by dementia and other debilitations in any form. I cannot help but praise those, too, who are attempting to unlock that puzzle of Autism that is affecting so many lives. I also ask that you might keep those loving folks living with Down Syndrome in your prayers. And all of you suffering, and or fighting certain diseases: *Please recall what God did for you and me when He entered the darkness and brought that everlasting Light that we shall so feel at home in, as God will certainly wrap His strong and tender arms around us all. And we Him... what a huge group hug it will be!*

Then there's Dave, saved till the end, but in this from the start. Had it not been for my brother, David Lee, and his keen skills and unselfish ways, this book might not have been published. It seems the old Alzheimer's fella started getting things messed up on the keyboard. *THANKS SO MUCH, DAVE. Love Ya, Man!*

LASTLY, I again acknowledge and dedicate this work to those ordinary chosen men whose lives were touched by Jesus, including the one who doubted Him; the one who betrayed Him; the tax collector; the doctor, just ordinary men who today yet make our seemingly crazy lives extraordinary. Men that walked those dusty roads with Him; men that climbed hills and sat in an open boat upon storm-tossed waters with Him; others akin to you and me, who learned that life is sometimes a roller-coaster ride, rather scary, twisting and furious. We must, if nothing less in this life, strive to maintain the many fundamentals reiterated in our blessed Guidebook: God's Word. *It is here that we meet Jesus, Jesus who leads us to God; the One to whom this book is truly dedicated.*

Psalm 31, verse 3 contains words that dominated my thoughts throughout the preparation of this work, for He IS my rock and fortress, He has led me and guided me. (Or as the song's lyrics proclaim: *O, how He loves you and me*!) As you digest these words, always recall this, dear friend: *TO GOD BE THE GLORY!*

TIME ZONES (Slipping away…)
Wayne Glenn TERRY

Chapter 1

The Beginnings

—Alzheimer's, A Disease—

I'm not the same me, at least I'm not *'the me'* that I used to be. It is unfortunate that I cannot go there and return, yet I can tell you that Alzheimer's disease is a world all its own. I can also explain some good news from my current 'time zone' where I now exist.

As Christian friends and family doctors, Dr. Annette Reid, as well as Dr. John J. Hennessey, IV, have shared with me, Alzheimer's disease is a somewhat fluid disease. Fluid in that it is entered into as water slowly trickling forth from a spring. I'll always recall words that Dr. Reid once graciously shared with my spouse: *Mr. Terry will go down fighting.* That's true. **Never give up**! You'll hear that from me until your tire of it. That is, if you don't tire from the sheer exhausting excitement of each page of this work.

A year to 18 months or so after I'd written those words, I began a letter that started out: *I am in fear.* I had turned a corner, rounded a bend, begun a new heading of sorts. It caused me to wonder if *I'm Damn Scared* wouldn't be a great title for a work. But rather than go directly in that direction, let's visit other areas first.

Blessings all mine. Children and family, who (for the most part) seem to understand what is taking place within me, have been a wonderful influence in my life. They had for Christmas one year purchased dry-erase slates, puzzle games and other challenges that assist folks who need to work their lobes (brain) due to trauma and/or disease. They are gifts that assist me in attempting to keep the cobwebs out. My lovely Lucy, as well, had purchased some great books.

Word-Finds assist my brain in working akin to how it works when I am reading or writing, whereas other Wordbooks seem different to me. That is, I must more diligently work in order to find the word I am seeking. Yet, I could have that all turned around and be all wet as well. I must admit that from the very beginning.

The writing process, one of my inherent gifts, is something I have accomplished for many years. It flows more easily for me than when I am struggling to find a particular word within a puzzle. This gift, locked deep within (Dr. John might say), is for some reason easier for my brain to process. Usually it comes out in a fairly proficient manner. And that, dear friend, is as everything: by the grace of God.

Searching for a word, even when we know the words within the puzzle, used to take me a terribly long time, much focus and concentration. Lucy's (a favorite endearing name I call Donna at times) Christmas gift gave me a great laugh in the wee hours of a morning, as I was able to find my first word in a big puzzle. The find was *grandparents*. Interesting that I'd found the largest word first, perhaps it was easier for my noggin to spot. I know it was grand to me, for being a grandparent is one of the sweetest revelations and assignments in this life.

My friend and neurologist, Dr. John would say, *some days are worse than others*, or was it better? It is something I once again learned this very morning when in yet another doctor's office.

The young woman behind the desk wore a tiny police badge-replica around her neck. I had asked her about it. She told me her brother, her angel, had been a New York City policeman. My mind instantly raced to the barbarous and brutal, the unbelievable falling of the World Trade Center.

That event had been especially personal and tragic to me, as I had worked in the building next to where the towers would one day stand. I had heard the first of many pilings being driven deeply into the ground in the late sixties. But "No…" she'd continued through years-old tears, as I pictured the old Federal Office Building where I'd worked at 90 Church Street.

She explained how her brother and his wife had been police officers; that they had been cleaning their weapons when the horrible accident suddenly took her brother's life. Things can always be worse, I long ago learned. And it seems I'm learning it all over again.

My mind chooses to return to Steinbeck's, *Grapes of Wrath*, and for a brief moment or two I sense the smells, the pictures, the action he so vividly painted for us in his work. I picture fruit pickers attempting to make a living during that harsh, somewhat far-off time. I am indeed thankful for memories. What an enchanting world books can offer us. This one though, may not be as enchanting. Yet I expect it will paint a portrait or two.

I want to turn to another read, Joanne Koenig Coste's *Learning to Speak Alzheimer's*. It concerns rehabilitation, or as she calls it, habilitation, or a simple way to look more positively at one's life with dementia. Joanne had been her husband's caregiver for many years until his death in the late seventies. I was fascinated by many of her viewpoints and experiences. I could give her nothing short of *Kudos!* for her work in the field. Here then, is part of what she wrote about habilitation:

> Optimizes Function
> Minimizes Stress
> Maximizes Success
> Promotes Positive Emotion

Optimizing and promoting and maximizing are all grand; yet the one that boldly stood out and brought this writer to full attention was minimizes stress. How important that one seems to me. I'll continue:

Not long into my personal journey, it seemed easier for Lucy and I to cross swords. It hadn't been simply because we had been reared differently, much of it had to do with striving to maintain our own worlds, if you will. 'Okay' (as our 8th President, Van Buren first began), maybe it was half and half. That is, Lucy and I know we hail from different parts of the checkerboard. I had learned it, and as I approached her early in the morning, one morning, as she prepared for work, well, it just turned out that I had picked the wrong morning.

Lucy's getting prepared for work is not always a good time to approach her; she just isn't a morning person. It's simply something one needs to know for their own good.

I know, or should by now know, morning is her quiet time. Yet I had been in the middle of one of my devil-take-care, humor-filled and probably not-hitting-on-all-cylinders (or lobes) mornings. As I entered the bathroom, coffee in hand, I had been rambling on about something. Yes, I've learned that I sometimes ramble. Many with AD do.

Lucy quickly turned to me to say something. In so doing, she jerked around and bumped smack into my coffee cup. As macho-tough as I am and as tightly as my hand had been wrapped around the cup, its contents still warmed the arm of my sweet Lucy's pretty blue sweater. *Oh, Man!*

It had not started out well at all. It had started out rather poorly. Donna rinsed her sweater's sleeve in haste, and then reached for the blow dryer, oblivious to my almost inaudible apology. I got called a name; probably one I'd deserved. It's much worse than learning your cat has once again left one of her play toys inside your boot. (Why do they do that?) It can be loud, hard to take back, those words sometimes issued in haste. I've learned it's not all Lucy's fault, but sometimes that's hard for a guy to admit, even a 'normal' guy.

Not long thereafter, the caregiver out the door for work, I began calling folks to tell how Lucy had called me the name; how she'd stripped me of my dignity and so on. Well, the part of me remaining here (at the time) had forgotten, back then, that I had been the one who'd intruded into her space, and I had been the one whose hand held the hot coffee. (And by the way, this wasn't later told to me, I processed it all on my own. It is something I'm rather guarded about now, what I can yet process.) (Oh, you noticed?)

Needless to go on and on about it, it had not been a great morning. It made it very difficult for me to tell folks that it was the 'best day I'd ever had' as had been my custom. It used to be one of my goals. In fact, that morning had been a rather nasty beginning, me wondering where 'Doll Face' would live, and Lucy (same person) receiving unexpected phone calls now and again throughout much of her workday (thanks to the AD patient: me). It was a stress-filled, loveless, somewhat selfish day on my part, at least for much of that day. (By the way, one doesn't need to call the National Alzheimer's Hotline number for everything. There is a national help line number (another number for dementia information: 1-800-272-3900.)

- 4 -

At long last, day limped into evening, for me near six p.m. of late. We had begun communicating. And communicating, whether with a friend, a loved one, or just someone close to you is a balm on the wounds of a dementia-filled person's life. Communication is not only a skill that I am convinced assists us in remaining in earlier stages longer, communication is also a necessity of great import to the caregiver's world. I'm saying the caregiver has a world and the patient also has one, as if they were two different worlds. Sometimes, it is just that they are very disconnected, much the same as 'normal' couples, whatever you might define as normal.

Thankfully, during that particular day, and because I'd reached out to various supporters, many people I later learned had been praying for us, I again learned what a blessing and power and grace there is in prayer! What many blessings are realized from good friends and a great support system! What precious grace flows most freely from God in our times of need, or when we're not in need. But back to the end of a rather havoc-filled day, as I share how I'd been (back then).

You see, I had been thinking about Lucy's residing at a different location. At the same time, she had shared her honest emotions of feeling lost and out of control. Scared. At last, she even looked sad. Now I was the one who wanted to be secure in telling people to 'cheer up' or that things will be all right, but the fact is, I have never been trained to do that. I have been trained to go with the person's feelings/emotions, that you are not to cause a heavy heart to sing. I therefore encouraged her that not only are tears good, but I had also encouraged my Lucy to cry. And cry she did. She did even better than that.

As she sobbed; as I held her in my arms, "I'm sorry for you," came out from her. And then, "I'm sorry for us." And finally, the one most fully charged: "I hate this disease!" Years of loving can easily turn into this hating hiatus, at least temporarily, longer if we're not being careful and concerned.

Now there's this. Between my combat world dilemma, Posttraumatic Stress Disorder (PTSD), and this new world unfolding before me: dementia, even these worlds sometimes merge quite easily. I was stunned the very next morning, the morning of words hardly yet dried on paper, to find myself bumping into soft flannel pajamas in the darkness. You're correct, depending upon where your noggin is: I had bumped into my sweet Lucy. Lucy, who'd told me she'd been awake since 2 a.m.; Lucy, who accompanied me on a chilly early morning walk; Lucy who so loves me! No matter what stage you find yourself in, in life, isn't it grand? Isn't love all that really matters? And don't you believe it is how God began, with love?

Whether we feel that we have the world by the tail, or whether this world attempts to control us, I remember what another friend long ago had shared with me. *You may not be able to carpet the world, but you can fit yourself with a pair of slippers.*

Alzheimer's disease may be one of the worst, scariest, loveless, most relentless worlds we may ever encounter, but there is good news: we can attempt to fight it! We can fight it spiritually, emotionally and physically as well. *It is my suggestion that you fight like hell!*

Good luck to you, if you're one of the prospective fighters. Many of these words have been prayed over and written specifically with you in mind. Never give up! Recall God's great love, and that it is always with us, and remember, God never gives up.

So thankful am I for a God who can and does enter any world. He will come when you call upon Him, and guess what else? He doesn't even need to be called. He's always here. He seeks the lost, even those in confused states of mind. All praise to our most Wonderful Counselor. *Thank you, especially for being with us, Lord, when we are tired and not feeling like ourselves.* Maybe we are as this cob-webbed-ensconced old author's brain, and where I seem to be at present. Place this in your heart, friend: "AND GOD SHALL WIPE AWAY ALL TEARS FROM THEIR EYES; AND THERE SHALL BE NO MORE DEATH, NEITHER SORROW OR CRYING, NEITHER SHALL THERE BE ANY MORE PAIN: FOR THE FORMER THINGS ARE PASSED AWAY." – Revelation 21:4

It is by God's grace that I am much th
horse, galloping with bit in mouth, excitec
dominance and yet freed at the same time.
again by His grace, was dumped several tim
the wrong striking of a key (by a person ill: n
sometimes floppy disks are not the best thing i
when doing this type of work (I've been told).
as if I am off at a gallop, during the many rewrit
polishing and more polishing, not only do I feel t.   .vork was
beginning to take shape, I also learned from various publishers
that it will one day come to fruition. That in and of itself is a
dream many writers never get to behold. I cried when I had first
landed a book contract, and I was all of fifty years of age at the
time.

The reason I report that it will come into being, is because
of these editors' words to me whilst I had been in the midst of a
draft or two: One editor, on 5th Avenue in New York, was elated
by its potential, but backed away because they do not do
'religiosity' he said. I swallowed at that and moved on. The next
editor stated that it had broken her heart not to offer me a
contract, that they were short on time and lacked resources as
well. I did note that they managed to get a young nurse's story
out though, one who'd just returned from Iraq.

I don't know whether that house was looking for a
contribution, but as this work is a total work of philanthropy, I
cannot work that way. What is earned from any royalties will be
turned over to the Greater Richmond Chapter of Alzheimer's, in
Richmond, Virginia. I have placed it in my will. And I don't
share that as a pat on the back for me, but I share it as a friendly
reminder that there are many ways you can help, even as you
plan your departure from this visible world. And lastly, there
was the editor who had stated: Your work deserves to be
published, even though it does not suit our list. But I highly
recommend you keep submitting it until you find a home for it.

There is nothing that compares with affirmation, other than
God's grace and love and wonders realized. So, if you happen
to be a struggling author, I'd like you to tuck this away back
inside the rear part of your healthy brain (I pray). The only

…a published writer and one who is
…that one of them gave up! Keep striving, keep
…keep dreaming, a friend of mine so wisely advised
…d I must add. Keep reading and writing as well. They
…ul do your mind a world of good! Indeed, it is a great labor of
love.

—There Are Times—

No matter how deeply I feel about remaining positive,
Christ-centered and loving (about this work), there are times
when I feel utterly lost. Indeed devastated. You are not realistic
if you do not sooner or later face some facts: and they are not
candy-coated facts. AD patients eventually forget how to walk.
If they live long enough, they become bed ridden and therefore
need to be attended to more and more, i.e., turned every couple
hours and so on. There is always the danger of bedsores, and of
course there are many other complications as well. Since they
usually no longer know who they are or where they are (latter
stages), it doesn't take long to discern: they just end up (we end
up) being or already are, someplace else, on our way out. I used
to use this line as one of my jokes: No matter where you go,
there you are. It just doesn't sound as funny any more.

It unfortunately did not take a long time for me to begin
thinking more and more of suicide. Sorry. This is how you get
to know someone, so hang on. What I am now sharing with
you, reader friend, is beware of any drastic mood swings! No, it
doesn't necessarily mean you are suddenly bi-polar, but now
and again we all have stressors, or just enough bad stimulation
to put us into dangerous tailspins. One weekend I had talked
with my friend, Dr. Reid. Doc, I'd begun, is my sexuality all
messed up? Are my anti-depressants messing things up for my
wife and I? (I am convinced sometimes that our various
medicines interact differently with us on occasion, I am sure
there is plenty that we probably might be better off not
knowing.)

†

Fortunately, as my doctor is much wiser than me, and as the next day or two proved better, I had learned a valuable lesson: Sometimes we just need to deal with whatever is going on. To hang in there if you can. We need to be of courage. Or as we used to say in the service: Tighten up the old bootstraps. Follow me, men, and all that. More on that later.

Whether you are a caregiver or a patient, forewarned can be forearmed. If you ever hear someone speaking about giving up, or worse, I hope you will respond to such emotion. Or at the very least, get him/her in touch with someone who can appropriately assess the situation. (And put this in the mix as well, friend, our Lord can bring about peace. The One who commanded winds and waves to be stilled? Remember?) Let me add one more thing. Sometimes we can get so very far down that it seems the good Lord has moved very far away, I want you to know that that's just not true. And most likely you know it to be untrue as well. I'm just saying, don't let a moment such as this one pass you by. I've been privy to some terrible tragedies in my lifetime. Never, ever look too lightly upon a person's emotions and/or words. Never. And never desert them in their hour of need.

I shared with Lucy how much I'd appreciated the way she had helped restore me one evening. I had been particularly low. She had turned toward me and lovingly touched my arm. "Don't give up, Wayne," were her reassuring, encouraging words. I had felt an angel in the room with me that night. She had once again stilled my hurting soul. Is it not all we often seek in life, someone to still our troubled soul from time to time? Someone who will simply love us as we are?

There are times when *Keep a stiff upper lip*, or even the famous, *Hang in there*, just no longer work. There are also times when I picture myself not at home in my comfortable surroundings, in my daily, somewhat calm routine. Instead I picture myself surrounded by others who have ridden the big wheels of the same train, or at least one similar. We all know of those times. We all have times and different trains we must sooner or later embark upon.

(Together we sit, practically huddled, most of us asleep. It is nine-thirty in the morning! We may get a 'change' before lunch; then again we may not. If we get up from our seat for any reason, which we probably don't know why we have, we may be rudely and loudly assaulted with "Sit back down!") You may have correctly assumed that I am mentally, at least, a patient.

I am seated in another realm. If one of my friends dares to turn in the opposite direction or chooses not to listen to the earlier given order, she/he may hear, "There's going to be big trouble!" And yes, I know this is not always the case, but all too often it is. I've heard it.

There are facilities in this Republic you would not want to place an enemy in. Yet are we not taught to love our enemies? We are taught to be forgiving, even as the Father forgives us. It's something to seriously ponder. Actually, it is something that we are to live. What I am telling you, once you've heard the aforementioned drama as I have, you know there are locations out there that you would not want to be a member of; not at all, not ever. Not even for a few minutes!

I cannot erase the puzzled look from behind clouded eyes of an old retired Navy Chief Petty Officer. I remember hearing a twenty-plus-years-young woman as she shouted at him, "Don't get up!" I did the natural thing: I pictured myself in his awful predicament. Mr. Jones (pseudonym), probably in the middle stages of his disease, must have utilized everything remaining within him so he would not go for her jugular vein. Either that or my old friend had already boarded his train. The latter would be my guess.

Now that's not a gentle, God-filled thought. But sometimes, that's the way it is. That's the rubber meeting the road. When I am realistic, Spirit-filled, or just wondering where God's moved to, I look the disease squarely in the eye and ask the question I've heard many times before, especially when I was ministering to folks: Why me?

Now I had been taught or heard, somewhere, yet I could never bring myself to utilize it. It is the *Why not you?* response. It is supposed to be followed by how our Father suffered and died for you and me, and that's all true, and truly wonderful, but for me to talk about someone's pain when I'm listening to the one in pain, it's too much to endure. I learned early on, sometimes the best thing to do is simply to L I S T E N. **Listen.**

I confess, it was much more palatable if I could say, if I had to say anything (and sometimes you don't): "THE LORD IS MY SHEPHERD, I SHALL NOT WANT." Can you imagine telling someone dying, or who for all practical purposes has died, "Sit down and shut up?" How and why is it that our society seems unable to provide counseling, training and especially a good caring ear to those who tend our elderly population? I strive not to say it, yet my very soul proclaims the plight of Mr. Jones, for these are the ones who now sit, half awake, half asleep, totally unable to fend for their lot. Ones who must not only endure a lack of dignity, but must also have indignities hurled at them! Just sit back for a moment, and imagine yourself in their place.

It seems to me from the number of places I've visited, and sometimes reported to authorities, today's nursing homes, retirement facilities, whatever you wish to call them, sometimes just either do not have, or are not capable of the one-on-one care and/or focus needed for persons suffering AD and other similar maladies.

I'm beginning to understand why my noggin has ached for the past day and a half. I do not feel that it has simply been my hairnet-like-covered brain. I believe my subconscious has kept working its way through this very point of this very segment, this very complex and often sad subject.

Wondrously beautiful, our God-formed minds; not only are they complex and ever working, they are practically unstoppable. Now there's the scariest part: for we know even our brains can be stopped. They can be stopped as surely as the tick-tock of the old grandfather clock, or the disappearance of a gentle smile.

Alzheimer's disease is a long and slow decline. In the mind, the hippocampus is eventually destroyed. The job is then slowly finished off by the destruction of the brainstem as well. The brainstem is what controls involuntary hard-wired functions: breathing, heart rate, sleep cycles, and so on. It regulates many of our organs. But remember this, even if you are one similar to those of us: who sleep very little, there is always hope. **Never give up! Never!**

Just as God has been our hope in the past, He will be our hope for eons to come, even unto forever. Or one I like almost as much: "AND YOU WILL SEEK ME AND FIND ME, WHEN YOU SEARCH FOR ME WITH ALL YOUR HEART." –Jeremiah 29:13. (All being the operative word.)

Although there are times, friend, I encourage you with everything left inside of me to hold out for the miracle. Trust in God! Might your daily song be: "It is well, with my soul." Might this be your truth, even if the miracle does not take place.

Savior Friend, no one knows our troubles and tragedies, every bump in our winding road, not the way You do. You are there whether we have following seas or find ourselves smack in the middle of a super typhoon.

Whether we are knee deep in the clouds atop one of Your majestic mountains or down within the deepest recesses of one of Your mighty oceans, You Lord, are there, too. Continue with us, no matter where we are, no matter where we might wander. Father God, especially be with those suffering tough times, times of challenge, times of change, times You've known about long before the beginning of time. Guard our troops, gracious God, guard our sweet loved ones who wait. Guard each and every tender heart that turns to face You. Keep us ever from the evil one.

—Childlikeness—

In my early onset days, I learned that assisting Lucy in certain tasks was good for me, yet I no longer felt that I needed to do it all myself or any longer take care of each and every situation, as a husband might normally desire to do. I believe it had been the beginning of childlikeness for me. It had begun in spite of the fact that we like to do many things all on our own as adults, or even when toddlers, or how some of us now say, *me do.*

Perhaps that will be bothersome for some patients and/or caregivers, but as I find writing an urgent matter for me just now, even in this umpteenth rewrite, I also believe I should share how I sense the process at this time; viz., how I feel the must share soon proclivity that I am sensing. It is part of my fear. Although I am somewhat fearful of not completing this work, I find I am more fearful that it will not be considered *good enough* to come to fruition, even when a publisher takes into account that I am suffering these debilities.

Childlikeness to me is allowing oneself to become a kid again. AD, as does age, enables us to relinquish; to be more in line with who we would have been, had we been more natural. In other words, it is a time when we are really more naturally ourselves. We are not as concerned about playing the role of intimidator, or having to worry as much about putting on for something or someone. We become peeled. We become stripped of any fear. We may even learn to love more deeply, more simply.

I am attempting to be objective about this. I had first become aware of childlikeness when an older, more thoughtful and wiser psychologist had advised me that he understood my PTSD. At that time I recall that he had muttered something about how he was not sure of that tone, there's something about that tone. I had never bothered to ask him, though many times thereafter I wish I had. Yet I had sensed that he was speaking of a change within my countenance, my voice and perhaps even my mannerism. It is much more clear to me now. Of course I could not totally grasp it back then. It had been a change that I had already unknowingly embraced. And I believe it was part of my *me do* way of saying that I was moving on. It is difficult to know the when and why of it all, but I do know I am moving on. The good doctor was telling me also, that I had AD. He hadn't come right out and said it, but I sensed that he was on the brink of it. He was older, again, and this time it meant he was wiser as well; you could tell he'd hung around that desk and space of his for a very long while. To me, it was as if he could see right through you, without staring right at you. That is a wonderful gift. It is discernment.

I am hopeful this changing back and forth between different times is not too intrusive for you. As we encounter change, and/or when it is forced upon us, does this change not begin from within? Are we, dear friend, not all changing as we trod along? Yes, of course we do. We are. We change with the movements of time's hands. It so reminds me of the rotation of the earth, and how I often see the same star patterns in the same locations night after night – this of course depending upon what time I stroll outside. (More on that later.) It also depends upon the changes of seasons.

†

I used to drive, all by myself. It has always puzzled me, the way some of us behave when seated behind the wheel of a motor vehicle. I am unable to place my finger exactly upon the pulse of it, yet today it seems accepted by most. That is, it seems that folks are eager to show their skills as poor drivers, continue to show rudeness, and for some reason utilize a devil-take-care wheeling of their machines on today's roadways. I hope it's a sign of healthy competition, but sometimes I think it might be that we sense we're at war one with another.

Is it because we're back to a wartime feeling and thought pattern that continues to hang over us? Or is it that we simply feel that we're passing through, therefore our childish play becomes part of the new us? Is that it? Is it the me do again speaking from deep within us?

My mind's eye recalls times of distress because of the manner in which I have often been out-maneuvered, or sped past at high speeds (back when I was yet driving). All of it seemed to make it possible for the other player to arrive in front of me at that next traffic signal. I have often wondered since my diagnosis, if these perturbations might also be assisting us in our mental disorders later on. Might our way of life perhaps be sending many of us to maladies earlier in life than necessary? I believe there to be some truth to that.

When the aforementioned players arrive at that finish line: that traffic signal, I sometimes look over and seek that typical emotionless-looking face that seldom stares back at me. More often it is they who continue to maintain a forward look, so they do not have to meet my gaze. In many ways it is that they seem to act as if nothing-at-all has taken place. Why is it that we often seem to become someone else when we find ourselves in the driver's seat? And why is it that we continue the facade that we are not being controlling and childish when in fact we're attempting to pull all the strings? I sometimes laugh at the one who speeds by me, cuts in front of me, and finally, once stopped, sits at that finish line (traffic signal) as if life were just some sort of video game, and yes!, they have just scored a hundred-thousand points being rude.

Is it our embracing childlikeness, or childishness? I would surmise that we are simply embracing what we've been taught all along: for how many times did we hear, *Big boy!* upon taking our first steps or when we first cleaned up a spill without having been told to do it. So engrained it becomes; so much a part of our early psyche.

I of late feel this childlikeness more and more. Somewhere there are words written about our being as a child. Yes, here they are: "VERILY I SAY UNTO YOU, EXCEPT YOU BE CONVERTED, AND BECOME AS LITTLE CHILDREN, YE SHALL NOT ENTER INTO THE KINGDOM OF HEAVEN. WHOSOEVER THEREFORE SHALL HUMBLE HIMSELF AS THIS LITTLE CHILD, THE SAME IS GREATEST IN THE KINGDOM OF HEAVEN. AND WHOSO SHALL RECEIVE ONE SUCH LITTLE CHILD IN MY NAME RECEIVETH ME..." –Matthew 18:3-5

Reflecting now, I picture friends singing in an Alzheimer's unit. I study their shining eyes, their sweet happiness (if only for a few fleeting moments). It is sharing their childlikeness as we together shared the twinkle-twinkle tune or the one about Jesus' love; those old songs so many of them recall. The songs seem to revive them, and they seem so proud to be recalling them when they do. The songs are somehow indelibly stamped deep inside of them. Those memories are therefore deep inside each of us, are they not?

Routine agrees with me. Not only because it goes along with the affectations of AD as I court the veil, but also as it is easily seen (to me) how as children we were easily cast into routines, liked or not. How childlike I often felt, sometimes carefree, other times as now, not at all in control. The simple surrendering of your driver's license does that to you.

Perhaps it is why I so love Paul's calming words: "BE ANXIOUS ABOUT NOTHING, BUT IN EVERYTHING BY PRAYER AND SUPPLICATION, WITH THANKSGIVING, LET YOUR REQUESTS BE KNOWN TO GOD, AND THE PEACE OF GOD, WHICH SURPASSES ALL UNDERSTANDING, WILL GUARD YOUR HEARTS AND MINDS THROUGH CHRIST JESUS. FINALLY BRETHREN WHATEVER THINGS ARE TRUE, WHATEVER THINGS ARE NOBLE, WHATEVER THINGS ARE JUST, WHATEVER THINGS ARE PURE, WHATEVER THINGS ARE LOVELY, WHATEVER THINGS ARE OF GOOD REPORT, IF THERE IS ANY VIRTUE AND IF THERE IS ANYTHING PRAISEWORTHY – MEDITATE ON THESE THINGS." —Philippians 4:6-8

They are words for adults. Yet how childlike we often feel when we think of being without worry, about prayer in everything, about being thankful. How it frees us up. Besides, did God not humble Himself when He came to earth as a child? Did He not come to die upon a tree so you and I might march into His forever kingdom? And there we will praise Him, worship and adore Him forevermore. Now it's honesty time: I have fallen very far short of all of that! I have never been one to be patient or without worry, and I have often been the gear that made the loudest possible noise so I could get the grease. I don't know if I'll ever be able to fully embrace those 'be not anxious' words. Yet I do keep striving to embrace them.

Sometimes, I see it when I'm very tired, at the end of one of my daily segments. Sometimes I cannot tell where my day ends or where the next begins: to me, it's two or three hours of rest here, an hour there, and many, many more hours of being awake. At the end of a segment however, when I am near total collapse, as I draw my Lucy close to me, it is then that I recall how childlike I really am. And perhaps later still, out underneath God's vast and glorious night sky, in the stillness of His all, I am once again childlike. When I'm in a quiet place and enter into serious prayer with God, childlike. When I crawl to Him, asking if I can merely stay with Him; childlike. When I beg Him to take away my heavy burdens; childlike: "WHEN I WAS A CHILD, I SPOKE AS A CHILD, I THOUGHT AS A CHILD, BUT WHEN I BECAME A MAN, I PUT AWAY CHILDISH THINGS. FOR NOW WE SEE IN A MIRROR, DIMLY, BUT THEN FACE TO FACE. NOW I KNOW IN PART, BUT THEN I SHALL KNOW JUST AS I ALSO AM KNOWN." –I Corinthians 13:11-12… The seeing dimly part: any pastor worth his salt will share with you that seeing the reflection is just that, a reflection, not reality. It so jogs my memory about the realness of AD.

Childlike. Manlike. And yet, dear friend, when I am told what I ought to do, or when I am feeling controlled, the wonder of childlikeness often flees. Alas, I desire to have some say about things, to be adult, to have my own way. Isn't that rather sad? Growth does not always bring about maturity. Sometimes it brings back the *me-do* attitude as well as a not-so-grand example.

The world of dementia is an emotion-packed world as you may have already gathered. It is difficult for the caregiver. Sometimes they forget their main task: that of listening. And when you are one fortunate, or not so fortunate to have been schooled in the art of listening, who has focused on listening for the major portion of his adult life, well, it can be just plain frustrating that others seem to fail to live up to your 'listening' expectations. It causes me to be anything but childlike.

So what about childlikeness is deficient? I can't say that I really see much at all intolerable about it. Is it not true that we revere our children and grandchildren in their innocent childlikeness? Do we not hold them up knowing that they are our very tomorrow: our hope that we somehow continue our earthly existence, even after we've departed? And that their existence will lead them to Heaven, to home, as is every Christian's hope? Lead more folks home?

"O how He loves you and me..." The lyrics leap at my heart, my head, as if they are receptors like a divine lightning rod. I recall not long ago, one of my grandsons had a situation on a school playground. His mother later asked, "Nathan, what happened? Why did you hit that boy?" Without hesitation, 'Small Fry' as I longingly refer to him, responded, "I guess my arm just didn't listen to my brain, Momma." The words were transmitted with little delay, without so much as the crack of a thunderbolt's warning.

Four years old! In a sense, Nathan had entered that world usually dominated by adults: a simple prevarication, or a moment of not wanting to admit to the truth. Yet the more I studied it, the more I concluded that Nathan had simply shared his faster-than-lightning reply in sincerity and childlike truth. I often thank our Lord that I am yet able to observe my hand responding to what is yet coming from my brain; my lighter, thinner, perhaps more entangled and fragmented brain. God's gift. Can I not yet call it His gift? Most certainly, I can.

"BEHOLD WHAT MANNER OF LOVE THE FATHER HAS BESTOWED ON US, THAT WE SHOULD BE CALLED CHILDREN OF GOD!" —I John 3:1. (in part) Whether my gift has been distorted, or is in some other way undergoing drastic change, we do not yet understand. I am still a child of God. And so thankful am I for that knowledge. Part of that is that unfaltering trust we sometimes sing about.

†

Thank You, Master, for allowing me to yet put pen to paper. That I might yet share with others preparing for their grand exit, too. Thank You for allowing me to sometimes embrace childlikeness. Your ways are so complex and astounding, beyond belief. I pray I'll never forget how You first loved us. Perhaps the seeing dimly words are coming more clearly now, or soon will be. I so look forward to that hour of full awareness, of ceaseless praising in Your Holy Presence forever, that time of no longer hungering, but only the 'drinking in' of Your love. Might I love You more. "I WILL REMEMBER THE WORKS OF THE LORD; SURELY I WILL REMEMBER YOUR WONDERS OF OLD." —Psalm 77:11.

—'De-Cluttering'—

'De-cluttering' had not started out as one of the spokes of my Ezekiel's Wheel Vision, which I will later share in greater detail. Alzheimer's disease affords us an unusual, many times unappreciated, not-looked-for sense of confusion. When I begin to tire, or what I call getting my hairnet fog over my brain, that is one of my confusions. Recently I was in touch with a caregiver whose spouse claimed she has glue inside her brain. I must add now, however, since I've been wearing the fairly new time-released patch I do not feel bombarded as much, at least not as I had when taking pills only by mouth twice daily. The 24X7 release (of the patch) is a definite plus for me. I am so thankful for the rewards of research, and Father's allowing us to make new discoveries.

Regardless of the name you give it, or how it affects you, most of us feel confused and have difficulty expressing ourselves (at one time or another), and that includes those of us in early onset. It is different for each one.

I need to share at this point, many of us are quite capable of singing, dancing, and playing piano, writing, and doing other tasks that we have been able to perform throughout our lives. It is one of the reasons that dementia is difficult for the general public to understand. Sometimes it is difficult enough even for people close to us to understand.

My main purpose at the time I had begun the 'de-cluttering' process, had not been fully deciphered until I got further into it. It had been a time of giving many of my prized personal possessions to ones close to me, although that is not yet finished. This grandson and that one, a couple of granddaughters, including extended family through marriage, each one received early presents from me. There was a commissioning photo, a telescope, military medals, some neat sculptures, an old Bible that I had studied from and utilized for many years as I ministered.

Some of the more bulky, yet attached to my bedroom wall items will no doubt later follow, names have been placed on the bottom and/or back of each item. I learned during this act of housekeeping, if you will, that as I released some of the treasures I had a sense of being somewhat freed up. It was as though I had begun streamlining my room, and had therefore streamlined and simplified my life as well (to a certain degree). So much seems to hit the AD person all at once. And soon more is on the way.

Sooner than I had anticipated, I began feeling as though I had relieved a good amount of pressure from myself. It is my hope that the children of course will maintain and preserve those mementos (the giving away of which helped lighten my load). Of course that might be up to the adults for a while, kids can lose a host of stuff along the way.

The giving process that I sensed also lighted that perverse darkness one encounters when first diagnosed, and when you later receive the *Ugh!* prognosis. It is in a sense also a freeing up which one who may have been divorced (and after having adjusted) can attest to, or you may feel as you might have felt when you shared a secret with someone close. I call that scratching the surface. It seems as we gradually begin to talk about the loss of a close loved one; often this freeing up, this sharing, occurs more rapidly.

This act of liberating not only lightens the load, it is somewhat akin to my anti-depressant's mission. It takes the edge off, and assists in eliminating some of the confusion. And confusion, friend, is one of the worst parts, perhaps the main threat to those of us with AD. At least it's a huge threat until we decide to turn it over to God. God can help. I believe it. I share it, and I am hopeful you might be one allowed to share that knowledge, too.

During this realignment of sorts I thought about priorities in my life, and soon, very slowly at first, I took back an old item or two that we had heretofore-stored elsewhere. Some items that I had previously fallen out of love with re-entered my life. And sometimes I hung some of them back upon my walls again. I found this process to be somewhat of an act of taking back control of my life. We all too well know, at least those of us with dementia, we are no longer in control of our lives. Yet control remains a very important issue to us. I found that I was able to carry some of that control forward as I reacquainted myself with my old possessions. Things from the past.

But I must share this; turning over control of my checkbook, which had in all reality become impossible for me to track, was a huge undertaking. I felt as if I had waved the white flag of surrender. Later on I realized it was the right thing to do, and that it would happen sooner or later. And then, having had to turn in my operator's license, well, there's not a whole bunch left that you really control after that. Those matters are tough ones. However, the more we 'de-clutter', the more we ready ourselves for new possibilities and new realities (or not).

Since many of us (patients) have a tendency to isolate, socialization is one area we do not always look forward to. Even heading for an Alzheimer's Association meeting can often be difficult for me, at least until I arrive and get started there. New surroundings are also tough for many of us.

All of this is a part of *time zones,* part of the subtle and not-so-subtle changes we endure as we traverse this new path, this direction taking us to Who-Knows-Where Land. It reminds me of a journey akin to Alice's. It is a challenge with more impact than I recall, more monumental than receiving military orders for a change-of-station move. In service to our beloved country (military personnel), at least we knew where we were bound. Most of the time.

In my travels with God, I strive more and more to keep Him at the bull's-eye. I know God goes with me, wherever I go. Still, I am very saddened for my sweet caregiver, Lucy. My Love is losing someone special to her, and she has started grieving early. She is traveling a road that is unfortunately sometimes very long and rough for the loved ones of dementia patients.

'De-cluttering' I therefore declare can be good. It is the door that opens onto your next garden (if you will), your next inevitable yet exciting journey. And that's not a bad idea: adopting the attitude that you are simply preparing for another one of life's journeys.

†

Almighty, Collector and Comforter of souls, allow our care partners to sense as we 'make our way' that they, too, are prayed for and not forgotten. If we're unable through language, help us to touch them with a friendly hug and smile. Enable us not to fear looking into their wondering, often questioning eyes; for the caregiver, too, is searching, scared, and sometimes just as lost as we. Though we love You, Lord, most of us also fear You. And sometimes we are simply afraid to approach You. We find it a dilemma, often running from the very One who shelters and guides us. When in fact You are the great and wonderful Comforter. Speaking of being scared, and wondering and lost, it merely leads me to my next portion: about a tough position.

"FOR YOU WERE ONCE IN DARKNESS, BUT NOW YOU ARE LIGHT IN THE LORD. WALK AS CHILDREN OF LIGHT."
—Ephesians 5:8.

—The Toughest Job—

It's awesome, the way things work out and we just don't get the why or the how of it. Not right away. Now and later on I'll share that ministering to senior citizens at nursing homes has been valuable preparation for this layman's work, his walk, this realization that I have very little control over any of it. I am the caregiver's dementia, and I'm not sure she likes it. I realize that's not funny to everyone. Sometimes I don't find it humorous myself. And I am certain that Lucy does not.

Having had conversations with a multitude of caregivers over the years, including my spouse, I soon learned the major complaint or fear that they faced almost without exception is when the patient finally looks the caregiver in the eye and that caregiver realizes that the patient no longer recognizes them, no longer seems to reflect that knowledge in any way whatsoever. It is most likely the most haunting recollection for the caregiver: whether the person is a relative, or friend, or their lifetime partner. Whether they have only spent the last 30 days or thirty-plus years with them, only now to watch them leaving on the next train: How soon his or her charge will become, or already has, someone else, indeed living someplace else.

That one happening is akin to death, akin to the losing of a mate, or a brother or sister. Some do believe that folks with AD simply have trouble (their brain has difficulty) sorting out who people are, that we (the patient), often recognize loved ones but that our damaged brain is simply confused, so that it appears that we no longer recognize loved ones or friends, not even our mate. And naturally, this is very sad indeed.

Even as I write of this losing of one from the patient's perception, I realize that it is never an easy thing to endure, and it can also be a factor that involves the development of caregiver's rage. Basically, I believe many caregivers, especially those angry or in the rage stage, are saying it without voicing it: I hate this so much, the terrible thought of losing you. Said or not, they think it; they believe it. We all wish it would simply go away.

The caregiver is running so fast, so scared, each responds somewhat differently, sometimes dramatically so. I recall many mornings, as the one with dementia: I might turn to Lucy's shouting direction and ask, "Are you enjoying the raving you're doing this morning?" She would be in one of her tirades over this or that. To me it was often a 'woman thing' such as, 'Why is it every time I arrive home there are dishes stacked in the sink?' But to me, then and now, I believe it is all part of their rage over the disease, and perhaps lack of understanding the patient as much, not understanding the changes taking place within the relationship. It is not easy. Not even for the optimist. Okay, it is easy for no one. I'll say it again, most everyone wishes it would simply go away.

Nevertheless, I am excited about these days (most of the time). I early on had decided that each day would be the best day I ever had; those close to me will verify those words as they've heard them from time to time. At least when I was feeling fairly well and not too clouded and/or tired.

I realized during my early onset that maintaining control is very important to the patient. Indeed, I will go so far as to say that attempting to maintain control seems essential to the patient, at least it has seemed that way to me. That said, I return to the caregiver: the toughest job.

To me, the caregiver, who is often far more fearful about what is taking place than is the patient, can easily disable the patient. In fact, it is this patient-layman's opinion: the caregiver can exacerbate the patient's condition, and here's how I got there. Indeed, I felt outmaneuvered when I had to relinquish my driver's license. Although it is natural for the care person to be concerned about the future, money, safety, and so on, to this patient that 'stuff' is rather transparent, that is the caregiver's early desires to 'get on with it' (as far as the taking care of the patient and planning for the eventual future), is a two-edged

- 23 -

sword. The caregiver is (rightly so) concerned about control, watching bank accounts, keeping a driver (the patient) and others safe, so my heart of hearts flashes to me that the caregiver may well be making a prognosis zoom ahead possibly earlier than is necessary without even realizing it. So again, instead of being concerned mostly about the patient's quality of life and dignity, and the patient's input, the caregiver might unknowingly and unintentionally be debilitating the patient!

The other edge of that sword: good friends and others may also, unknowingly, convey the caregiver's concerns to the patient. Family and friends can also be in denial about what is taking place with the patient. This reverberation, this second jolt of the same message, often makes the patient feel either outmaneuvered again, or just plain thumped upon. (I say that out of love, not to hurt anyone's feelings.) And I say it as a patient who has managed by God's wondrous grace, to remain somewhat lucid for the past 4 to five years.

This sounds too much about the patient, and it is. Yet it is important for caregivers to focus mostly on the patient. Focus on the patient's needs, as opposed to whatever the caregiver can control and/or dictate. And this is not easy territory to cover. I'll not forget attempting to explain that to my sweet Lucy, only to hear her scream out at me how tired she was of having to focus on the care receiver all the time, or of being told of that importance. Even when a caregiver wants to, or does say, *I just get so tired of hearing that patient stuff,* they need to know that they are hurtful words.

So if you are a caregiver, try to remember, along with everything else, the feelings of your diseased partner. Yes, it is a tough job! The toughest. What I would encourage is that the caregiver find a pastoral or an empty open area where they can scream about all of it at the top of their lungs, or somewhere they can yell at God. And don't worry about that: God has the broadest shoulders anyone can ever imagine.

It is another one of my opinions that patients likewise, should be concerned about their caregiver's feelings. Yet often that is all but impossible. Sometimes care receivers (patients) do not understand it. And I am not fending for the patient side, I am simply trying to explain what I am envisioning/sensing from the patient's point of view.

Sorry. It is again natural for one who loves the patient to do all they can for that person, only to learn that their best intentions seem to thwart a patient's ability to live well, or said another way: sometimes it just doesn't matter how it's handled. Yet I would prefer both sides handle the situation with love, as good as they can. Sometimes patients feel that caregivers can seem rather oblivious to patient longings, and I am sure that is easily seen on the other side as well. What we all need to concentrate on most of all is how is it we can retain dignity and a loving influence as long as possible.

Patients need to be able to express their personhood, and to be involved as well in maintaining their dignity, even when they are no longer able to verbally express these important factors. The more scared and perhaps shocked the caregiver becomes may well, once again, cause caregivers to focus on what we all realize is up ahead, and therefore may signal, I need to take action, to take control, and I need to do it quickly. It is all part of the initial shock and the sense that a lot has to be accomplished, and quite frankly, they (the caregiver) may well be in a condition not too far from shock. Yes, I know that sounds somewhat unfair or perhaps hyperbolic, but plainly speaking it can be a mess. And sometimes a power of attorney is a necessity. Sooner or later, it is without a doubt a necessity. Yet it can also be a decision entered into by the patient and caregiver as a team, early on. This is said to aid the caregiver and others, especially those who may not or do not ever venture into the reading and/or learning about the disease. For in so doing, they never fully learn the inner workings of their most important role, enough about that for now friend.

It is a substantial amount to take in all at one time. Some of this will need to be passed on, and dished out to and by various facilities and facilitators. It is valuable information.

—Inappropriateness—

Some of us, (patients), are yet aware that we say inappropriate things in public. Caregivers and patients are relentlessly linked, it is all connected. They must know one another better than ever before. That is: it is an optimum goal. One of the caregiver's major roles therefore, is a thankless task: sometimes having to explain to folks that the patient is being inappropriate and that she/he cannot help it. Many Alzheimer's Association chapters maintain small cards the caregiver can carry and show folks. The card reads that their 'friend' has the disease. It also asks for the other person's patience. It is a silent way of heading off an otherwise sad scene. Unfortunately, my chronic PTSD and/or panic attacks do not aid this situation. I also need to add, Lucy found it just as easy to get close to the third-party person enduring the patient's obvious inappropriateness by simply saying: *He has Alzheimer's....* It works just fine.

One good thing has been that my very long days may well be one of my greatest assets if properly utilized, that is, unless the day/night is interrupted by a combat 'mare, which usually throws my entire routine in another direction. It is also an area that I am trying to keep somewhat in the background of this work, yet am finding it almost impossible to do. You see, all things are connected.

I also live on oxygen during times of rest. My brain doesn't get enough oxygen when I am in a resting mode. It is one diagnosis I would have much preferred years earlier. Trust me. I have, however, managed to pass it on to several people, those who snore, so I feel good about that possibility for them.

—Other Impairments—

Another battle, is attempting to ensure that the caregiver gets enough rest. This is very important to the whole facilitative process. Because of my strange hours, I walk around on eggshells a lot, particularly during the wee hours. But I must confess that an oxygen-making machine's constant drone can be quite helpful. If the caregiver's life is too much intruded upon, it is naturally more difficult for them to properly function, so once again, the dreaded two-edged sword. And its point can be razor sharp! If the caregiver's ability to be patient is not maintained, then the caregiver's flexibility and understanding will also be greatly diminished. So it happens, both partners become more quickly impaired. Sometimes an abyss is created too early. What a shame that is.

I am more than thankful that my long-term memory remains intact. Of course that is consistent with most AD patients. It is where we mostly live. And one does get to the point that you appreciate anything you are yet able to accomplish the way you used to. So there is again, always something to be thankful for. **Never give up!** I feel compelled to also share with you that through much of my reading as well as lifelong experiences, I have learned, finally, it is of almost no value whatsoever to tell the caregiver or receiver (patient) that things will turn out fine. Simply put: we do not know that.

And although much is being said here, it is also important as you live with Christ to realize, often someone telling you that *things will turn out fine* may simply be their God-faith-based words which often ring true. For we are to know Who is in charge, are we not? All praises to our God and King.

Yet by and large it is true. Much of what we say when attending to/ministering to folks in need is not what they need to hear. Yet those may be part and parcel of words that should be the opening for an entirely different novel. It is true: many of those more scholarly men and women than myself are often God-led scholars. I am, by no means a scholar.

On the other hand, it would be a total ignoring of facts if I did not share what a good friend had shared with me: *sometimes you simply have to play the cards you're dealt.* I prefer this though: *"More of Thee, and less of me."* Those are heavy words, especially for the one who is former self and present self, wherever that is. For now, I am grateful to know that it seems it is the present for me, at least for now. Actually, the present is where each of us is, no matter where that might be. Really deep, isn't it? That's sarcasm in case you didn't get it.

It is vitally important again, that we allow the caregiver the freedom to talk about their fears, their floods-of-emotions. Sharing is often cathartic. Please do not make the mistake of keeping your caregiver 'tied up' unto yourself alone, for they need space, too.

As one passing through these *time zones* I realize that there are many people in similar circumstances. And now they are forecasting many more of us with the next wave of senior citizens. It is also fairly common knowledge that all researchers know is that most of us are pretty much plaqued-up, that we have 'stuff' that not only gets into our arteries, but for some of us the brain as well. After all, our blood travels throughout our body.

Naturally, there are other factors involved as well: strokes, surgery, and so on. There are many folks in other categories, or suffering differing maladies who are also predisposed to becoming members of the AD club sooner or later.

†

Ministering in intensive care waiting rooms has somewhat prepared me for this work, as has God. I have learned that it was easy for me to get the ear of those grieving, as long as I asked God to go with me, and then I could invite the grieving ones closer to Him. Sometimes I would be working with one or two, then later on perhaps an entire room! During these times, as well as times to come, God is the One Whose grace will soon tug at a publisher's and/or editor's heartstrings, and this work will be on its way to press! He has taken all my doubts away!

—Talks—

One-on-one talks between care partners and patients are not entirely different. I one day simply asked Lucy what were her chief concerns. This never really became so vivid until during a time close to a Christmas event. One of my daughters, unwrapping my Vietnam Service Medal (one of my treasures) read, with my Lucy over Amy's shoulder, words that telegraphed that they would one day see me in the stars. It was not much later, I discovered my caregiver out near the back door, her tired head in her shaking hands. She turned to me and blurted: *I hate this disease*! She went on to say she hated what it was doing to us. It readily explained where 'Doll Face' had gone, where she was going with the myriad of unfriendly and mixed emotions. I had hardly ever seen my Lucy cry. That day,

- 28 -

she cried a great deal. She literally sobbed for me, for us. That, too, can be very rewarding and relieves folks of dreaded tension.

†

By His love and grace, one day we will see God's loving face. O tender One, might this forever be to You my love song.

Thank You, God, that my Lucy was able to stay with me that day. That she walked and talked and listened to my innermost thoughts; that afterwards she attended an Alzheimer's meeting with me. Later still, she promised, as You have to never, ever leave me. How great is that? How great is Father's love, especially when we are troubled?

Chapter 2

Introspection

—Never Lose Sight—

I'd thought of it over lunch with my good friend, Billy Moran. He was always thinking, willing and able to do whatever he could to further the greater cause, the Lord's cause however or wherever God's call might lead him. We don't know how He'll lead us, but Bill was always on the road, dedicated, attentive and working. I admire that. I revere this dear friend.

NEWSFLASH: CNN, on this 28th day of July, 2008, (some Chicago doctor and a national study group) just announced what your humble writer has been saying for a couple years now. Exercise (and drugs) will slow the progression of Alzheimer's disease. How about that? Being as suspicious as I am, I can't help but wonder whether the publisher that held my manuscript (with interest) for 7 months had leaked my paradigm: you'll see it in chapter 13, that paradigm, those ideas of what may be beneficial for those of us who look within.

It hadn't struck my noggin hard enough until when I was being afflicted by dementia. I then realized that I had allowed the old world and its circumstances to mire me down. I had completely abandoned what I had once so loved to do, write. I had indeed lost sight of one of my grandest dreams and joys. Not only had I lost sight of it, it had completely disappeared from my radar screen. Fortunately, a couple siblings, boys and gals and Momma, as well as my sweet Lucy, had encouraged me to *go for it*. My neurologist as well had recommended getting back into living life. So that diplomat in neurology, the guy who had written my Foreword, I am finding to be completely correct. Correct about the living of life.

In a sense, the being mired down, had reminded me of some of the 'stuff' that Colonel Charlie Beckwith had endured to get Delta Force, not just a book title but also a unit, off the ground, and of how General Meyer had eventually thrown him the golden ring which enabled Charlie to charge ahead, in and outside of other rings of the puzzle palace, er, I mean pentagon. (This is a world I can sometimes read and think about, at other times I have difficulty exposing myself to it. So, often I just leave it alone.) Such is the world of one who lives with chronic posttraumatic stress. Not only had the obvious: the now and again correlation between Colonel Beckwith's undertaking and my current life given me valuable insight, they had ignited within me the long lost desire to strive to do better at what I'd felt born to do, to write. Of course, that might not happen very much longer with AD at my doorstep, or me at its doorstep.

With my regimen for AD in front of me, that of exercising, proper nutrition, attitude, support systems and prayer, and more, a revamping of my life, I forged ahead with new dog-eared perseverance in spite of my quickly-sapped strength. For now it seemed, I could only work in spurts, in segments, if you will. But what God-led segments they have been! What a feeling, knowing that He leads me, that with Christ on our side, who can be against you or me, friend?

I am really striving not to lose sight now. I have typed and retyped this manuscript so many times, I am beginning to wonder if it is the albatross that will eventually drive me across the line and into that veiled world that I know so very little about. I get about a hundred or two-hundred-plus pages into it, and then something happens. I push the wrong button and before you know it, I am pressing too many of them, and my Lucy is telling me to just type: that she will fix it all later. I cannot do that. I have to have headings and page numbers and, let me just say, it has to be just so. But I am beginning to wonder if I'll ever finish the work before it finishes me. You ever feel that way? Part of that is introspection.

But finally, approximately one year after I'd finished this work, long before this rewrite, Lucy and I learned that the Alzheimer's documentary we were featured in, one directed by a Ms. Roberta Fountain and entitled NO WAY BACK: Coping With Alzheimer's, had been awarded an Emmy! That is, Roberta won an Emmy. Not only did I picture myself jumping up and clicking my tired old heels together, I got started thinking: Perhaps the work I had been working so diligently upon, this TIME ZONES, also stood a chance at being beneficial work. And suddenly I began to believe what so many houses and editors and publishers had been telling me: One day you will find a place for TIME ZONES (Slipping away...). What a wondrous thing it is, when you begin once again believing in yourself. It is indeed my prayer for you as well, whether you are a new caregiver or an AD-affected brother or sister.

Thank goodness I have had great support. My grand siblings, children and neighbors, my church fellowship, and an old friend, Doctor John, the good doctor that often speaks to this devastating battle. And there was another gift from other friends, an older vintage of a computer that later flew the coop, if you will. Thanks, Ron and Suzanne, how I love you both!

Now and again God places people and rewards and more treasure before us than we deserve in order to bring His work to completion. I believe this work to be God-led. Really. I have believed it from its very conception, as He believed in and knew you and me long before He ever formed us!

_\

—Goals—

Do not lose sight of your goals. Often times there may be a break, a separation, an interruption, a disease. Yet there is a time when your goal is to be revived, made whole and new and fresh! Or you might not call it your goal, but your labor of love. After you find yourself 'back on track' you will be more content. I have actually named labor of love one of the spokes of a wheel that I describe in more detail later on. (So try not to get too exhausted over these exciting pages.)

I am convinced that God never leaves us, that it is you and I who forget to be open, sometimes we forget God. I must offer this: Had I not been brought down by certain circumstances and trauma in my life, I might never have looked back and therefore never bothered to look up.

Yet for some wonderful reason, God has allowed me yet another chance. And it is all so very humbling. What else reader friend? He will offer you another chance, too.

—Getting Lined-Up—

Get things lined-up within your sights, so you might once again understand God's great insight, God's purpose for you. At the time of the original inception of these words a terrible wind had struck central Florida, once again taking many lives. My eyes upon that devastation, a scene that will always play in my mind was the picture of a man standing next to what had once been a beautiful church. The man's immediate words, "It will come back again." Do you not see what God can do? How many lives He can touch, so deeply, so quickly?

My neighbor's love and his work with the church have indeed inspired this cloud-enshrouded mind, this head in turmoil. Part of my inner strength comes from good friends such as Billy and Debbie, yet most of my strength naturally comes from an amazing God, and the sometimes fear-filled yet loving one I live with, my Lucy, my 'Bug'.

When I 'signed on' with Lucy, I recall my words: "forty days or forty years, I'll take it." Donna was and is a high-risk gal, especially in the health department. But my love for her is akin to God's love for you and me. As soon as I got her in my head I realized that I would not be able to get her out of there. I knew she had to walk with me, talk with me, touch me and love me.

I didn't realize until much later, she would be the one assisting me, and not I her, as I struggled back to my other great love, that of writing. Writing and walking with our great God; and yes, I sometimes assist my Lucy as well, as I can.

†

Loving Lord, thanks for Your revisiting, although You are always here. We know You don't just come and then go, or hide, or forget us. You have not left us on our own. Yet Your ways are so complex to us. Even though they are also plain and more comprehensible when we avail ourselves of Your love and Your assistance, Your loving leading. Creator God, One ever present, be with us today in these troubled times of saber rattling and shouting voices from various corners of the globe. It is my prayer that many more will turn to You, before You return again, indeed before Your glorious and gracious Son returns from the East!

Never rule out the great expectation and wonderful possibility, that of a miracle, even against all odds. When we consistently, consciously and continually flirt with believing and only believing the prognosis, we may be closing a door to Someone and something far greater than anything we have ever imagined, ever experienced. As a Christian beyond milk, one who has tasted and sometimes eaten of the meat of our faith, I truly believe in miracles and have seen and been part of many of them. Thankfully. Your background, persuasion, and/or denomination have little or nothing to do with the receiving of a miracle.

Whether you have been a 'good' person or you have failed to do your absolute best, or even when your peers fail to accept you for who you are, all have absolutely nothing to do with whether you will be the recipient of a miracle. Trust me. Seated with as many as 80 or 90 different denominations, I long ago learned that we cannot or should it be said 'should not' try to contain our masterful, infinite, unblemished and loving God. He is not to be contained; God is to be worshiped and adored—lived-for. Amen?

Then there's the clincher that some will no doubt have difficulty with, for I have witnessed those who are either in total disbelief or who just continue to turn their backs on God, even they are privy to His grand miracles. I've seen it over and over again. Who can explain it? Those words cause me to recall lyrics of a song: "Who can say, just how great You are?"

†

It has been said thousands of times by doctors, "I don't understand it, Mrs. Picklesteimer, there is now no sign of the cancer." Is it not superbly awesome that God is willing to forgive us as well as those who may have led some of the poorest examples of living, and even heal them, and further, that He will give even the lowest example a second chance; or as with the thief on a cross, next to Him, who heard the, "THIS DAY YOU'LL BE WITH ME IN PARADISE" words? Might it be because He had already forgiven us all, and made paradise possible for all, by His grace? Certainly! (I hope the Picklesteimer didn't throw you off. I had placed the name there for my Grandson Jacob.)

It often seems for us so incomprehensible. And yet I sense the meaning of God's "YOUR WAYS ARE NOT MY WAYS." We are just so far removed from Him, so far from God's amazing grace and power and love. It matters not where you hail from or what you have accomplished, or again, how good you think you've been. He loves enough to forgive us in our conniving, even in our loathsomeness, in our ways that are nothing short of 'down and dirty'. I am a sinner, and so are you, friend, period. And just for the record, We are all conniving and disturbing to God at one time or another. Yet God forgives us all, and He does it time and time again!

Why? Why would God do this for us? Part of that mystery is in Paul's words: "HE HAS DELIVERED US FROM THE POWER OF DARKNESS AND CONVEYED US INTO THE KINGDOM OF THE SON OF HIS LOVE, IN WHOM WE HAVE REDEMPTION THROUGH HIS BLOOD, THE FORGIVENESS OF SINS."– Colossians I: 13-14.

In other words, let love, which binds us together do its perfect work. That is not such a mystery! It's God's inclusive, unending, perfect love for each one of His creatures! Further, not far from Paul's words are more of His in Philippians, "...NOT THAT I HAVE ALREADY ATTAINED OR AM ALREADY PERFECTED; BUT I PRESS ON, THAT I MAY LAY HOLD OF THAT WHICH CHRIST JESUS HAS ALSO LAID HOLD OF ME. BRETHREN, I DO NOT COUNT MYSELF TO HAVE APPREHENDED; BUT ONE THING I DO, FORGETTING THOSE THINGS THAT ARE BEHIND AND REACHING FORWARD TO THINGS, WHICH ARE AHEAD, I PRESS TOWARD THE GOAL FOR THE PRIZE OF THE UPWARD CALL OF GOD IN CHRIST JESUS. THEREFORE LET US, AS MANY AS ARE MATURE, HAVE THIS MIND, AND IF IN ANYTHING YOU THINK OTHERWISE, GOD WILL REVEAL EVEN THIS TO YOU. NEVERTHELESS, TO THE DEGREE THAT WE HAVE ALREADY ATTAINED, LET US WALK BY THE SAME RULE, LET US BE OF THE SAME MIND." —Philippians 3:12-16.

The goal of Apostle Paul's career is beyond this world. He proceeds. He presses on. He strives for the mark, to reach the goal of the calling of God. The prize? The prize is the Heavenly life of the redeemed! He never looks back. He strains with everything within him to reach that goal. If only I had that tenacity.

Miracles are often illusive to us because we do not look for them. It is also true, they are not always allowed. Sometimes God's plan includes another way, another direction. Sometimes the going must be rough, and we do not yet know the reason why. Yet when that miracle comes, what a great light appears to one and all. What great everlasting joy, or it should be. And it should always be remembered, and should change and affect the rest of one's life. It is difficult for me to admit: I am not the scholar I should be.

I've never been on the Christian jaunts that my brother, David, has led. Often times he'd go and build churches and other buildings outside our country for ones less fortunate. How I always recall his testimony and that of his sweet (nurse) wife, Andrea, how filled they were with God's joy and blessings upon their return home.

Why? It is because they had been with Him, and He with them. Often we overlook the fact that we see them (miracles) daily: Baby's first breath, the sun rising in its fullness once again to warm us, God's gift of allowing us yet another day. I have also seen growths removed; person's saved by strangers; people who will die for someone they know not. Are they not all miracles? You bet they are!

You need to know not only that I believe in miracles, but also that I believe that God may well have a miracle waiting for you! Do not rule it out. Do not merely dismiss this amazing possibility. I learned of one humbling human trait when serving in Vietnam, years ago. It is a saying from an earlier war, yet it applies to all wars: *There are no atheists in foxholes.* When we get weak in the knees, drained and forlorn, at the end of our rope, that is often the time when we look to our Blessed One. It is however, purely out of His love and grace that miracles are allowed. They are not granted because of our human piety or hand wringing or because we've been particularly good. They are granted out of grace, by God's grace, and partly because of your faith. Is it not written that we are to believe? Believe in those things unseen?

Miracles are a result of His pure, constant, unfailing love for us. They are an example of God's mighty power. Why are so many miracles illustrated in His Word? It is to show His absolute sovereignty, that there is no power above His. God is ruler of this world and any worlds to come. He has already placed the prince of the air under His sovereign control. That was accomplished on the cross, when He said, "IT IS FINISHED...." I do not even allow the prince to be placed in large letters, that's because he has been downgraded. And he can get over it!

So friend, look for the miracles. Be expectant! Keep looking up. They are happening all during our days and nights. Somewhere someone is unexpectedly assisting in the delivery of a baby; at another place someone is catching one who is falling from a window. On and on it goes – around the clock. (For God there is no clock.) There is a marriage being repaired; a drunk is slowly being restored to health in body and mind, a brand new life; one who has slipped to unforgivable depths has just been redeemed. All by God's loving grace!

The miracle can be for you. Count not yourself out of this great possibility. If you are downtrodden or afflicted, diseased in any way, look for the miracle. Is not John 3:16 a miracle? "FOR GOD SO LOVED THE WORLD HE GAVE HIS ONLY BEGOTTEN SON, THAT WHOEVER BELIEVES IN HIM SHOULD NOT PERISH BUT HAVE EVERLASTING LIFE." Believe the miracle!

Beloved Teacher, thank You for Your miracle of life. Thank You for the priceless gift of Your Son – our only way to Your throne. Thank You, that we not only see and believe in miracles, but that indeed there is a chance that we may be given yet another personal miracle, other than the one You have already granted us: life. We look forward to fulfilling Your holy will, Your awesome way – for we believe. We believe in miracles!

—Best Day Ever—

Attitude plays a huge role in the habilitative process of persons suffering AD. I continue studying and working my memory mirror, a special place for me, in a special room where daily I gaze at faces of family and friends adorning a large mirror. It is an almost sacred place now. The center portion of the mirror has a rectangular space reserved for the patient – me. I yet stare into that space from wherever I am, wherever I've traveled to. Stare into that centered empty space. I could go on about the day when the face in that space might frighten me, or become unknown to me, unrecognizable. Instead, I choose to focus on all the angels positioned around me. They are kin, friends; those who care. What warmth and love they offer me. If your face is missing, and you were invited to send a picture, or you were somehow overlooked, or I ran out of room, please don't take it to your grave. My mirror is after all, only so big.

"See how they love one another?" The words reverberate within my being this very morning. How can any of us look upon God's grand words and not be impressed? Is it not refreshing to know and believe His promises? He goes before you and me. He will never leave you or forsake you. Here's another portion I so love, "BUT THOSE WHO WAIT UPON THE LORD SHALL RENEW THEIR STRENGTH; THEY SHALL MOUNT UP WITH WINGS LIKE EAGLES. THEY SHALL RUN AND NOT BE WEARY. THEY SHALL WALK AND NOT FAINT." —Isaiah 40:31.

It is not my intention to overwhelm you, friend, especially if there are those reading these words, ones with little hope or waning faith. Nor do I wish to inflame you. I would much rather inspire you.

I cannot help but picture another portion of God's Holy Word, one so convincing, so comforting, "AND THE LORD, HE IS THE ONE WHO GOES BEFORE YOU. HE WILL BE WITH YOU. HE WILL NOT LEAVE YOU OR FORSAKE, DO NOT FEAR NOR BE DISMAYED."—Deut. 31:8. It is repeated elsewhere in our glorious Guidebook, too.

Why so many references of comfort within the pages of our Guidebook? Is it because as the Babe and then the One crucified, God so identified with what is up ahead for each of us, for you and me? He not only shored us up with a Comforter, God also shares words beyond our expectations. They are words of comfort, of hope, of glory! You see, in feeling as we do, and as He always does, God is able to fully show us that there will be bumps and certain dangers and catastrophes that befall us throughout our lives. He has been there. And this is one of the reasons for His comfort, and largely the reason for which He came here to earth. He came that you and I might one-day march proudly into His loving, eternal kingdom. Therefore, the words amazing grace.

It is possible you and I will never sweat great droplets of blood, yet God knew we would one day find ourselves somewhat the way He found Himself in the garden, alone, with even His friends sleeping, instead of keeping watch. He knew from day one, even before this day of soul-wringing, there would be times of total abandonment, times when we would also feel that God is so very far from us. Yet in His grand love and out of special concern for each one, God allowed Himself to suffer and die. And it's even more dramatic than that: He willed Himself to suffer and die. That even when we were less than we ought to be, even then, He made the atonement not only possible, He placed salvation within reach of our very weary souls. How great is that?

†

How many of us have not heard of Him? How many of us will not turn to God at one time or another? Such abundant grace flows from Him. I often consider AD groups, and family and friends to be much akin to God's grand love, His comfort, and His unending care. Could it possibly be that in our various gatherings, we are emulating Him, His awesome grace?

—Another Best Day—

"Best day I ever had!" It's an attitudinal reply. Yet I find it rather strange. I am thinking of how wonderful our lives are and of that little dog Lucy so loved; how I had not wanted Cleo to suffer. Sorry, I can't recall whether I've already told you about this happening. That's dementia. When you love something or someone so very much, and yet you're willing to give it up, that's even more powerful than attitude. Is it attitude in action? Some. But that's not the description I seek. Attitude can make enough of a difference to call it love in action.

When attitude allows us to give up something in order that someone might be better off, that's the attitude part of the love description I seek. No. No my friend, it is more than that. It is being able to ache, to cry, to suffer and often to be willing to die for one we so love, or one we hardly know perhaps. Like a hero in battle with no thought for her/his own safety, one moves

- 40 -

ahead with vigor and determination, running into hell in order to save another human being.

Heeding not the din or smoke of battle, or the noise and utter confusion, the unselfish one moves forward, eye ever on the prize. He is disciplined, dedicated, and selfless. That's love. That's the greatest love: the agape love. That's the love that causes us to be willing to give up something, without question. "BUT WE HAVE THIS TREASURE IN EARTHEN VESSELS, THAT THE EXCELLENCY OF THE POWER MAY BE OF GOD, AND NOT OF US. WE ARE TROUBLED ON EVERY SIDE, YET NOT DISTRESSED. WE ARE PERPLEXED, BUT NOT IN DESPAIR; PERSECUTED, BUT NOT FORSAKEN; STRUCK DOWN, BUT NOT DESTROYED – ALWAYS BEING ABOUT IN THE BODY OF THE DYING OF THE LORD JESUS, THAT THE LIFE ALSO OF JESUS MIGHT BE MANIFESTED IN OUR MORTAL FLESH." —II Corinthians 4:7-10.

—Choices, And The Invitation—

Who could possibly argue let alone understand the depth of those long ago words? Words once and now again penned. They fire a mighty melody into my troubled head. And then words seeming appropriate for this very moment: *"Have Thine own way, Lord, have Thine own way. Hold o'er my being absolute sway..."* Can you sense what God has done for us? What others have done especially those so young and tender, during the recent wars? How I hate the current war, and that our leaders will soon debate it no doubt in haste. (That too, written some time ago...) And is it not true all these many months later, now years?

It is by Your grace, we come to You. It is all by Your loving grace, Lord. How is it some will take an entire lifetime to fully appreciate Your gifts? I do not believe in accidents. I am wholly convinced as we traverse the paths of this planet, dusty and rocky, or clean and smooth, You Lord, know our every foothold, our every thought and deed, or lack thereof.

Although it is true (what my Marine friend, David, says), "We all have choices." It is also true that God had our way planned long before our first breath. I have been very fortunate to find myself surrounded by a blessed cadre of informed, loving, encouraging people most of my entire life – people willing to scratch the surface, willing to talk not just of the ball game or the weather.

Part of that, the reason for that has been allowing God to have His way. It is our precious God being invited into our daily lives. Or rather, our making His Presence the center of our lives; God is invited into these often shattered, crying, lost and lonely shells. Sometimes we are broken, yet it is He again, who puts us back together. For this to take place requires a receptive vessel. That, or one that is so broken, one that cries out for the Master's help. This is why I suspect that many of us are broken long before we invite God in. It is the brokenness that causes the crying out, is it not? I believe it. Have you yet had to be allowed to be broken?

—His Being With Me—

Often I have prayed on my way, before ministering to folks in nursing facilities or hospitals. This practice stills my soul and opens my vessel to God's Spirit. It allows our beloved One to enter in. It is this invitation that makes such a valuable difference. And it can be felt. I believe He's always near, ever present. Much of me believes that there must be this invitation, this special stillness within us; this openness to receive God in, so He may freely work and flow through us, so we may be His very hands and feet upon this colorful gem of a planet.

This disease, AD, is one that often makes you feel quite alone and desolate. It is very intense. It reminds me of when friends desert us, when we are most in need of support, yet they sever us. It may be with good intentions, but sometimes, it is just that we do some really crazy things when we think we are doing what should be done to one another. Father, forgive us. But back to the disease that causes me to cling to routine, much the same as a leaf clinging to its mother, the branch. For me, being open to God plays the grandest role in my life. Though this disease-laden part of my life has been so lonely, even when people are around, it has also been very abundant, very Spirit-filled. A time of great joy! A time of finding once again, people can be so very gracious and loving.

Ordinarily being alone can be a rotten thing. It should be how modern-day preachers describe what happens when we fail to call upon God, how your end might be because you were never receptive to Him. At least that seems to be part of the new concept being 'dished up' as what happens to those of us who do not make the grade so to speak. In learning this is 'the best day I ever had' I have found that God is always with me, always present. He is here through the rough times and He is with me when everything seems calm. What blessings God has to offer us in troubled times. What a blessing for each of us, at any time, forevermore!

†

Lord God, thank You for Your eternal comfort, Your promise never to forsake us, that You will go with us wherever we go. You are such a divinely comforting Father. Thank You for loving and forgiving even me. Allow me Father, to forgive those who I have felt poorly about, for I have carried that burden far too long. I pray for Your healing touch in the lives of others as well. I would never attempt to disrupt Your mighty plan, even if it meant that I am not to be healed. If in my daily distress these words might help one other person, then let them sound afar. If during this venture, these words assist just one other person to a better understanding of Your way, allow them to be read. If they will indeed draw just one soul to Your precious side, allow them to keep flowing from me. I am aware, Lord, it is important to recall one of our earthly song's lyrics, "There is healing in His grace, healing for the soul." Is it not what our entire life should be about? For if we are not willing to come to You, and learn of Your grace and example, could it not be that You might get our attention through allowing a dilemma to enter in? I certainly accept that, Father. Accept it as part of Your plan to reach the hard-to-reach soul. By Your grace, Your love, might we one day see Your loving face. O tender One, who urges me on, might this forever be to You one of my love songs. Thank you, too, Rabboni, that my Lucy was able to stay with me, even after I had to surrender my driver's license. Thank you that she has walked and talked, me in tow. She has promised to never leave me – even as You also promised. She stayed with me, listened and cared for me. Later, she cared enough to attend an Alzheimer's Association meeting.

- 43 -

It was a place where I learned of the love of others who are facing the same situation, the same questions.

†

Many years ago, I worked for a man named Vernon. Everyone called him Sam. Sam and I were a hoot for that place. We spoke directly to one another, and tried to be as honest as two crazy guys can be. He shared as much as he could with my shrinking brain. Since I have never seemed too mechanically inclined, I learned many things from this old boy, and it wasn't long until we became fast friends. It was a second-time-around experience for me at that establishment, so it made it easier still for us to become good friends.

I presented Sam a picture of one of the submarine tenders I'd served aboard; I even inscribed it for him. Sam was sort of a hero to me. He was, and also is a hero in the sense that he worked diligently to see to the needs of his patrons. He saw to it that each one was served as quickly and efficiently as possible. Yet his bailiwick didn't end there. One really neat quality about him, I never heard him grumble about his job.

A most helpful thing I had learned from him was "Remember, there is a trick to most everything." I was recently reminded of those words as I lightly brushed the filter of our clothes dryer, a clean dry paintbrush in hand. To me, it was a Sam-ism. Heretofore, I'd always done it the hard way, clawing at the dust and dirt particles on the net-like filter, then banging it up against whatever happened to be handy. This way I made a great mess. It had been Sam I am sure, who'd taught me the trick, the easy, efficient way to clean a filter. It was one of our many secrets. Something only Sam and I knew about. Unfortunately, the company Sam worked for will never understand how great this guy had been for them, to them. Indeed, there will never be another guy like Sam there. You see: some guys can never be replaced.

Whether one needed help with a closet door, or their heating and air-conditioning unit; something small such as adjusting the leg of a table or completely renewing an entire wing of the building, this, one of the last good guys, got-her-done.

Sam had a keen sense of humor and a way of prodding this person and that one, silently, behind the scenes, so eventually they might at least attempt to get along better; Sam was and is a peacemaker. I should have known back then that I was having trouble socializing. I was not always easy to get along with. In fact I was often a pain in the neck, maybe lower.

I remember when I first attempted any kind of painting around the place, it was Sam who had showed me how to angle my paintbrush so I could eventually paint the straightest line you ever saw, without so much as kissing the ceiling. It was another trick he had shared with this old sailor boy.

Sam and I often grieved the passing of this one or that one, almost in silence, as if it'd never happened. But we always felt each one's passing. At times he would share personal things with me, and likewise, I would tell Sam things that no one else had ever heard from me. You see, Sam was and is a friend for life. You don't get many of those, even in an entire lifetime.

When in the midst of unpleasant situations, it was Sam who'd stuck by me. He would watch out for me and do whatever he could. During times when I felt as if I might 'pack it all in' Sam knew how to back off and was able to ever so gently assist me in making the better decision, often he'd help me to just plain keep on keepin' on. Little did I know, something was amiss.

Even after I'd received my diagnosis: dementia, he remained steadfast and loyal. He was much more than a boss to me. He had the greatest gift of never letting you down. When my back pains worsened (Now I know about bone spurs and other ailments that burden our bodies), it was Sam who had pulled me away from the moving and lifting of heavy furniture. Sam cared. And as I believe I have shared elsewhere herein, when I began having trouble finding the right word, it was the same Sam who would fill in the blanks for me. He was being a caregiver, and didn't even know it. He was a natural for it. He was a great listener.

The amazing thing about this talented, caring friend: Sam seemed to have enough love inside of him, that he could be patient and helpful to many people at the same time on any given day – even when he (himself) wasn't feeling so hot.

They'll never replace Sam. There will, simply put, never be another Sam! Everyone ought to have a Sam. *Thank You, God.*

✝

Helper and Keeper of our eternity, thanks for the Sam's in our lives. Special people who know how to listen, how to be helpful, how to be as You'd have us be. There seem to be so many doubting, distrusting folks today, Lord. Might You allow us a few more akin to Sam to come along? Allow us ones more akin to You. Ones who take us for what we are, where we are, and gently guide us along our daily way, even during times when we seem rather contrary, or hurting inside and/or physically. (And dear God, be with another Sam, in Iraq, even as I type these words. Keep him safe and at peace in the midst of the horrors of war.)

—Music And Trains—

Thankfully, in the beginning of this work I learned why my church worship team nearly caused me to 'jump ship' if you will. By studying and sensing the disease, you early on learn how much 'on track' you are, that is, why it is that you're doing or have done many things that you're doing. I had become over-stimulated; bombarded by noise, that is, to me it was noise. No offense gang.

Now don't look for anyone to volunteer that information to you, there is of course an exception to every theory. There's one to what I just told you. If you have a good support group, or groups, a system, you will hear and learn many things that others have suffered, are suffering at the same time as you. And there is healing. Remember that. It causes me to reflect upon these words: *"THOUGH HE SLAY ME, YET WILL I TRUST HIM."* (First portion of Job 13:15). Thus enters the thorn, the set-me-free thorn.

Or in a neophyte layman's terms, had I been created to come to this time zone, enabling me to share this information with you? It makes God's purpose for me more abundantly clear now. I am totally convinced of it. Everything has led me in this direction for some time now.

But again, do not wait for anyone to share with you how noise overload or bombardment may affect you. I have since learned that the noise overload situation I most feared is usually a short-lived process for early onset folks. And indeed, it may be one of those affectations that you never experience at all. That is, if you're a patient, you may never suffer noise overload.

Some of this is as in other diseases, not carved in stone. AD groups are relatively new to this nation, having been started only about forty years ago. So a lot of this is relatively new territory. And as for me, since drums and bass guitars often remind me of war noises, overload may not be over. The sounds often trigger thoughts of long ago; thoughts I cannot erase.

Yet I must return to music, music the joy of the soul, music that makes me feel whole, music that is now one of my daily goals. Music revives me.

The why and how of music's blessings upon us is one of those realms that I did not ask the psychologist or neurologist about. I didn't even contact Doctor Reid, one of my favorites. She is not only a caring Christian woman, she is also one who would do whatever it takes within her means to make life better for a patient. She is indeed unique today. She is a blessing.

Knowing when I hear the lyrics and melody that profess we are standing in God's Presence, I yet get shivers up and down. It awakens my very soul! And, it reminds me of my friend, Doctor Reid. It reminds me because she cares. She knows His Presence! She daily lives with Him. It is something that I, too, am learning more and more. Recognizing more.

It should never escape me, for when I entered a local dementia-filled unit, still fortunate enough to minister then, and as I slowly and softly witnessed to mostly ladies there, I again and again learned the greatness of the simple words and melody of the 'Yes, Jesus Loves Me' song. There is no need to further explain that melody or those words. But it's not simply the singing. It is smiles and gentle rocking back and forth, eyes shining for a moment or two. There is something about music and Jesus that restores life, if only for an instant. It is a connection traversing a chasm, sometimes a very great chasm.

Surmising is not particularly one of my fortes, but here I go: Suppose one of the trains that I've had waiting on the track of my life is my combat train. Now I cannot explain to you or anyone else why it is that my train has been fairly quiet until wars began starting up again in the early nineties. Don't get me wrong; the train had been there all along, maybe they had kept her fired-up just enough to keep the old embers glowing within her, but I am going to surmise that the train waiting upon the track, with the exception of an occasional combat nightmare, had been waiting for me twenty-four years before the early nineties! My combat train had been there ever since my 'visit' to Vietnam and the Mekong Delta. And, as sure as that train's movement has again been triggered by old memories, I have learned AD has triggers as well. It is after all, those triggers that enable trains to have their fiery souls revived not only by a voice from the past, a memory, or a smell (and so on), but by our up-to-date, up-to-the-minute news media. The fast reporting force that 'shoves it all in your face' and often goes right to your stomach, to your very core! Many cannot comprehend it, for they have not experienced it.

Suppose for a moment, train number one let's call it, suppose the wheels are turning and the mighty noise and smoke revive feelings deeply seated within us similar to my combat-revived stuff. Suppose the train regurgitates its rumbling sounds and begins as well to spew out beautifully billowing white steam clouds. Suppose it is as vivid as when my mind's eye visualizes a chopper landing in my front yard on occasion, and when this happens during one of my short sleep cycles, I bust off a tooth. (It is by the way, the only crown I'll ever see. And one I no longer need to worry about paying for.) And actually, Someone else paid for the other.

What kind of force is this? It's the same question I'd asked my neurologist. "What kind of 'stuff' is this?" Of course the writer of my Foreword, Doctor John J. Hennessey, IV, probably said something such as this: "Think about landmarks, Wayne." And I might have returned, "I'd love to, but when you can't recall what's in front of you or what's behind you, well, landmarks aren't real helpful, Doc." Little did I know I was tipping him off to giving up my operator's license.

Some of this I can work through; other parts of it are more difficult. Now that this intimidating train has been around so very long: it has become a chronic train for me – my chronic combat train. (But convincing people of that has been a whole 'nother book, trust me.) I realize it will always be a part of me. A very discomforting, ready to roll, hyper-vigilant train, a lot like me. It sometimes causes panic, and actually, I sometimes see it with other AD patients.

Then there's train number two. Are you lost yet? Train number two is my dementia-laden train. I might call it my AD train. This train was also loaded long before I had ever been notified. It was loaded without so much as a whisper to my ear. Secretly, I guess. This train is normally a slow moving, somewhat sneaky train. Picture that, a sneaky train, and part of me does surmise as that old song, *My Child Is Going Home.*

For although we become childlike, it's that loaded AD train, loaded long ago with old memories, that train now slowly pulls away from the platform for Who-Knows-Where Land. So the train is either noisy and mighty and smoky, or it's sneaky and slower. Are not those trains somehow tied together in my memory bank? Or, as I say from time to time as I make my way along, are the trains not all of a piece? Is it all not somehow connected?

Just as my locomotives chug along, their loads trailing behind them, is it not possible that music could also be a train? I don't believe I'd give it a number, but I might name it. I am picturing 'Joy Train,' or a 'Happiness Train' name. But no, to me it must be 'Memory Lane Train.' Simple, descriptive, appropriate, 'Memory Lane Train...'

No wonder the gals at the facility rocked ever so gently from side to side; No wonder their eyes were so wide; No wonder it had been a moment or two of pride. Somewhere from deep within, no matter what stage they've entered, somewhere, huge wheels have begun to turn, and slowly, ever so slowly, that huge old 'Memory Lane Train' has begun its forward momentum... bound for Who-Knows-Where Land.

Music makes me think that our spirit does not leave us, even as we endure these vast changes in life. God's grace. Remember how He cares for you? Read Psalm 121:3-8. It's a grand reminder of God's care.

†

Thank You, God, for enabling me yet to write. Thank You, I am still able to converse, to think, to share thoughts with others as music continues to revitalize me, too. Your depth, Father, is beyond our comprehension, Your love fathomless, Your grace ever flowing. To me, Father, Your mighty power is world shaking. Thank You, God. And thank You for music; those mysterious melodies that make it possible for lost ones, if only briefly, to become able to join the ranks of the here and now. Thank You so much. How we love You, no matter how many trains we face in life - no matter where those trains are bound. For Father, we realize that You are the Engineer - that You always will be, and it is You who takes us to our final destination, home.

Chapter 3

Affectations

—Fear—

The subject of fear and how we approach it is different for each of us. As we plan our way through life, we sooner or later discover that life is what happens whether we plan our way or not. And sometimes that means we will be facing fear of one kind or another. It causes me to recall the publisher who asked for my work (with interest) and held it for more than half a year, and upon returning it never bothered to say why.

I suspect that how we react is according to experiences that we have gathered along the way, in part, and yet with many of us it seems that we often invent unnecessary fears for one reason or another, or as we wish to. There are also times when fear comes from who knows where, and comes in many different forms for different reasons: psychologically, chemically or physiologically, or as Doctor John might say, pathophysiologically. (Doctor John knows those bigger words.) I have noted persons very calm in emergencies, and others who go to pieces it seems when baby gets his first gash, bump or bruise.

As I begin to ramble along, I am entirely out of my league, only reaching for what I think might be proper words to explain a complex world few laymen may ever understand. Fear is not only what happens to us; fear is not only something we may help form; fear is sometimes thrust upon us. Fear is akin to what C.S. Lewis once wrote or was quoted as saying in '*Shadow lands*': "…Lands we sometimes don't understand, nor wish for, or hope to endure…"

Yet somehow, for some reason, part of me realizes that deep within my heart of hearts, fear is also part and parcel of what makes us human. It is what erases all presumptions, all foolishness, and enables us to realize how delicately fragile we really are. For me, the worst part may be continuing to be alive, yet concerned about being lost. But I promise you this: If you put on the helmet of God's salvation, and carry your Sword with you, and realize that you are God's, then fear can and will be lessened to a great and grand extent. Trust me. No, trust God.

Fear is very real, very human. And our Lord certainly understood that kind of being lost, fear: abandonment. Fear can be so demoralizing and can quickly bind you into a shock-you-into action world like none before. Fear is what saved many of my brothers and sisters in battle. Then again, not to freeze, but to be able to work in the face of fear for the love of a comrade or a group and country (or as the Marines say, The Corps), is one of the noblest goals I can think of at this writing.

Other dementia-laden folks have shared some of what I will also share with you, that I am experiencing. It is a different kind of fear. For example, I've had very vivid dreams of playing, wrestling with my grandchildren. It is as if they were here with me, tumbling and giggling and climbing all over me. There is nothing but laughter and screaming in my ears. Then upon awaking, it is so very sad, for sometimes I wonder if I'll one day lose the cheerful playful dreams: even those grand yesteryear thoughts of such playful delight.

It's difficult imagining how those cheerful, loving images can suddenly seem worse than any combat dream. Perhaps it's just the thought of losing the good stuff, even though you know your traumatized dreams will never end, never go away. (Now there's an area that I would not mind ditching.) And yes, it is one that I have often spoken with God about.

A Diplomat in Neurology, Doctor John, was right so many months (perhaps years ago). "Two trains are headed for you at the same time," were part of his fateful and insightful words. Words that not many others could grasp or decipher. I really believe that some agencies don't want to know what we are living with/through. Some of the workers seem to act as if it is their money they are taking out of pocket to help you. How sad. Too long in their chairs I'd guess.

†

I have a friend who was a door gunner aboard a chopper in Vietnam, and the other day I learned that his primary care physician advised them that they have been denied assistance for PTSD because he (or she) claims that it is not connected to his current situation: Alzheimer's. You talk about going into a rage. Yes, I'm talking about me. I yet have not decided what to do with that. It shall not die though, you can count on that.

It's one thing to forget a word now and again, or to over and over forget why you've entered a particular room, or to forget the name of someone close to you. But the grave realization that what is up ahead may be so drastically unknown to you starts one to thinking, how much longer do I really have? And maybe it's not how much longer do I have, but, when will the quality of life become so diminished that I will no longer realize it is quality of life?

How much longer can I remain with ones I love? I have wondered when will it come about that I will no longer recognize my safe haven, my home, friends, my beloved church family, and especially, how long until I can no longer recognize my sweet wife, my children, siblings and acquaintances. And for some unexplainable reason the worst pain: the idea of never again knowing those innocent, loving grandchildren. I guess that's the crux of it, because they're just starting out and we long to know how their entire lives will progress. I don't want to say that all we can do is pray for them because I know the power of prayer! Prayer is as God, limitless, at least sincere prayer is. It is because God can do anything! That, my friend, is worth repeating: ***God can do anything!***

I remember fear from my younger years. All that fear seems somewhat incidental now. Some of the fears at least. Fearing where my next duty assignment would take me; fearing whether I could 'pass muster' during my military evolutions; fear of failing period.

We create so very many often-needless phobias for ourselves, and yet I recall Paul's wonderful words: "FEAR NOTHING, OR WORRY ABOUT NOTHING." St. Paul seemed so steeped in his love of God that he seemed to have no fear, either that or he was so committed to not showing fear (for the love of his brothers and sisters) for the strength of his convictions. What a bastion he had become for Christ, for Christians everywhere.

†

On the other hand, in our younger years we don't seem to fear as much, do we? I had even felt that I'd played the part of a crusty old pirate of sorts on my way into Vietnam (at least until I departed the airplane), only then upon deplaning to learn of and see men lined up on either side of us, rifles at-the-ready across their chests. Welcome committee? Hardly. We were actually receiving incoming fire. It was something I was not real familiar with. I guess it was then, 'boots on the ground' when I first became aware that I was no longer just a lad. Could no longer afford to be a boy. Put that in your PTSD files!

I had thought: What a place to grow up in! No, I simply pretended that I could shoot my way out, alongside the best of them. I wasn't there for any birthday party. I had, after all, been a volunteer; I had wanted to serve. There were many more of us back in those days it seems. More pride it seems, perhaps more longing to be of service to a promising Republic.

But I now have an even deeper, more repulsive fear; to me it is worse than combat's fear. Is it possible, and I'd gamble it is, when one enters that very innermost part of the sanctum, is it possible that he/she might forget those memories of long ago, especially the good ones?

One night I had the strange sense that I was the 'old me' and the ' new me', yet I was aware of my sweet Lucy's presence, too. You tell me.

In the dream, I thought back to carefree childhood days on a farm, of how when I was barely able to walk, each time I'd approach this one particular Billy goat, how I would once again learn that he was disinterested in my standing up. Ever. Each time I did stand or make my wobbly way toward him, he'd knock me down again. I can yet hear Momma's laughter behind me. That feisty Billy though, he had been the adversary that had made it possible for me to always get back up, again and again. To keep on keepin' on. Never give up! (I had first learned it from Billy.) Yes, it's worth repeating: Never give up!

Would the long ago embedded memories be torn away from me? Fear. There it is again. Then there's that always-haunting thousands-of-years-old line out of China: 'No one knows what goes on in a man's mind.' How true that is. Yet remember this, friend: God knows.

Would I forget the day, hand in hand, Momma had first walked me to the school bus stop? Would I forget long before I had ever learned much about military discipline, that life had been quiet and I had been so lovingly surrounded by smiles and warmth and love, all of it so NOT akin to military life, at least in the beginning.

What a fear it can be for some of us, just growing up. Little did I know on that first scary day of school, a young mother feared for me, too, as she let my tiny hand slide out from within her hand. There's a certain amount of reluctance within most adults when one of the little ones takes his first steps out of their parents' tender care. All right, for many of us it is/was apprehension, fear. No, more like trauma: sheer and very real trauma.

It had all been as clear as burning white phosphorous, (flashback), that I'd better fear it when my second wife and I began to watch life's situations escalate before our eyes. It was another white-hot fear recalling the success rate for Vietnam veterans on their second time around in marriage! A little knowledge can be dangerous indeed, or helpful.

The reason for the beginning of that fleeting thought about my wife and I, especially for those of you who revel in minimization, is because I'd started to share with you that fear can be a good thing. Fear can and sometimes does save us from unexpected endings, sometimes even death, or at least some less difficult situations.

Someone once penned that ninety percent of what we worry about never takes place. This patient believes that for the most part, or as we say in Virginia (now that I've been transplanted a while) *right much*. Sometimes all that's needed is to communicate, as my wife sometimes does, lovingly, standing before me, making eye contact and repeating: "Take chicken out of the freezer for dinner," until I finally get the message and/or acknowledge her.

—Uncertainty—

I'm not totally sure what stage I've progressed to at this point, for that matter, who is? But I note with AD that I yet open the refrigerator door now and again upon hearing the microwave's "I'm ready" beeping. My wife could more readily tell you where I am, trust me. Yours, too?

Here's hoping that you are not one of those folks that laughs and says, "I do that all the time." Well, chances are if you've made it into your 70s or 80s or beyond, and can yet laugh at dementia, I reply, God bless you! He loves you! Keep on laughing. Seriously.

†

No one knows his or her own fate, or exactly what waits up ahead. Not unless they've been terribly bad on purpose their entire lives. Yet I do know and believe in a Power above and through all. One who helps us along the way. Praise God for His eternal comfort to us. Praise God, who turns fear into love.

And Lord God, thank You for loving us, even though there are times we do not deserve it, are certainly NOT loveable. When You first set love in motion for us, Father, it indeed caused the world to go 'round, at least Your wonderful world, the unseen world. And that is (for me) the only true world in existence, the eternal world, for all others mock Your loving ways. All others fall dreadfully short.

(My sinful self, my only shame, my glory all the Cross…)

—Sameness—

This AD patient early realized the sharing of 'sameness' of issues for the patient and the caregiver. It is without a doubt important for both caregiver and receiver (the patient) to prioritize his/her life if at all possible. It reminds me of how 'de-cluttering' had assisted me in encountering less stimulation, enjoying cleaner simpler lines around me, and generally giving me a sense of calmness. Both giver and receiver find the simplifying and ordering of their lives important. This is a time of emotional overload, during early onset, a time that tries all our senses. It is a time when we begin to focus on basics, on the stripping away of nonessential games of life, detractors, anything that gets in the way of what is real.

Keeping yourself in good physical condition (as mentioned in our *Newsflash*) only pages ago, as well as working the mind, are areas my caregiver and I have found to be common areas.

There is much to be said for being physically fit. It is an area that I will later address more thoroughly. Remind me.

I've found, as I visited Alzheimer's facilities, or places that house AD folks, these precious people are often sequestered away, almost totally lacking in any exercise regimen whatsoever. Trust me. I would counter this immediately to border on maltreatment, not only because it (exercise) has such great advantages for us in many ways, but also because it promotes longevity of life. And I realize that may be contrary to the thinking of some, but I am certain of this: Exercise makes quality life/living better for most everyone.

Sharing emotions with friends and family is another important area to the caregiver and patient alike. Much of that is due to the huge volume of stress-filled data, as well as stimuli that daily bombard us. Thankfully, I have observed and noted that patients seem more at ease conversing the more they attend and adjust to their meetings, their gatherings, and their sameness.

Allowing others to realize how we feel and 'where we are' is rather cathartic. If you can't do it with someone close, find an acquaintance with a good ear. As the patient, much of my daily life is spent in routine, and that is something very important to me. Naturally, as the caregiver allows himself/herself to also bring others into their circle, some relief is likely to take place for them. It is again akin to our assembling, all of us in similar situations. We find ourselves not only drawn to one another in our commonness, but also we are more easily bound together by our common dilemmas and situations. Any good facilitator or pastor will share that with you.

It is not wallowing in our pity when we gather, but rather a way we begin the process of healing (as far as possible), and or adjusting, or at the very least a better understanding of our condition. Whether you are the patient or the care partner, being able to share your thoughts, fears, desires and hopes is surely on the plus side of the board. From a brief conversation I had with Nancy, a neat lady at our local Alzheimer's Association chapter in Richmond, I was thoroughly convinced that I had shared and been heard by a very caring, loving devoted person. She is a family care coordinator, and they have the right person in that slot. What a blessing it is to meet someone so attune to what the patient is facing, to what it is that consumes patients during this most devastating journey.

This is an area of considerable concern for both partners, as they traverse the path leading to a place where only God can go, it seems. It reminds me again, as I'd shared the 'Yes, Jesus Loves Me' song with other patients. It makes one wonder if these old, so loved songs are one of His ways of assisting us in being transported to the new, rather unknown world. It would be one of my prayers that I never forget my wife's sweet voice and way, as we often sing praise music as we travel along in our vehicle or sit in God's glorious house. We get so pumped! And that's the way it is with God. Sometimes it's as if we've already been to His eternal home, even before we get there. You can... you can go there, too. Music so stokes the embers of our very core! Music involves many of our senses. Music may be one of the areas far underdeveloped during the habilitative process. It is why I have also placed it as one of the spokes of my Ezekiel's Wheel Vision paradigm. More on that later.

†

Then there's the breathe perspective. Please breathe, and breathe deeply. Do not allow yourself to share the worst of the worst with yourself, that is, do not convince yourself that the worst thing ever has come into your life. **Never give up!**, and breathe.

When we start believing that our situation is so poor or unyielding in any way, we are allowing ourselves to relinquish to this disease even before it's time. (Then again, I'm not sure I feel that everyone should be fully made aware of his or her new life, and I believe it has much to do with what stage they are in, and other medical conditions and considerations.) This, my friend, may well be doctor and/or counselor parley territory. That one's free.

That awareness mentioned above, is akin to the person I will tell you about later, who lost a toe and gave up and died! Now I hope and have every good wish and prayer for the abandoned-feeling person. I only wish I could have influenced that life more. Earlier. What I'm getting at is: I'm not certain that it's always proper for everyone to be fully cognizant of where they are/what they are up against. Sometimes again, it is a doctor's call. (The family, and/or loved one may need to consult with the doctor. An old minister's opinion.) See John 15:16. It's a comfort to me.

†

After the release of my first work, *GIRLS CAN DO ANYTHING!*, I happily opened letters mostly from young readers. Their sweet words of one day being a writer 'like you' soothed me.

There is sameness in this, too. All of us desire to be emulated in one way or another, to have a kind of legacy. It is not just to be emulated though; it is that hope that we will have embraced something worthwhile in life, something that someone else might embrace that makes a difference in his or her life, a difference in the lives of others.

One thing I sense in my bones, more important than most of us may realize is our veracity. And some folks might think this is much to do about nothing. Well, dear friend, this is a time when I refer you to Romans 1:18. It speaks of mankind suppressing the truth. It seems that we often overlook one of the vital tenets of our Lord's foundations as we turn away from truth. I am not about to launch into a dissertation on it, but will say: sometimes we pay little attention to an area that requires more focus, more concern, especially in the lives of our little people, when they are developing. If we do not teach them honesty when they are young, later on they will be even more conniving. Of course all of that comes from a person with dementia. Yet I stand by my statement, and God's truth.

Speaking of dementia, have you ever looked closely at words listed under dementia? Here are a few of them: 'insane, stark-mad, crazy, sick, psycho, lunatic, of unsound mind, deranged, deluded, unhinged, unbalanced, out of one's mind, cracked, brainsick, not right in the head', at least, those are a few. It is not the vocabulary one would pick for his legacy, is it?

If care partners and receivers are honestly able to make an effort to move the situation in a worthwhile direction, what a change this might cause! Both sides, partners in the disease, are scared out of their wits! Understandably so. As you sit on the patient side of meetings about dementia, you learn that there are many different sides to the disease. It seems no two people are alike, at least not a lot alike, yet I have noted that most of us (patients), are rather docile in that we are caring and loving. We seem to fit in with one another. Usually.

There is no model for the disease; and sadly, there is yet no cure, only the wondering, the waiting, and hopefully a great attitude to help us get by. The attitude of a fighter, that *Never give up!* attitude. This is the fight of your life, you'll hear that again.

On the care partner side of the meeting, they too are devastated, grasping for straws, for hope, a new sign perhaps. A big new neon sign on the horizon that flashes that he/she is coming back. I've heard it said in my wife's exasperated times: "I wish I had my old husband back." (It is quite possibly why I sit here today, typing alone at my keyboard, while my caregiver enjoys her grandchildren's birthdays, as if I were something or someone to keep hidden away. You see, often the care receiver can be an embarrassment to caregivers. It is not always a joyous love circle.) Fortunately, that is not the case here. Not normally.

Just for the record, Lucy has always been good to me, but as everyone, she sometimes needs a break! So don't be too concerned about my 'left-alone' words. They change with the wind, just as you and I sometimes do.

If you have not already read it, it is the single most horrific part of the disease, when your partner no longer recognizes you. It is something akin to death. (Although some say they (patients) actually do recognize folks. I'm not sure how they've arrived at that, and I haven't asked the 'experts' about it. I'll leave that one for your research.)

Caregiver and patient have sameness in that they are striving for identity and understanding: a chance to speak their mind. Maybe it is a hope that they will get a glimpse, even a tiny glint that there is yet hope up ahead, maybe not as far off as the 'guesstimators' claim. After all, who enjoys saying "Goodbye" early? Who wants to be the first to say, "It was a great run," or "I have so loved you?" Really.

On the opposite hand, that of being hidden away: There is often a 'drawing together' almost exclusive to spouse and patient. It becomes apparent that there is more caring, more tenderness, perhaps a stronger commitment. Whatever it's called, anyone with any feeling for another human being suddenly realizes just how short and fragile our lives are/how very little we really control. Sometimes that even includes we (ourselves).

Kid yourself not, this roller-coaster ride, this little dance the caregiver and receiver do, sometimes separates us, and yet at other times in our separateness we become more alike. In what we sense as 'isolating' we become more bound together, inexorably bound. It causes one to not want to be left, the other not wanting to be left alone. And of course that can easily be switched around.

A sad statistic: fully 30% of caregivers die before the patient. What does it say concerning the love of a partner who must take on responsibilities for both persons? No wonder so many caregivers eventually give up, or are forced to depart early, good fields of work.

Then there's the difficult decision about how long the caregiver can continue on, or if their patient must be maintained elsewhere. To me, it seems to depend upon what stage the patient has entered and/or his/her physical wellness, as well as the ability or non-ability of the caregiver to care for the patient. In the final analysis, there remains nothing but care, and more care.

As you have probably surmised, these are heavy, emotional, difficult times and decisions that no one else can make for the caregiver. When? How long? How much? Is it any longer important to my loved one? Did I see to the wishes of the individual? Have I honored him/her? These things can turn one inside out in a very short period of time. An intelligent caregiver may even have to consult his (or her) doctor about some assistance.

And always there's the "Why me?" part of it all: in the beginning, in the middle, in the end. Just as in any good writing, three specific segments, even if they are considered fragments. If you know anything about this disease, you know that 6 out of

10 of us wander. We either lose our sense about where we are, where we belong, or merely become more and more confused. It brings about much sadness and/or danger.

Some say once the declaration is delivered, that one 'has it'- the disease; the caregiver loses his/her life, the focus so drastically changes. There is however, believe it or not, an upside to that, too. It is aptly captured in Matthew 16:25-27: "FOR WHOSOEVER DESIRES TO SAVE HIS LIFE WILL LOSE IT, BUT WHOSOEVER LOSES HIS LIFE FOR MY SAKE WILL FIND IT. FOR WHAT PROFIT IS IT TO A MAN IF HE GAINS THE WHOLE WORLD, AND LOSES HIS OWN SOUL? OR WHAT WILL A MAN GIVE IN EXCHANGE FOR HIS SOUL? FOR THE SON OF MAN WILL COME IN THE GLORY OF HIS FATHER WITH HIS ANGELS, AND THEN HE WILL REWARD EACH ACCORDING TO HIS WORKS." Please be not concerned for yourself here, friend, fight that urge. Works are grand. But remember, eternity is made possible by God's grace! His grace alone; then again, do not abandon the good work that you might have done because you rested solely upon the grace part, they do, after all, go hand in hand. There is a balance. I often thought how this portion of the book could have easily been entitled: *Balancing Act*.

The last judgment is what the reward part is referring to in the above passage. But never dwell on the rewards portion. It reminds me of closeting ourselves away in prayer, a good practice (not one of puffing ourselves up about what good we do or say). Yet be not pious. I fear that I have started preaching too much here. In reality, our churches (he goes on), fall far short of anything God expects of us; most of us in the pews have a shortsighted idea of what we are to be about – and many of us are content to allow our church worlds to become clubs of a sort: busy in this and that. Clubs where we pay our weekly attendance dues. What a drastic shame.

We can miss so very much in our 'busyness' it seems. I'm afraid too many of us think that 'being busy' is what it's all about; no wonder so many of us seem to be rushing around to be first to arrive at the next traffic signal. Where are we all rushing to? It's not simply a Western question any longer.

And the real question, the crux of it all, my friend: It is found in I Timothy 2:1-4: "THEREFORE I EXHORT FIRST OF ALL THAT SUPPLICATIONS, PRAYERS, INTERCESSIONS, AND GIVING OF THANKS BE MADE FOR ALL MEN, FOR KINGS AND ALL WHO ARE IN AUTHORITY, THAT WE MAY LEAD A QUIET

AND PEACEABLE LIFE IN ALL GODLINESS AND REVERENCE. FOR THIS IS GOOD AND ACCEPTABLE IN THE SIGHT OF GOD OUR SAVIOR, WHO DESIRES ALL MEN TO BE SAVED AND TO COME TO THE KNOWLEDGE OF THE TRUTH." –NKJV, Zondervan

There is great richness and strength in our working together. Indeed the church is not about the pastor alone, or about this one or that one. Always, we are to be centered on Christ! Let's not allow our 'busyness' to be considered what we are all about. Recall instead the words in our Guidebook: SEE HOW THEY LOVE ONE ANOTHER. I wish I had written them first. Please save one another has much to do with these words. Love and honor one another, as God has loved you.

†

Almighty Creator of all, thank You for the wisdom You have allowed us to visit. Assist us as we mine Your word for truth and wisdom. Thank You that there is a brotherhood even in the sharing of disease and what You allow us to endure at times. Not only does it draw us closer to one another, trauma often draws us closer to You; it draws us to a sameness, an awareness. What a gracious, loving, all-powerful God You are. What an inclusive God You are! We ask You to forgive us for our childishness when it comes to the ways of Your kingdom. Nothing we desire compares with You! Nothing.

Speaking of sameness, you should see my nephew's twins: Grace and Olivia. Talk about sameness? Congratulations Chris and Betty, and grandparents, too.

—I Didn't Realize It Until I Read About It: Sexuality—

"You would have died laughing," I laughed as I had shared with my Lucy that very morning. The description I'd earlier read, and why I therefore encourage you to continue to read about AD as long as you can; it had fit me to a T!

… "Call the cops!" I'd said aloud not many days earlier. "Lock me up!" I'd been standing almost directly behind an attractive young woman in a drugstore line. She had caught your humble servant's eye and I was being very mundane and saying something about the great things God makes, and I'd almost added that He had almost kept 'it' to Himself. It was indeed, very inappropriate. Scary. Yet what scared me more about it is what AD researchers and care partners have written about 'it', what they have observed.

I do confess to old friends and kin as well. Yes, I know I've always been somewhat confused in the sexuality arena, alright, I've at times often said this: "Terry genes are some of the most powerful genes on the face of this planet." That can be a curse as well as a blessing. I'm not going there. Be thankful.

But guess what, old friend, I also had felt God's awesome Presence in my home at nearly the same time I had been writing those words. And it wasn't much later, as I hugged Doll Face (Donna), as we sang the *You are worthy of my praise* words to a song we so love. What a graciously amazing, forgiving and compassionate God!

Here is what some writers and other thinkers say about sexuality. One, it is often apparent that we become hypersexual (AD folks), and we sometimes make inappropriate advances. (I last year returned from a cruise to the Bahamas, trust me: we *do* know how to have fun!) Caregivers may wish to think about obtaining a letter or small card that states why their charge says stupid things, or worse, does stupid things. Some Alzheimer's Association chapters have such cards readily available. (I think that may be reiterated herein elsewhere.)

Patients become frustrated, eventually, due to the inability to talk about intimacy. A back rub can often help us (patients). (I know it works for caregivers, too.)We sometimes do express sexual interest in other parties. (Much to the chagrin of our partners.)We sometimes do not get the meaning of jokes; nor do others get the meaning of ours. Remember, intimacy can continue, and perhaps is needed more now. Trust me!

The sexuality situation does nothing to calm me; if anything, it simply confirms the doctor's diagnosis; confirms his 'you have it' words.

†

I had always had an eye for/on the 30-year-young group of women, but for a time I'd found myself practically seeking them out. Now, much of that can simply remain playful badger, but there is yet enough sense in what is left of my brain to know that you may not always get that trickle of laughter and gigantic smile response. More importantly, you may find one day that you've just used what you felt was the perfect line, maybe: "My, I haven't seen you for so long," is a good example. You might use that, and learn her (or his) guard dog is standing nearby and has just overheard you, and is not aware you are a patient of dementia. He may beat the crap out of you! Needless to say, this keeps your caregiver, and/or close friend on their toes!

—Struggling—

Yes, I had struggled with the thought of approaching my family doctor, requesting medicine for the situation (Notice I did not call it a problem). Instead, I prayed heavily and heartily and long about the situation – and yes, God provided an answer, as He always does when we are sincere. Unfortunately, I must not have prayed hard enough, or my genes were stronger than my faith. But I did read these words from our Guidebook which helped. They are especially powerful for me: "...WITH HER FLATTERING LIPS SHE SEDUCED HIM" "...AND ALL WHO WERE SLAIN BY HER WERE STRONG MEN." (Refers to the under-world). (From Proverbs 7, a portion of verses 11 and 26.) Next, verses 16 and 17 from Proverbs 9: "...WHOEVER IS SIMPLE, LET HIM TURN IN HERE; AND AS FOR HIM WHO LACKS UNDERSTANDING, SHE SAYS TO HIM, STOLEN WATER IS SWEET, AND BREAD EATEN IN SECRET IS PLEASANT." The forbidden is often attractive, unfortunately. So if you need to be, beware. And ponder this, please.

I have also learned during my study of AD persons, such as myself, we have other problems with sexuality, such as inappropriate sexual activity, exhibitionism, and unrestrained use of sexual phrases or even promiscuity. (W. Malloy, *Alzheimer's Disease,* A Firefly Book.) It seems everyone needs to be touched and hugged and held, even folks with illness. Unfortunately, some of us are unable to express our needs in socially accepted ways. (And inappropriate grabbing can be a problem!) A big problem.

As expressed before within these pages, as I walk mornings, evenings, whenever, I often spend time with our Lord. It is after one of these 'segments of time' I call them, I read this in God's

Word: "I REMEMBER THE DAYS OF OLD; I MEDITATE ON ALL YOUR WORKS; I MUSE ON THE WORK OF YOUR HANDS. I SPREAD OUT MY HANDS TO YOU; MY SOUL LONGS FOR YOU LIKE A THIRSTY LAND. ANSWER ME SPEEDILY, O LORD; MY SPIRIT FAILS! DO NOT HIDE YOUR FACE FROM ME, LEST I BE LIKE THOSE WHO GO DOWN INTO THE PIT. CAUSE ME TO HEAR YOUR LOVING KINDNESS IN THE MORNING. FOR IN YOU DO I TRUST; CAUSE ME TO KNOW THE WAY WHICH I SHOULD WALK, FOR I LIFT UP MY SOUL TO YOU"... —Psalm 143:5-8.

It was this portion of our Guidebook that helped hammer it home, my inappropriateness. As you may have guessed, I don't mean that I haven't thereafter noticed the beauty of women, and I also admit that I have not always been back on track, but God is helping me, showing me that I do not need to comment, or linger long in thought concerning the beauty of any other than my sweet wife, my Lucy, my one and only, Donna.

Now I've gotten down to the very serious task of asking for God's forgiveness, of realizing and facing my obvious weaknesses, and of asking our Lord to lead me in how I am to go. I know it sounds simple, and in a sense it is. To me, however, it is mostly an attitudinal thing, a commitment to one who died for you and me; One who wants the best for us; One who expects nothing less than our best. Or as Oswald Chambers' book title so aptly declares: *My Utmost For His Highest.* (That one's for you, Favorite Daughter.)

†

Thank you, God, for enabling me to be bound more firmly to my wife's loving personhood. Thank You for helping me realize that You bound us together, and that You did not mean for either of us to stray, not even when we find ourselves greatly tempted. And thank You, Father, for that portion of Your Holy Word that describes how a man is to treat his wife: even as Christ cherishes the church. Father God, offer us that healing, so even those of us diseased, may readily recall Your words early on in a heartbroken prophet's words, "HEAL ME, O LORD, AND I SHALL BE HEALED..." —Jeremiah 17:14. (in part)

—Sometimes I Do It: Ramble—

This segment, and what it is about, often drives Lucy mad: my rambling! The strange part about it: I know I ramble. Usually, I know. Is it because I have so much to say, or is it something about my temporary feeling of well being that causes so many different senses and emotions and ideas to spew forth from within? Is it because I fear forgetting what I have to say?

It is possible that I should have collaborated with my neurologist-friend, Doctor John, for I am certain that he would have wisdom heretofore unknown to this pea brain. Yet I automatically and quickly apologize to our Lord for the pea brain comment, for He has created such a beautifully complex and otherwise unobtainable work: the brain. The brain and our complex vessel it is housed in. And if I did collaborate with doctors on their opinion about everything, then the work would be more from the medical point of view and less from the patient's perspective. How unfair would that be? (Not to mention sometimes boring to most everyone as well.)

Yet rambling is what I do. It has caused Lucy to *Shush!* me more than once. I often feel guilty about what the caregiver endures. It almost rivals the guilt of being able to return from combat, when so many others do not/did not. And my PTSD-affected brain often flies to ones all busted-up and/or limbless. Pictures I really don't want to see or recall, yet ones that haunt me all too often. Sometimes I wonder if it'd been better to have died in combat. Sorry, Lord. (That one's for you, John McAllister.)

The rambling often begins early in the day with AD, and I'm not usually even aware that I am engaged in it at that time, not until it's brought to my attention. And yes, sometimes it occurs late in the day, when I'm very tired. When my cobwebbed brain feels 'fried'. That's part of dementia, at least for me.

†

On one occasion, our sweet neighbors and Lucy and I were on our way somewhere. Debbie had turned to my wife and asked, "Is he always this way?" Yes, often I am. Part of me wonders, since it's often early in the day, or would that be four or five hours after my first awaking, I wonder if I have read my subconscious thoughts and my mind merely continues to 'roll ideas out' even when I am at rest. I wonder if it's what has recently been processed, and has just begun to come to the surface again. Sometimes I do not sense what's taking place, as if everything's in autopilot. Or is it merely a confusion of a sort?

That, too, could be misinterpreted, that is, sometimes it seems the 'rambling' has something to do with what I've recently dreamed or thought while in a dream state. Still, another part of me wonders: Can the subconscious be running one work and your dream state occupy a totally different area at the same time? Or do we only recall what we were last somewhat consciously or subconsciously exposed to? Were I not so busy surmising, I might search for a text or two on dreams, or on the brain. Instead, I am going to ramble and leave all of that to the experts, and/or you, friend. I find that last line interesting. It is the first occasion that I have ever considered whilst in the stillness of night, and the stillness of me, without voice, perhaps I ramble as I write? (All right, who said that?)....

Does rambling even serve a purpose? I fear that I have learned little about the subject and therefore this should be a rather shortened portion. Part of me initiates yet another thought: I ramble mostly when I'm agitated or when I'm over-stimulated. While in the docile state? Well, we all know how we seem then. We seem calm and collected, or cannot for some reason bring ourselves to speak. At other times our brain is confused and therefore we cannot speak. Sometimes.

I've had a few pretty weird dreams where it seems that I cannot speak at all. I know Lucy might have kept sleeping with me, years ago, sharing my bed, had I had more of those, and fewer combat dreams. I really don't believe my ex-wife ever realized any of that. I'd kept it well hidden as good as I could; until I restarted thinking about it (war), and what it's done to you, or when you up and run into a wall as I did one night in Brooklyn, 1969.

But back to rambling, what may perhaps not set us apart from other creatures walking this life-filled sphere. I sometimes wonder if rambling is the beginning of the gibberish that later often follows. I realize the laughing hyena must ramble. How I wish I could be more of a laugher and less lost. (*Sorry again, Lord: for You have promised that I am not lost, and I readily realize and admit it, and am so very thankful for that knowledge!*) This nocturnal mammal (the hyena) sometimes does seem a grand example of myself. And then there are the gibbons. Have you ever listened to this Asian ape? (Speaking of rambling, I am going to give up on what I had started, placing names of loved ones herein. Let the acknowledgements or some other portion of the work speak to my love for each and every one of you. I am in fear that placing a name here, and a comment there, might be too disconcerting even for me.)

I could continue on about ramblers, about ones who are lonely, ones who may perhaps only be rambling when they have the opportunity. Ones who obviously not only ramble, but also utilize that gibberish I mentioned a moment ago. This rather obscure language, I so look forward to, and the animation and affirmation, the smiling of those (who are usually unfortunately left to themselves); to me it is all rather charming. Perhaps another gift from God.

To the places that often confine and ignore these sweet people, I say: These patients are not persons devoid of meaning; they are not people who mean nothing to us any longer.

Each life is significant! Then again, I'm not sure that reporting anything today will be that enlightening to many. I pray that I am totally incorrect. I am hopeful one day, facilities will change, that there will be a total reinventing and breaking away from what we now know as the wonderful world of care giving. *Our nation, in many areas of the country today needs a reformation of the nursing home system,* and we need it now! (Of course we need bridges and roads now, as well.)

We need it for seniors, and some younger ones who deserve it. The folks, who were as some have written part of *The Greatest Generation,* are deserving of nothing less than our best.

Are you one of those that realize that God knows your every need, every longing, and every whimpering? That He also knows the needs of those lonely and lost and ill-treated? What do you think God's response is going to be to the secretive maltreatment of our patients when we arrive wherever we hope to arrive? Will there be a Great Advocate awaiting you, or will there be the total absence of anything filled with love and grace and power and might, all-forgiving, all-knowing?

I cherish the words just before The Lord's Prayer: "THEREFORE DO NOT BE LIKE THEM. FOR YOUR FATHER KNOWS THE THINGS YOU HAVE NEED OF EVEN BEFORE YOU ASK HIM." — (Matthew 6:8). Christ's words ring true even as I write these observations. As I have ministered to and worked in many facilities that would cause your stomach to not feel very good about man's inhumanity to man, I yet am able to share with you His words yet ring true, despite our brutality to one another.

Of course the living of His words are above all else; yet we need to understand God's words in order to live them. It is why I recommend that those who study might seek Bible commentaries. Seek all the help they can get their hands on before sharing with others.

Prayer is not to inform God of our needs, as the heathen think, but that we may have conscious communion with Him as His children. That is a solid spoke, **prayer**. It may be small, yet it is golden and essential. More will be shared about it in chapter 13.

Is part of the gibberish that I've observed out of the mouths of fellow AD folks used to commune with God? I surely hope so. I do know, as I have entered a space and come upon the gibberish-speaking person, the beloved *Yes, Jesus Loves Me* song always begins them once again to sing, or sometimes they go into their rant. Either they'll go for the rambling, or they stop and join in the singing! Whichever they do, it is always as if they look forward to the one who will listen to them, one who doesn't need to be there, but does come, because he/she cared enough to visit them. Who doesn't enjoy a great listener?

There are not as many good listeners left in most circles today. There are some who are shaking their head, or planning a reply even before your sentence has been completed. Yet I maintain hope, hope that goes along with faith. "SO THEN FAITH COMES BY HEARING, AND HEARING BY THE WORD OF GOD." There are on the other hand, many places you can yet find good listeners, people trained in the art of listening. Seek them out; learn their ways, there is something very cathartic about telling your story to a good listener, especially ones who do not have to 'be there.' A good listener accomplishes much! I challenge you to learn that art, that wonderfully sharing gift. It may even be from God.

The bombastic speech may only be the result of the patient's laying their eyes upon my personhood, or whoever it is that comes to call. No one knows, not that I've ever heard or read. Okay, you know the exception to that one. There are many subjects such as this, subjects that may never be revealed to us until God wishes them revealed, until He allows them to be discovered. That is, "if God allows it before the dimness is made clear."

†

Father Friend, thank You for Isaiah 55:1-2, for the promise of that which satisfies, that which is good. I do not wish to ramble merely for rambling's sake, but thank You for so much that You have allowed to be revealed, or allowed us to stumble upon. I know those things are not by accident. I recall the story of a young lad who crashed through a glass door on his bicycle, and of how it led mankind to learn that the cutting and re-shaping of the eye could bring about clearer vision. You so amaze me the way You often reveal miracles to us, God. I thank You, too, that all is not rambling and/or gibberish, not a tower where we cannot understand one another. Thanks for: ... "ONE JOT OR ONE TITTLE WILL BY NO MEANS PASS FROM THE LAW UNTIL ALL IS FULFILLED." Matthew 5:18. *Thank you for commentators and translators and interpreters who have helped reveal the meaning of Your world and Word, Your way, i.e.,* "THE RABBIS TAUGHT, 'NOT A LETTER SHALL PERISH FROM THE LAW FOR EVER.' 'EVERYTHING HAS ITS END: THE HEAVEN AND EARTH HAVE THEIR END; THERE IS ONLY ONE THING, WHICH HAS NO END, AND THAT IS THE LAW.' 'THE LAW SHALL REMAIN ETERNALLY, WORLD WITHOUT END.'" (*The One Volume Bible Commentary*, Reverend J.R. Dummelow, Queen's College, Cambridge)

This being improved upon, or in Christ's words fulfilled, explains that the prophets of old were fulfilled by Him in a most comprehensive way. Christ was not content simply to carry out their idea of the Messiah, as wonderful as that is. He improved it. He improved the words, for He is the Word!

Something inside me, tells me that even gibberish has meaning. I know that God understands it all, whether it means anything to us or not.

—Look Back, But Live! The Disease—

As we entered our eighth year of loving marriage, I noted that Donna, otherwise known as Lucy, now wore a bracelet. It was unusual, for I'd never seen her wear a bracelet for any great length of time. This one she now wore daily, nightly, always.

When Lucy first sported her 'Safe Return' bracelet and I'd spotted it, I could not help but think, *Now that's living for someone!* She had put in on for me. Only me. If she had gotten in an accident, for example, and ended up in the hospital, folks could tell by the numbers on the reverse of it that Lucy was/is caring for someone else, someone alone, someone who might otherwise not understand what is or has taken place.

Unless you're in some way connected with or involved in this disease, most readers might not have heard of these materials or devices. *Safe Return*, an Alzheimer's Association program, reminds me that people working with AD are marvelous people. They know you can either merely 'exist' with this disease or choose, where possible, to *Live! with it.*

The phone number for the Safe Return folks is contained within these pages. By the way, these people who work with AD folks are normally magnificent as well!

Never would I purposely ignore that a person can be in one of many stages, that the way you are able to live could be different from the ability of the diseased person seated next to you. The more I read, study and write about AD, the more God's grace flows through me. It enables me to understand and to savor this, at least in the early onset of dementia: we *can* live with this disease. Thankfully, I have thus far lived a rich and full life. Please bear with me during the following autobiographical sketch. It is set forth to show you what kind of life can be changed/touched. If you are one who lives with AD, you, too, are in good company.

†

Yours truly, has performed in many plays. He's given Memorial Day addresses in various communities, and has sung with the Bluejackets (Navy) Choir in the early sixties. He's had so many wonderful experiences during his lifetime. He's met Mohammed Ali and Ben Kingsley, Gregory Peck, and many other famous people. He will later talk about Maxie, who died with his Japanese friend in a horrible balloon crash as they attempted an around-the-world flight, 30-plus years ago! Then there was fishing with Fred, a friend. (Fred used to steer the Presidential yacht, Sequoia.)

He's waited on a former Commandant of the Marine Corps; rubbed elbows with General Westmoreland; and admired an associate who turned out being fairly famous, a conversationalist (to date yet on TV); Ollie had been an Intel guy like him. He relieved a young fellow at an overseas location who was chosen to travel the world with Dr. Henry Kissinger. He's known presidential bodyguards; men who have dived aboard our deep submergence vessels; and he was in and out of a war before his twenty-third birthday. It was a war that shall always be with him; one he sometimes attempts not to recall.

Seated in an Intel class in late '79, he was one of those briefed by Dr. Brezezinski. He knew then as a young Chief Warrant Officer, he had no longer just fallen off the old turnip wagon. (That's a modest joke.) His skipper aboard a guided missile destroyer, USS Dewey, DDG-45, recently ended a distinguished career as a three-star Admiral. He had the distinct pleasure of serving with Colonel Robert "Bob" Mountel, USA, one of the 'snake eaters' who was a classmate of Colonel Charlie Beckwith. Colonel Beckwith developed Delta Force, an elite counter-terrorist unit for our great nation. Actually, Bob Mountel is no slouch; he, too has known presidents and other people of high regard and authority. You will read more about Colonel Bob later on.

Once, when stationed aboard a submarine tender this young warrant officer was there when the ace fighter pilot Jimmy Doolittle, visited an alongside submarine. (Did you know Doolittle once was forced to ditch his B-17 bomber, and became a sailor for a few weeks?) He was at another occasion onboard when the father of the nuclear Navy arrived at his site. So many famous people. Often they were special people. People like the founder of Stephen Ministry: Rev./Dr. Kenneth Haugk. Ken founded a wonderful listening ministry in the seventies, which is yet alive and well and thriving! (And he has been an inspiration and a friend, as well.)

He's sat only feet from Nancy Sinatra as he listened to her youthful 'boots' song, as Bob Hope 'cut up' with his troop before *the troops.* How he admired Bob's love and respect for people in uniform, his lovable sense of humor. Bob made it possible for a soldier/sailor to forget where he was, if only for a few moments. (Bob Hope, as far as this writer knows, is the only civilian to ever be named 'honorary military' by JFK.) He looks forward to meeting Bob one day again.

In a four-star hotel, he met the gal who sang *Don't Cry for Me, Argentina,* in a 1960s Cannes Film Festival. He's been around the world and back again. He has lived in places where education didn't matter, and in other parts of the world where everyone wanted to be there and be part of it all, all were vital, caring, well-educated, well-mannered folks from scores of countries and backgrounds. He's lived on an island with B-1 Bombers at one end and Fleet Ballistic Missile Submarines at the other. He has frequented churches large and small; and he has had the pleasure of serving in the pulpits of many of them. But his New Hope Fellowship, in bucolic Powhatan, Virginia, possesses more love than any one person or congregation could possibly contain. It is a church *on the move for God*! A church that cares about people; a church that remembers Christ is the head of The Family; a church that has indeed prayed for this very work.

He's communed with some of the toughest commandos in the world; some with Inshore Underwater Warfare groups, others who had been point men or Recon men in some of the bloodiest battles of our times. The real thing (commando) has been his companion, as well as men who were legends in their lunchbox. This young chief warrant has walked in crowds of over a million people, where all one can see as far as you can see is an ocean of faces. He's known men who lost their lives as spotter pilots, and not long ago lost a uniformed nephew in a chopper accident in the waters off the coast of East Africa. One of his biology teachers served briefly in the battle on Okinawa, and several older friends were in combat in the South China Sea, the Philippines, and one quite long ago, now deceased, had served in the Fields of France. Another fine man he knew, when serving with Mobile Technical Unit Twelve had been on a bobsled team in the U.S. Olympics. Then there was Danny, a friend who had taken his life because of the terrible back pain that he could no longer endure. (What a shame I could not have done something for this veteran.) He later learned that Danny had been a purple heart Marine. Danny was no sissy. Those men and others yet, and he himself, lived very full lives. He's known tough guys and even tougher gals. And what's even better yet, he's known men that so reminded him of Christ; they were nothing less than great shining examples of how we should live our daily lives!

Serving in some of the most beautiful places in the world has been one of his greatest privileges and honors. He's watched whales spout-off in waters enveloped by majestic snow-capped mountains, a gentle breeze at his back. At times he'd pictured one of his (at that time) modern ships anchored in such a fashion that it spun slowly and freely around an anchor buoy in South American waters, seemingly without a care for anything; yet it had been outfitted with nuclear missiles that had the capability of reaching thousands of miles away, on target.

He's biked in North Africa, and carried a machine gun in Keflavik, where he was part of Iceland's Ground Defense Force. It was so cold in Iceland that your milk carton's contents would freeze in your beard. That's back when one could still wear a beard when serving in uniform. He could go on and on about places and people and scenes and experiences yet catalogued somewhere inside his tired head. He is so thankful for those long-ago memories. Some fond, some not so fond.

(Tired of hearing about me yet?) His children and siblings and Momma, know and love our God – and it doesn't get much better than that. We (collectively) have had so many victories and miracles in life that it would impress the likes of Billy Graham; Billy was once invited by his one sister, Mary, to a church she had served at, and Billy came there! He is so proud of his children and grandchildren, nieces and nephews and extended family, perhaps you gathered that when you first saw this book's cover.

And he loves this nation! Sometimes he feels as if we live in a nearly perfect world. What he could proudly write about his family, close-up and extended, would be a book all its own. He loves Lucy's kids as if they were his own; he indeed claims them. And he knows they feel the same about him! And he is thankful for that.

He has been a proud member of the Veterans of Foreign Wars, the International Kiwanis, and the National Ruritan Club. He is an active member of the Military Officers Association of America. He's been invited to serve in other organizations, but knows it is not fair to belong to too many. Another great privilege is a recent one: that of being asked to serve in an advisory capacity for his local Alzheimer's association, of the greater Richmond area. One cannot do it all and do it well, not if he belongs to too many outfits. (Yet I could not turn down Mary Ann's special request. Lucy and I love you, too, Mary Ann Johnson.)

He's served as a chaplain and he's been a brig counselor, later he was the brig officer onboard another ship. He's accomplished duties for this beloved nation that he is sworn not to share the description of with anyone. Yet it was his great pleasure to carry out those duties. Through it all, he's always kept in mind that if it takes a thousand points to get to Heaven, all the aforementioned 'stuff' will add up to One point. Okay, he readily realizes there are no points, that points don't matter, and we don't always get points. Even when we do our best, we sometimes don't get points. Nor should we seek any points.

He's served as a department head with prestigious organizations, and he's swept floors in small quiet places. (Now that doesn't sound so high and mighty, does it?)

One year, he had work published in a national poetry anthology and he holds numerous writing awards as a young fellow, for this essay and that one. Indeed, he's lived a very rich and full life. He has been so blessed and privileged.

His first book was published in 1993; and five hundred-plus loving Christians at a Stephen Ministry Leadership Training Conference sang a song he had once written. That singing sound put a lump the size of a walnut in his throat. Not a pride-lump, but *a love-for-God lump!*

But this story is not about him, or about his fading away, or having been at all. It's not about all the talented and vibrant people he's known and met and/or served with, and it's not about his adventures; though much of what remains of him is yet part of an adventure. It's not intended to be a story about him. This segment though, smacks of the fullness of living that he's been privileged to be a part of, to have lived, and now the talk concerns how we can **live** with disease.

Naturally, he had not felt diseased during all of the aforementioned. Yet dementia-affected folks can often do many things well, even after being diagnosed. That's one thing that causes folks to have difficulty spotting AD folks, because some of them are yet able to sing, or play piano, or even dance! How gracious is our loving God! A God who challenges us to dance! He is a God of second chances. (Thanks, Max.)

†

"I know Who holds the future, and I know Who holds my hand." Have you heard those words before? I surely hope so. Father has led me not only to my every word upon these pages, but He has supplied my every need so His will might further be delivered, with this story or without it. Yet I am certain it will be shared.

Is that not a loving Lord and Father? King of Kings, Prince of Peace? I have not made Him into some kind of errand boy. It works not that way. You can make Him do nothing! Yet as I have been open to Him, and as He leads me, He has communicated in this way, "AND MY GOD SHALL SUPPLY ALL YOUR NEED ACCORDING TO HIS RICHES IN GLORY BY CHRIST JESUS." —Philippians 4:19. God's wealth contains all sorts of treasure. (The previous quote, after the Biblical words, comes from *The One Volume Bible Commentary,* MacMillan Publishing Co., Inc., Reverend J.R. Dummelow.)

Just as God supplied Lucy's huge hope chest that I often utilized for a writing table, now he has provided me, me with the already rich and full-lived life, a better way to proceed with this work, God's work. I have located a nearby library. Such nice people work there, too, in Powhatan, Virginia. They greet you, and love you, and serve you as well. Thanks so much Kim and Mary Ann.

It only once again serves to make this work, His story, for you! It is God's way of saying: *Live! the disease!* Similar to the way God has offered these words, last portion of John 10:10 – "...I HAVE COME THAT THEY MAY HAVE LIFE AND THAT THEY MAY HAVE IT MORE ABUNDANTLY." They are transparent words, or at least should be to one and all. God's gifts are His way of offering us abundance as we are moved to do His will. And it is not a big stretch for me to add, it is God's desire for you to *Live! your disease*, where possible. Accept it, capture it, modify it, or totally reject it, but above all, *attempt to live it*!

I confess that I love a piece that Helen Steiner Rice wrote, years ago:

The Bend In The Road.
Sometimes we come to life's crossroads
And view what we think is the end,
But God has a much wider vision,
And He knows it's only a bend,
The road will go on and get smoother,
And after we've stopped for a rest,
The path that lies hidden beyond us
Is often the part that is best...

So rest and relax and grow stronger
Let go and let God share your load,
And have faith in a brighter tomorrow
You've just come to a bend in the road.

How jealous she makes me! As I walk and talk with God in the midst of certain distress and trauma, and as I go with these *bends in the road*, I attempt to maintain a regimen inclusive of exercise, proper nutrition, attitudinal motivation, prayer and appreciation for the past, present and the future. Yet the most important, things eternal! Those amazing unseen things!

A little bit ago I said something about REJECTING your disease. The reason I say reject your disease, is because one of God's gifts, a miracle, may occur if you are able to reject the idea of the disease in its totality. If we reject the idea that we are diseased, there is always the possibility, whether we are open to it or not, yet more likely when we are open, that God may well work a miracle within you. Yes, even you. After all, has He not died that you might live? Did He not sacrifice the closest, the most Beautiful One to Himself? Has He not sacrificed the greatest Gift, so you might know of His mighty love and that you might have eternal life? Has He not walked with you and behind you, gone on before you, all for a reason? Yes! A resounding yes! to all the aforementioned, He did! He does! He will!

†

Gloriously wonderful God, Omnipotent One, although we cannot fully understand Your never-ending desire for us to partake of Your abundance, Your love for us, we come to You now. We receive Your Word; we heed Your Word; we BELIEVE Your Word. What more is there for us to say than thank You, God?

Read the twelfth chapter of Romans, friend. Read it and savor it, study it, take it to your heart; my brother and friend Reverend Michael Lamm, once again shared it with Lucy and I, and others. It was and is another one of God's miracles this very day! For if we are open to God's miracles, there will be many more of them, over and again. So many miracles. A life of purity is mentioned therein (in Romans again). Words one of my brothers, David Lee, recently shared from miles away: "I strive to live with purity..." They are so much more clearly convincing now. Thanks, Dave. *Thanks, God.* (And yes, you're correct. I can do better, Dave! Thank you, again....)

"AND WHATEVER WE ASK, WE RECEIVE FROM HIM, BECAUSE WE KEEP HIS COMMANDMENTS, AND DO THOSE THINGS WHICH ARE PLEASING IN HIS SIGHT." —From I John 3:22

If only
I could...
have that much tenacity.

Chapter 4

Discoveries

—Reading And Experiencing The Disease—

Overstressing the importance of learning as much as possible about AD cannot be done. I never realized how many books there are on the subject until I was diagnosed. So much can be gained by learning where you are headed, if you're yet able to read and consider it, and have an idea of where you're headed. I pray you are one yet able to process that/this.

Fortunately I have a couple letters from publishers stating what thorough and detailed study has been accomplished. Now if one of them will step forward with the magic contract so its words might assist others...

"What changes do you see in yourself?" a close friend inquired of me. That had been tough. I hadn't really thought much about it. Thanks for the question, Bill. It has been helpful, in fact, I yet think about it every now and again.

Our Guidebook was given to us to assist us in this walk on earth, and books on AD can be a wonderful gift as well (both to patients and others). Often those answered questions helped me sooner or later to answer a caring friend or neighbor's question, or one of my own.

†

The knowledge of Alzheimer's disease began for me with pointing at objects, making signs for something I needed at work, as I was having great difficulty verbalizing words for tools that I needed at the time. I would make a motion, a question-like look obvious in my eyes.

"Hammer?" my boss Sam would ask in his patient way. At that time I was also mad and confused, not knowing exactly what was taking place inside of me. I just could not come up with the word, and as time progressed there would be other words I could not recall as well. It had been the beginning of many following signs. Different signs. Signs not so obvious to others. Not accepted by some.

Next, I noted I'd be driving along and go beyond the point of my destination, or suddenly could not recall exactly where an office building or store was located. For those of you who are quick to reply, I'll do it for you: "I do that all the time." Do you do it daily? Do you now carry a dry-erase slate with you wherever you go? Have you told your spouse you'll meet her, depart ahead of her, and end up arriving late because you drove several miles beyond the meeting place? Well, multiply all the things you do by a hundred!

Yet believe it or not, some will never understand or comprehend or even believe that you *have it.* (By now, I more clearly realize it is one of the things that loved ones do, for they do not wish to believe you have arrived at where you are; they don't want their heart to be aching for someone close, and therefore, they do their best to become involved in denial. And for the record: some of them will die that way, never believing that their loved one ever had the disease. That's just the way it is, folks.)

Bill and readers, the progression is different for each patient. I share words later about 'walking the leash…' Yet what scared me more, more recently, was when I had swallowed the allotted number of prescribed medications, had finished washing them down, and then spent frantic moments wondering almost immediately thereafter where I'd laid the pills, whether I had indeed taken them, and/or wondering if I'd simply lost them! Do you take them again? Who do you call? And how many different answers will you get about that most unusual question?

My sister, Mary, who I often refer to as an angel, suggested after that, that keeping my pill box in one certain place, and then immediately upon the washing down of the pills, the taking of them, that I should right then, before doing anything else: write it down on one of my slates (which I now faithfully keep beside my medications). "Write breakfast, or breakfast pills…" she had begun, "…follow that with a little checkmark." That one suggestion has been a great answer for a frustrating problem. And frustration is one of the big items for the AD-affected person. Thanks, Mary. It was an item that I would later share during an educational television documentary about AD.

To others they may be seemingly small items; to us, they can be a very big breakthrough. Sometimes these frustrations are so pronounced within and without; we seem to magnify them to a proportion much larger than they need to be. To me, at times they seemed as huge as His grand galaxy! And you know how huge that is. Okay, at least you can imagine.

A word of wisdom for care partners and friends of the patient: One of the greatest things you can do for the diseased person is to simply LISTEN to them. Listen intently, with care and concern. (Recall fellows, how you had leaned-in with interest and asked questions of that prospective girlfriend and/or date? How you would back off when you sensed that you were not making any significant progress?) It's somewhat the same with this and many other caring relationships. Go with the patient. DO NOT GIVE THEM THAT "I DO THAT," SONG.

It means nothing to us; is often not realistic. Point in fact: you might really tick off the patient. Lastly, never tell a patient (or anyone experiencing trauma for that matter) that you know how they feel. You have absolutely no idea. Patients can be very sensitive, and I am one of them. The best thing you can do, I'll repeat: Simply listen! Some folks never get that.

Did you know that even the supposed 'experts' can let you down? In today's world of distrust, later discussed in more detail, well, suffice it at this point to say: you need to know that there are those who specialize in looking for phonies. Why do I bring it up?, one might ask.

I bring it up because of outfits that spend months and months delving into the same ridiculous questions over and again, as they attempt to catch people at something they are most likely NOT doing, or in other words, to ascertain whether or not you are one prevaricating. But getting back to where I was before rage started to build up inside of me. Those of you who may be referred, in order to ascertain whether or not you are sincere, honest, and/or diseased or not, referred to ensure that you are not some idiotic manipulator, may well be referred to a psychologist or psychiatrist who watches for those little tricks they might spot: body language, positioning, how you react to their questions and baited words and so forth. And I have another newsflash for you as well, these same folks with the somewhat hidden agenda, are also in no great hurry to address your welfare. Indeed, they attempt to make some of their clients not only look foolish, but they are also happy to drag out their mediocre experiment on you while they at the same time line their pockets to the tune of $150 an hour or better! Does it sound as if I am rather tainted about this topic? I am!

I do now, however, understand some of this, once I got through my madness about it. We do live in a penny poor, pound-foolish society. And there are those who are fakers, frauds. Speaking of government. No, I should not do that....

Can you yet see the sight of our 'leaders' debating back in March 2007, whether or not to fund or not fund the Iraq situation right in the middle of the war? Were they really serious about whether it was to be or not be a part of a budget proposal? Were they really serious that since they believed we should 'pull out' that we'd just up and stop the flow of money to the very men and women who are saving our butts right now? Do we have trouble revealing and/or realizing that what it will cost to take care of our returning veterans will amount to a much greater figure than the money they are currently funding for our current venture?

And yet, they attempt to keep passing packages that hardly anyone besides JFK could read because of the sheer volume of pork contained within them. Do you believe the general public really knows how many troops are wounded for each one who is killed? Trust me, ask twelve different people and guess how many different answers you'll get? Yet there are folks saying that we must pull out right now! We must pull out and once again be recognized as a country that has blundered again, a country that starts something they do not have the stomach to complete! **My only apology is to our troops and their loved ones, especially folks left behind.**

In fairness though, yes, I'm big on fairness: some of these 'investigators' mentioned a bit ago, ones masquerading as 'concerned ones', can actually end up being friendly. That is, once you've proven to their satisfaction that you are for real. Fair enough? That's about as far as I want to go with it at this point; I could however, go much further, and it might not be any prettier. When it comes to psychology and psychiatry: nothing is cut in concrete.

†

Let's return to Billy's question for a moment longer: about changes. Although I've often said I've turned it all over to our gracious Creator, some days I'm not so convinced. You ever slip backwards? Slide across a greased pan, looking similar to a half cooked egg?

There are some strange things taking place within our kitchens. I note of late how much I love shrimp cocktail sauce on my beef patty. It is something that drives 'Bug' crazy. Yet my Lucy understands that I am evolving into something quite different in the kitchen. I am entering a totally new world it seems. I'd be remiss here if I did not warn you: especially caregivers, about the obvious dangers of allowing patients to cook. That part is not a joke.

I just found a cold cup of coffee: It had been made some time ago. I have an automatic shut-off-after-a-bit coffee brewer. This is an excellent idea for AD patients. I recommend it if you can get one.

As long as I have opened a safety issue, let me share that there is a wonderful home safety handbook for AD folks. It is NIH Publication No. 02-5179 of March, 2006. It was disseminated by the U.S. Department of Health and Human Services. Therein, toward the back, is also a listing of very helpful organizations. Under Alzheimer's Association is listed the Safe Return program, as well as others. You can get information at *www.alz.org* or call 1-800-272-3900. It will be worth your time and effort, and may even be a lifesaver. (PS – I recently heard they are merging with Medic Alert folks; that could be beneficial.)

—Decisions From Love—

This portion was purposely placed here for a practical reason. Over the years I've found, especially where strong emotion is involved, it is good to allow that searing note of those stress-filled words to be placed aside for a day or two, if you can allow it.

Leaving a dentist's office not long ago, I remember how a temporary tooth had several times been broken off due to my bouts with PTSD/bad dreams. I was quite upset and had actually written a rather nasty letter. In it, I'd included that they'd not only left my broken tooth in an incomplete state, but that I also could not believe I would need a crown to hold what was left (of it) to keep it together. I had penned words in haste: about a veteran feeling abandoned, and further had made a 'copy to' for Senator McCain, as John has come to my aid on an occasion or two.

Although the senator and I do not agree on everything, I know John McCain cares. He's been there, and he has a heart for the veteran. What greatness he and his family have meant to this Republic! God bless you, John.

The very next morning, or segment number four, I had decided that my letter to the dentist was filled with entirely too much emotion, that I should handle the matter in an entirely different way. I had taken time, fortunately, to let my emotions subside. I had allowed myself to become more aligned with a sane decision, not one of simply striking out at someone.

I have seen this time and again, with myself, with others. Not that I always do it, but 'slow down,' would be my best advice. Do not act in haste, or simply out of anger. That can be particularly difficult for one with either PTSD or dementia. Tied together as they are in me it could be volatile.

The writing of this section is therefore a challenge as it involves territory that I am very concerned about, and is released somewhat out of emotion, from what I have witnessed, and because I am curious concerning the actions of 'mice' when the 'cat' is away. If you are familiar with my mindset, you, too, may well be a fighter, one who never gives up, especially where it concerns loved ones, or those who cannot speak, or fear speaking up for themselves.

It is of utmost importance for families to make decisions from a common sense approach and not to be tainted by unhealthy guilt or a promise made perhaps long ago, or in haste. It is apparent, and I have seen it as I ministered to folks, that many people attempt to honor the patient's wishes, and that is good. However, as the patient's disease progresses, so may the severity of the patient's behavior. Sometimes it is bad behavior that can get her/him killed, or at the very least into great difficulty. That is: not something the patient necessarily intended, but it happens.

When we get into the heat of battle with a care receiver, where calm and logic no longer prevail, it is important to back away from the drama and emotion in order to be able to properly think the situation through. Do not argue with an enraged or combative patient. And do not waste your time preaching to them. DO ensure that they feel your touch and/or hug, your love. And if their attention needs diverted, it's time for the caregiver to step up, and step in, in love. And yes, there are other areas of concern, areas that can cause trouble.

If Grandma is leaving the pot boiling while she naps, she may well burn the building down. Believe it or not there are loving children and grandchildren who will argue to the death and/or challenge anyone in order to figure another way. They will do anything to keep from having Grandma moved. Yet when it comes to the safety of Grandma and her neighbors, it is definitely time to make a decision based not only on good common sense, but one thought through from the thought out/thought through point of view, not from heart alone.

Please, if you are a tired caregiver who has been fighting the good fight for years on end, you may be risking not only your kin's life, but others as well. Step back, take a moment, and rethink the situation. For not only can you die from an unjustifiable heart attack, you will also no longer be able to assist your loved one. You will not be around to do so.

†

The placement of Grandma or Grandpa is a time for surprise visits to facilities, after you've let them (the facility) know that you are considering placing a loved one there, and have advised them of what you'll be doing. Okay, so much for the surprise. Go at different times of the day, when management is present, when management has left for the day. You'll be without your care receiver of course.

Although some workers in facilities are keenly aware of everyone's presence, there may be one or two workers who will show their true colors, and this will enable you to move to your next choice, another facility.

You might think that since we have arrived in the 21st century that all is in automatic and all is well: this today is not the case. I have personally witnessed much gamesmanship, power struggling and bickering within and outside of the worker corps of various facilities. I would not dare tell you the name of one of those facilities. But what a shame it is that many of them continue to operate. They are antiquated, ill informed, and uncaring about anyone's grandma. So be wary of your selection. Be thorough in your investigation. I really believe if you find a facility whose workers are on their toes on the night shift (after 5 p.m.), the day workers should be even better. And by the way, I have a cadre of friends who will support my claims.

If you need to do so now, you may wish to turn ahead to *Healthcare Blinders and Blunders,* the next segment. It is factual and from the heart. Real. I do not feel that it is written from a mean-spirited point of view; I believe it to be fair and honest. Transparent.

Next, do not for a moment believe that the amount of money you expend monthly to 'take care of' your loved one will always make a big difference. As for assisted living, or elderly care or nursing homes, I care not what you call the place, for what is presented to you in writing may be far from the real thing. Again, things are not always as they appear. You may have noted that our *leaders* in Washington recently held a meeting (as of this writing) concerning the healthcare industry, ***and it was the first one in 30 years!***

Call the facility a few minutes before the staff arrives. Learn how the workers answer their phones, how they treat you and your questions. I have unfortunately watched workers pretending to be busy, while allowing the phone to continue to ring. Are the workers attentive? How do they treat someone they don't yet know? Do they seem to have time for you?

Any good facility will go to great lengths to ensure that each of their soldiers is schooled and carries out their proper duties consistently, not just between the hours of 9 to 5. It must be continuous, efficient, quality work. Caring. It must not be for show alone!

Check around your community. You may be surprised what person in your church or social circle knows of, or has had a family member in a particular place (home). Word of mouth is still the most powerful and effective advertisement for greatness and mediocrity as well. Again, check around. But don't forget to do your own reconnaissance. This is not just a decision; it is a decision worthy of extra attention. It may be solely entrusted to you alone. And that puts the pressure on even more.

Take your time! Do not decide on Thursday that this major change for your loved one must take place that very weekend. Explore, inspect, plan, discuss; look for and find that caring attitude. This is a commitment that you do not want to fail in. Do not expose a loved one to bedsores and mean-spirited people because you were in a rush for one reason or another; Set aside extra time if necessary. Remember this as well: some workers who act sweet and courteous in front of you/to you, may be altogether different when you go around the corner. We're talking about care for your loved one, not you. Pretend that it's a place we're looking at for you, for the remainder of your life. (Hang around a corner, you may learn something vital.)

†

Lord God, assist us in slowing down long enough to tenderly and clearly think of our loved ones and their needs. Help us to plan and be guided by You. Thank You for Your example, which we may sometimes have to search for to see in others. And if it's simply a matter of communicating, enable us to befriend those who will be with our loved ones day in and day out, when we cannot be there. Sometimes we need to spend time with the prospective caregiver, building a lasting relationship of trust and caring. Sometimes a less than optimal situation can be avoided by our initial questions and visits. Thank You for good healthcare workers and nurses, doctors and staffs that DO care. Yet give us the discernment to learn a facility's ways and true intentions before we enter into this important decision. Second chances may come very slowly, or not at all. And conditions may become worse once that final decision has been reached. We praise Your grace, Your Word, and Your way. We ask Your special blessings upon healthcare facilities everywhere, and we call upon Your special angels to assist any wrongdoers that they might become more focused upon You and Your ways. Cause them to choose to be more loving; there may still be that possibility. Great and loving God, watch over our loved one, as well as others; and assist us in making good decisions for our loved ones. "NO ONE IS HOLY LIKE THE LORD...." —First line of I Samuel 2:2.

—New Vision—

This was part of a newness that I hadn't expected; yet I must share with you how I now notice the world around me in more vivid detail. I call it my *new vision.* I spend more time nowadays studying pictures that I have not heretofore spent much time studying. Sometimes I spy a new house or part of a landscape that I had not before noted, though I may have driven that way hundreds of times. At first I figured it was just curious, but the more I thought about it, this newness, the more I realized that I was seeing in greater detail, with a new freshness if you will.

It is as if AD affords us a new pair of eyes, or glasses. Sometimes I am content to study more than ever the flow of our tiny creek, the bathing of a lone bird, the crisp outline (eyes allowing) of trees against God's canvas extraordinaire.

And actually, as one of my grandchildren might say, I often am more drawn to what people have to say as well. That alone seems rather peculiar, as I have always considered myself a great listener. Then there are other times when holding my attention, especially now, is not something anyone can do for a very long period of time. *Changes....*

Part of that, I am beginning to realize, is living in the present more than ever before; another part is living in the past more and more. The old familiar, the 'stuff' stuck more strongly to my hard-drive so to speak, is where I also spend much of my time. And something has been sparked within me causing me to more vividly view textures and colors and kaleidoscopes of everything around me, causing me to live for the moment. It is our 'real' living, is it not?

†

I am also sensing more and more that each moment of our life is to be revered. I often ponder if it's because of the *how much longer* thoughts. When does that final time of remembrance, of lucidness arrive? How long until I march or crawl headlong into that world we seem to know so little about? Yet I truly prefer a way a friend of mine has referred to it: "He will never let go of you, and His everlasting arms will enfold you as the two of you journey through the growing mist." The trick is: trying to hold onto those love-filled words.

I've heard and read bits and pieces about chemicals for the brain, which allow fear or the sense of euphoria to be felt. I often wonder how those tests can read things of that sort, or that is, how the people who read them, read them. How they explain what takes place inside our brain? More often than not, I suspect the brain yet remains fairly obscure, a rather scary unknown place, one of God's mysteries. Sometimes I wonder if we are dabbling too much or what areas God might have us remain out of, if any.

Often I spend time staring at my Lucy now, something that drives her crazy. It is a new look, too. I verbalized it one night: how I want her indelibly etched upon my very soul and what lies yet not entangled within my skull. How long do we get to hold on? Sorry, it keeps 'going off' in my head. As much as I revere words about God being my companion through the formidable mist that lies ahead, there is another who I will so miss.

—Changes—

It is somewhat akin to being caught between a patient and his family and the doctor(s), when one is ministering. It is not always an enviable position. Especially if you strive to fulfill the patient's wishes which may or may not be the same as the others' wishes; I've had to 'back off' and away from such drama before: to secret myself away in prayer. Okay, sometimes I liken it to being fear-struck, wanting to run away from the entire mess. That, friend, is when you have forgotten to call upon God, trust me. No, I mean: trust God!

A recent visit to the Richmond (local) Fine Arts Museum only confirmed this newness, this pondering that I am speaking of – even the newness of listening more intently. (Thanks, Alzheimer's Association and family.)

I wrestled some with how I could better explain these changes: this new vision. Do you recall the first time you caught a baby catching a glimpse of its own hands? How they study their tiny hands as if they were heretofore unknown to them? It is that way with my new vision. It is a beginning all over again, a grand new beginning. Sometimes I believe that is a good attitude.

In a sense, I now understand the stillness and staring that I had noticed with various elderly folks over the years, when I had been observing them, long before I had been diagnosed. It had always fascinated me, and yet I now feel that I had not focused upon it enough. I laughingly recall inviting a father-in-law to remove himself, suspenders and all, from atop a huge piece of vinyl flooring that I had once attempted to install in his kitchen. He had been eyeballing my work, as I had often eyeballed folks with AD.

Speaking of eyes, they have some great 3D books available that they claim may improve your eyesight. Yes, I realize that sounds pretty wacky, but sometimes I have to get to it while I can. The 3D books: Look for *Magic Eye Gallery,* Andrews and McMeel, Publishing, LLC, Kansas City. The pictures are grand, colorful and fun!

†

There is another interesting side of the disease. I discovered it as I talked with a lady who had for years been part of watching AD at work. Recently I was especially struck when she relayed how eerie it had seemed, watching folks who no longer know their partner, but who are yet able to walk and perform their old loves/talents, even writing, or playing piano! What a puzzling disease! No longer able to talk, yet able to perform, even amidst this terrible deterioration. And of course that is because different parts of the old machine are still working fairly well. (Oh, www.nfcacares.org is the National Family Caregiver Association's website, and they do care!)

In my new vision: as I readily visit and revisit places and pictures and people, I pray it for you as well. I guess this newness is one of God's special ways/blessings, one of His mysteries. I am not going to second guess God or His wonderful gifts to us. But I do praise Him, even amidst this disease: No, especially in the midst of it. It draws us even closer together. *Changes.*

†

Father, we praise the depth of Your wisdom, Your special love, the many gifts that You continue to shower upon us, even in our diseased states/stages. Forgive us if and whenever we think too highly of ourselves. We know that everything comes from Your precious hand. Might our new vision bring us to a renewed sense of Your love and hope for humanity. Thank You, God; I am yet able to write. Thank You, too, for this new clarity.

What joy! I love how Oswald Chambers explains it to us (in his March 30th entry, from years ago) from *My Utmost For His Highest*: ("Are we worshiping God or disputing Him when we say, *'But God, I just don't see how You are going to do this'?* This is a sure sign that we are not worshiping. When we lose sight of God, we become hard and dogmatic. We throw our petitions at His throne and dictate to Him what we want Him to do. We don't worship God, nor do we seek to conform our minds to the mind of Christ. And if we are hard toward God, we will become hard toward other people.") Thanks, Myron. Thanks, Oswald. *Thank You, God. Thank You for coming here for us!*

(And thank you, Connie and Bill for leaving the brand new grill outside our back porch when we were away in God's house. You two are something else. Something wonderful! Thank you, Levi Taylor, for all your help around our place, and for that gal of yours who brings her potato salad here on occasion; and I can never forget your 4 grand kids! Thank you Chuck and Debbie for your work around the old place when you were here on vacation; and you as well, James Scott and Amy Lou, Debbie and Bill. Blessings all mine: having friends and relations so very special. Anjuli, I can never forget you, or my buddies: Nathan and Victor.)

When the administrator of one of the facilities that I'd ministered in motioned for me to enter his prestigious office upon my arrival, and sat me down and asked me without so much as a pause to curtail my services to their residents, it more than ever declared: We do not understand how it can be important for an Alzheimer's-diseased person to feel useful, even if it is God's work. It further declared volumes about their care of/for the general population of the home: **What a shame. What utter gull, to cause one bringing joy to patients to be banished from their marvelous facility.**

Only a few days prior to that session, I had made the critical mistake of being honest and had as well advised the new young admissions person of my knowledge concerning several patients who had 'escaped' their facility, and that one of them, let's call him Calvin, was now in bed dying on the second floor of their 'locked up' realm. Calvin had made it through an exit door and fallen down a stairwell, it had not been a pretty sight. (It was their cutting edge idea of a loving habilitative environment.) Perhaps you think that's unfair, but it's accurate and honest. And I can confirm it. There is absolutely no excuse for this type of non-care!

Although the administrator had not directly attacked me, he did mention that I had worn a large-brimmed hat into their fine facility (Oh, my!), and further that I had sat on the edge of the bed of one of their patients. (I didn't bother to advise the administration or him that the resident had invited me, as he had little space remaining in his already cramped room.) Let's just cut to the secular chase of it all: I knew too much about them. I knew more about them than they felt comfortable with me knowing. That is what had not been shared.

To this date, I am saddened yet for those remaining old friends who I'm certain miss my visits. They were the ones whose faces lighted up when I'd enter the room, the ones who were able to make contact with someone who did not have to be there. How I miss them. I cry that that facility's leadership (?) seemed more concerned about 'situations', and that translated, they had meant: 'Don't be a problem for us, regardless of any good you might think you do here.'

Striving for objectivity and fairness, I now share with you that I had always worn my lapel pin that reads *Safe Return*, and I wore my *Safe Return* bracelet as well. There had been nothing hidden about my diagnosis, that I live with AD. What saddened me most and yet does today, is how healthcare workers and some of their *leaders* manage to shut their patrons/residents off, how they manage to lock them up and keep them away from people who are positive, folks who show concern for them. It seems some facilities are more concerned about keeping staff and workers happy; that is, the staff gets to watch 'soaps' while residents sit slack-jawed, heads bowed, attempting to avoid the everyday bombardment of gossip and the worthless, mundane entertainment. How wonderful is our twenty-first century cutting-edge healthcare system! How easy it is for us to turn our backs on others. Why should we hold the healthcare system to any standard? After all, we haven't been able to do it with the U.S. House or the Senate, have we? *Changes? Anyone?*

While I'm yet thinking of the *Safe Return* program, one day I had called 1-888-572-8566, and advised them that their *Safe Return* key holder reads safe return, but it has no statement anywhere upon it about the phone number that is provided. The phone number on their key holder is listed to notify police!

Since I'm not crazy about lawsuits, I will not go on to explain what interplay I had with those folks. Let's just say that their key holder, I suspect, yet reads the same, and the other side, which is totally blank, is still without additional information. The police contact is important: When an AD patient is missing and/or confused, there needs to be a system in place. Let me just finish by saying that I encouraged them to either provide the non-emergency phone number (previously listed by me herein) or to print something on the reverse side of the key holder, perhaps: *This number is for emergency notification only.* But as I said, if you call the number listed on the key holder they give out, you are getting a location whose job it is to put you in touch with emergency help. At least that's the case as of this writing.

"I just want to leave here and stock shelves for some company, oblivious to any day-to-day complaints from people within and without." His candid words stung. It had been a resounding declaration that perhaps someone SHOULD be moving on, but it was not I. Do I sound overly sensitive, friend? I think not. I know a few loving and sensitive Christian doctors. Even before they read these words, one of them will attempt to keep from crying. These revelations: that there are people in charge who are not really concerned about their patients, would make one particular doctor sick to her stomach. Why? Because she is a doctor who cares about people.

No names. clean, fair, objective. But dear friend, the whole truth, dare ask me? Anyone? I'll make a wager, and I'm not a betting man. I will never hear from that place again. I will never hear from a single worker at that facility; and not one will ever challenge what I have written here. You see, they are all seated in the same boat, each in their own way, paralyzed at its proverbial oars. And what do many of the workers long for? The tick of the clock and hands in the position that show their day is done. Their care completed. (*Wow! It's much the same as their supervisor had wished for.*)

It is more than a little sad, how it is today. I've played the games. I've worked for outfits that openly tell you, *don't bring us your problems.* What a sin when a few close-minded people rule the entire system. Does it not seem similar to our governing bodies at times? I can let go of the sense of being offended, but if I continue to allow it to roll around inside of what's left of my brain – it causes me to wonder what has happened to our ideals, our sense of honesty, our concern for those less fortunate? Do I stand alone? No! We are never alone.

And how is it that those actively working no longer sense any burden for the lost masses? Okay, I'll give you that one, I'd said it when I was a member of the working force, but I did not voice it over and over, like a cancer slowly eating away at me. The fact that part of the burden (cost) is on the backs of today's workers (to maintain patients and the less fortunate in our society), well, if that's all workers worry about, what a selfish · point of view.

Sometimes you can't blame folks. It seems our government has an uncanny way of continuing to spend while at the same time it cuts benefits and continues to whittle away at the middle class: targeting many for tomorrow's poor. What bothers me more is the number of folks making a lot more money, while the blue-collar worker continues feeling the squeeze. Did you realize that some companies are now paying gasoline expenses so their workers can afford to drive to work? What would be wrong with fixing the problem? Paying someone's gas, or a portion of it is a nice thing, but it does not solve this Republic's problem!

Somewhere it is written that giving is more, what is it, blessed, than it is to receive? Familiar? I hope so. I realize that I sometimes forget, too, shame on me. Sometimes I've given less when I should have given more. But it is easy to get into the '*I pull as many of them out of the hat that I can*' attitude.

It's what I call the Chevy point of view, for those of us who cannot afford the Lexus. It is important, that we think and act upon what we are to be giving back to God. After all, it all comes from Him; it all belongs to Him; and a portion of our money is supposed to be returned to Him. In fact, we're supposed to give God the first fruits. But when there is no one looking out for the common man, how is anyone supposed to contribute to the church? We either put Him first, or we put Him in the hat. And that is a disgrace! And that is an understatement.

I have as well been one who either pretended not to know of a need, or simply ignored the reality of that need. (Our sins of omission.) Will we ever be able to grasp the grace, power and love of God's heart? His inclusiveness. We are to strive to do so.

†

There are other folks who'd 'gotten out' of facilities. Some states are now passing laws that levy fines on facilities when a resident gets out on their own. It is a good idea: Too bad that many of these 'escapees' go unreported. These places can hush up a mess like this quicker than the U.S. Senate can sidekick a bill.

God placed me at one of those particular 'escapee points', one of those crossroads, three to five years earlier. My wife had been with me on that sizzling day. Just as we prepared to round a corner leading to a road that enters a shopping area, I spotted the elderly woman walking along, shopping bag in hand. She was shakily preparing to cross a busy roadway. It had to be nearly a hundred degrees that particular summer day, and the lady was practically a hundred years old!

When I stopped my vehicle and addressed her, her question to me was: How did you know my name? And later, in front of her temporary home, as I helped her down from the vehicle: My, but this place **does** look familiar. Although reporting of such incidents may seem a bit humorous to you and I, that particular event could have turned into ugly and sad tragedy real fast.

†

It is at this juncture that I invite your attention to a favorite AD work, *The 36-Hour Day,* Warner Books, page 261: 'Since the confused person may not be able to tell you about the care she receives, *you as caregiver must know about the quality of care the program provides.* Many of the agencies that refer you will not have reliable information about the quality of services they refer you to.'

Lastly, remember that assisted living homes are NOT licensed for skilled nursing care, something those with dementia often require. And yes, whilst I'm pondering it, more than one publisher has published *The 36-Hour Day,* mentioned above.

Your public library's shelves will lead you to another work or two, about finding nursing homes with care for folks suffering dementia. This is a question that you DO NOT want to allow to be glossed over. Unfortunately, behind that great guy or gal's friendly smile, there also lurks a great sales person for the prospective nursing home. Be aware of that. **I cannot overstress what has just been relayed to you. It is surely one of the most important duties you might ever fulfill, checking out a facility before you place your loved one there, if you must.**

As for data presented in writing at facilities today, as you are no doubt aware, such data may not always be as it seems. Lastly, you may ask any facility administrator when it was that the 'home' was last inspected, and further, ask to see those findings. That perhaps can be a timesaver and an eye opener.

Watch to discern if there is any squirming or reluctance to share such a report. And if it's not available, ask them to have it for you the next time you drop in. (And if that's not answered, they are speaking volumes!) They may not be a real good read, either.

There are other stories: other names, other places. One year I approached a particular administrator and had given her my opinion (One of my unfortunate characteristics), that at least they could place the patient's name and address around patients' wrists, at least ones prone to wander. Just a phone number would be helpful. It was another request that would remain ignored. (Do not get the idea because you minister to folks, or to their residents, that they are going to look upon you any more favorably than anyone else. It doesn't always happen.) The dark side of today's truth in our visible world: some facilities don't like fresh eyes around.

I to this date am a friend of the daughter of one of those residents who 'got out', one no longer with us. When her daughter sees me, she runs to me and places both her arms tightly around me as if she's not going to let go. You see, even though I had been practically a stranger, I, too, loved her mother. I cared enough to visit her. Getting up from the bench is the beginning of the real game.

There were others: other patients who 'made it out', most of them fortunate, some not so fortunate. How sad, when our medical facilities cannot provide security to keep these patrons from harm. And it's not simply the healthcare workers. Often it has more to do with who is running the establishment, and how it's being run, who cares, and/or who is able to turn their backs so to speak.

We, too, often turn our backs today, do we not? If someone does stick his/her nose in somewhere: maybe they pull someone out of a burning house, for example, they are considered a hero. I would more correctly say that person was just being a decent human being.

The nursing home task is too large; the workers unfairly over-tasked and they are desperately underpaid. I'm not particularly happy talking about these matters, but the wages healthcare workers and aides receive are just another disgrace to our nation, our nation and its many senior citizens, the numbers of which are growing daily. Unfortunately, it is sort of *a la mode...* you probably know that's French for *in the fashion.*

I am hopeful that you are not passive about reading these words for you may one day find yourself 'locked away', too. (I so tire of editors and publishers whose notes to me concerning this work read: 'Your work is well researched and thought out, and needs to be addressed, but it didn't get the approval rating it needs to be published.' I sometimes wonder how much of this work they have really read, or whether they, too, care.)

Guess what happens when one working in one of these facilities voices their complaint, be it active or passive about the amount of pay they are receiving? Well, they are generally greeted with, "There are lots of folks lined up to accept your paycheck." What a wonderful, healthy, feeling communication, what a caring environment. *Right!*

Yet recall this, friend, we are led to be forgiving. He has MORE than asked us to do this. This is a challenge that I've mentioned before: 7 out of 10 AD folks will be able to live at home. Yet there are those of us who will see the inside of facilities far less than appropriate when one considers how unprepared many of us are, especially in today's shrinking middle class society and economy.

Another particular concern that needs immediate attention, has not to do with how patients are treated or not treated, but deals with this plain fact: It seems as fast and proficient as our researchers are (even amidst budget constraints) our FDA system is a cumbersome, antiquated system to say the least. There needs to be a process in place whereby we can balance our 'common sense' approach with one that may perhaps be a little more challenging, yet worthy of earlier release of experimental drugs, as is taking place in other countries. Some of our newer drugs need to be brought off the shelves!

I am thankful at this writing, to announce that certain Alzheimer's drugs are now in a time-released patch form, so the dosage is spread out more evenly throughout the entire day. That is a praise item, folks. It makes a difference! There are also some universities doing trial studies with folks on certain drugs. Sometimes it only takes one!

✝

Forgiving Father, it is easy for us to sit in judgment, to offer our opinions. Let us not forget those feeble ones cloistered away, practically defenseless. Mighty One, we ask You to enable us to both forgive and forget, but more importantly to be instruments capable of causing change where change is needed. For Your ways are so far above our ways, Your compassion we often cannot understand. Help us, too, to forgive if we are holding any grudges. Lord God, be with those lost ones who are confined to 'homes' where they are in need of Your safety, security and comfort – but above all, Your kind of compassion. Great and gracious God, be with all Your children, both day and night. Keep them safe from harm until You bring them home: To their real Home.

TIME ZONES (Slipping away…)
Wayne Glenn TERRY

Chapter 5

Different Warriors

—Soul Warriors—

A huge loving force surrounds me on all sides. It originates not only from a loving God, but also from a loving fellowship that I regularly attend. Although not mentioned by name here, it is mentioned within these pages, and constantly prayed for. And that is because it is His, and it is in God's hands, as is all else.

Without loving soul warriors, something one should be able to place in huge bold lettering at any time, the whole of this work would not only have been too difficult for me, the work would not have been possible. How powerful is prayer, whether en masse, or from our separate closets, in our aloneness, in our weakness.

Behind the scenes, even as the evil one roars about (and I'm not going to give him the benefit of capitalization), striving with all his keenness and energy to literally eat us, or at least to make life difficult for us, there is a Strength above all, within all and through all that shakes the evil one to the very core. It is the strength of God, and the strength of our collective prayers to Him. For the battle – the battle between good and evil has already been won, already paid for. And that being accomplished makes you and me victors, too. (That line is for you, Grandson Victor.) Prayer, our God-talk, provides us armor, gives us an Advocate as well, and much more. Finally, there is the sword, our Holy Bible, the greatest seller of all times, for all times!

Have you lately taken time to look at the many mighty miracles within the pages of our grand Guidebook? They are so numerous, so diverse, they will astound you. They are not only Christ's miracles, they emanate from Him now, daily. How boundless God's power, His love, His infinite work continued by soul warriors, each and every moment of each and every day. Prayers without end are indeed of limitless power, and so is our love conversation to God.

Soul warriors seek God in prayer, and then become prayer warriors. They realize that He's always there for them, here for them. They pray much, about much, much of their day and night. I know one who barely sleeps because she finds herself so often in prayer. She has to 'catch up' during the daytime, a catnap here, one there, to make up for her prayerful nights, her times of adoration. (How about it Mary Z?)

The numbers of soul warriors would cause the coldest heart to warm at the thought of all this collective prayer power. To me, it is akin to learning that there are stars even larger than our great sun. The sun warms us from literally millions of miles away, yet there are stars that dwarf our mighty sun! Imagine. Is not the power of prayer as mighty? Certainly.

There are, likewise, soul warriors who dwarf you and me, even on our best day. The times that I figured I'd had it altogether in life, as I looked back, I learned were often times that I'd been all wet! I had missed the entire ballgame; I hadn't seen the ball since the kickoff! (The only saving grace: Many of those around me had missed the game, too.) Yet that is exactly where you and I should enter in. God wants not one lost. Can you possibly bring yourself to that knowledge, that realization divine?

When I recall Dick and Gale, and the wonderful work they have done over the years with hundreds of foster children, I am at awe for this brother-in-law and sister who so remind me of Christ. So remind me that without Christ's touch upon this tough world how differently it would have been for so very many.

Soul warriors neither think too highly of themselves, nor do they contemplate themselves for extended lengths of time. Yes, there are times of sweet introspection, or unnecessary worry, and times when we must pray for spiritual maturity, often we are more properly out of ourselves, praying for others. We are out of ourselves because soul warriors are more into Him. Soul warriors are the hands and feet of/for God today. And sometimes, no, oftentimes, we are that Spirit. I believe we are to be part of that comfort that God promised to leave behind.

This is not hyperbole, that is, as we worship Him in spirit and in truth we become more Christ-like, more comforting to this hurting world, and hurting folks around us. Around the world.

Do you realize what a grand heritage that is? "'NO WEAPON FORMED AGAINST YOU SHALL PROSPER, AND EVERY TONGUE WHICH RISES AGAINST YOU IN JUDGMENT, YOU SHALL CONDEMN. THIS IS THE HERITAGE OF THE SERVANTS OF THE LORD, AND THEIR RIGHTEOUSNESS IS FROM ME,' SAYS THE LORD.″—Isaiah 54:17

Righteousness comes from God. Can you ever begin to catch a hint of that meaning? Soul warriors are much more powerful than we'll ever be able to grasp until we are seated nearer Him, or prostrate before Him. A caution might be good here, especially if you consider yourself a warrior, or are contemplating becoming one. I alluded to it earlier:

Be aware of the one who is always about, sneaking and seeking to take God's very precious ones away. The warning is simple, friend, *do not underestimate the adversary*. This is not about frightening anyone, yet it is about making you forewarned. The closer and/or more involved one becomes with the Master, the Mighty One, our God, the more devious and cunning become the ways of one that God has already placed His miraculous and mighty foot upon. These words alone the adversary will not like. But you know what? He can get over them! Really.

"YOURS, O LORD, IS THE GREATNESS, THE POWER AND THE GLORY, THE VICTORY AND THE MAJESTY; FOR ALL THAT IS IN HEAVEN AND IN EARTH IS YOURS; YOURS IS THE KINGDOM, O LORD, AND YOU ARE EXALTED AS HEAD OVER ALL.″—I Chronicles 29:11. Can you not hear the singing?

Pray for our entire world. Pray not only for leaders and fallen soldiers and crying widows; pray for an ambulance passing by; pray for the flood-infested lands far across the sea; pray for the fires, and the anguish and confusion of living in fear; pray for the homeless, the downcast, the hungry, so very many literally and figuratively hungry, pray for one and all. Pray for you, and thank you, pray for me.

†

Our Master, Jesus' last words in Scripture, "SURELY, I COME QUICKLY" (—Revelation 22:20), cannot come to fruition soon enough.

Holy Lord, thanks for Your Spirit yet alive, and thanks for soul warriors, too. Your good will continue long after we have departed; Your grace and power and love continue forever!

Here's to soul warriors everywhere. Keep on! Don't look back! Remember the evil one has already been conquered! Wear your armor, and your helmet of salvation; carry your sword at all times. Stay alert, for none knows when He comes again. Not one. It's in our glorious Guidebook. I dare you to read it! Be you in good health or living with certain illnesses: I DARE YOU to keep on, and to Never Give Up!

—Bad Days Pass – Routine—

Routine has and continues to bless me. My routine may be somewhat different from other patients, not only due to the combat 'stuff' that I endure, but also because I strive to push through some of the affectations that work on me. That is, sometimes I walk, even when I feel I shouldn't be walking. Sometimes I extend my days, when I feel I shouldn't possibly be striving to extend my day. (What little knowledge I have, I gladly share with you.) Today started out somewhat differently for me, then again, they all do. Do they not?

My first segment, as you probably know: I don't call them days much anymore. My first segment often begins at 2300 (11 p.m.), because I sleep little. Sometimes if I am real tired, I may sleep until midnight or a little beyond 0100 (military time). It was at 0100 or so, this day, I did NOT enjoy my nightmare of being buried alive, once again. It is one that caused me to break off the recent temporary tooth the dentist had made for me. (I may have written about it earlier…)

Hours later I can report that my dentist had become somewhat tired and dismayed at rebuilding the tooth, and the unnecessary cost to him. So he had advised me that he would have to do something different. Translation: "*Ugh!* It's going to cost you big bucks!" Back then, as I had been striving to get to a rating board for MANY months (I am closer at this writing as I have enlisted the aid of a senatorial and some congressional-types, something that does help). I, simply put, did not have what it takes to order/make a new gold crown. I thought I could live with the busted mess. (*Ha, ha…*) Think again, Mr. Tough Guy.

But once again, friend, I return to what is supposed to be routine. I have found abiding by my routine, my normal segments of time, or in a sense mini-time zones, it's far easier for me to simply abide by an old friend's advice: (The ninety-plus-years-old friend who I'd often ministered to in my younger days.) The old friend's advice was that when he was hungry he would eat; when he was tired, he'd lie down.

It seems when I rest, I often just rest until I awaken, or decide to stand, and sometimes that can be quite sudden. But simply put, it works better for me if I sometimes simply rest and pray when I cannot sleep. Part of me tells myself that I am often afraid to go to sleep, and that is not good. It doesn't allow peaceful thoughts to come any more swiftly. Yet God *can* help.

You know yourself that if you're over-extended, how it affects the entire rest of your day. I recall one morning years ago (my best recollection), before the disease, being very much out of my routine. I had been scheduled to lead worship at a fairly large suburban church, and had just departed the emergency room only two hours before. In many ways that happening years ago is akin to how I daily feel now as I live with dementia. Sometimes in this fog, or as though my brain is just plain tired out, I call it being fried. I recall mentioning at that service, way back, how slowly I'd felt I was moving, that I needed to take one day at a time. It was something I had worked into my words in the sermon. Or it may have been His working… Amen?

Routine helps us to remain at our best level of performance. It allows our system a chance to rest and therefore to be renewed, revived. Rest allows tired neurotransmitters an opportunity to become somewhat calmed. (Okay, I'm just rambling here; I have no idea what transmitters do at rest, or even if they ever rest, and now I am wondering what an editor will do with that entire line.) But I do know: *Rest is very important.* It restores us, as does exercise.

†

Routine has enabled me to feel more at home in my safe haven. There is something about the not so familiar places and/or new places and new situations that sometimes triggers certain 'dis-ease'. When I remain within my home base, my sanctuary, and this parcel of land that assists me in my daily contentment, it seems that I am better off in my usual, non-threatening environment, not one that is noisy or unusually over-stimulating. And that can change daily or from moment to moment. I remember several older friends whose only wish had been to be left to complete their lives at the *old homestead* because that helped them to feel in touch with life, more than death. I can easily identify with that feeling now. Their longing to remain with the familiar was a bastion for them, and had made it easier for them to face what was up ahead.

I do need to confess and report, however, when my neurologist advised me that it might be good for me to go on a 'fun cruise' with the rest of my relatives, and as he told me to live and laugh and enjoy life while I could, I did! There is so much I could say about that adventure. I plugged my ears with earplugs and danced the night away! I must tell you that it was good to feel twenty-five years young again! But a warning for other patients: You might need to talk this through with your mate; if yours is anything at all akin to mine, she may be one T-d off lady! A word to the wise.

Then again, she might have fun along with you! That would have been nice. My fault as much as Lucy's...

Routine's pattern also assists us in feeling in control. And once again, control is very important not only to the relatively healthy person, but to those afflicted in one manner or another. We **all** at one time or another, feel that we lead this parade. We pretend to be rather self-made folks. Yet the longer one lives, the more one begins to realize how untrue and unrealistic all of that is.

Sooner or later we grasp the truth: that we control very little; further, we are *anything but self-made people.* Perhaps we are attempting our last ditch effort at control, or having the ability to yet make our own choices. For right now, I prefer the latter. I'm certain that it assists me in enduring the difficult times.

Yet I'm sure that God is laughing at what we sometimes consider tough. We are not really so tough are we? *Not one of us....*

As I sense that I may be rambling again, all I desire to share is that routine suits most of us. That is true as well for those typically considered normal, is it not? Bad days, terrible times pass, and life continues on. (Of course, it may not be rambling: a good friend of mine, Steve, often tells me that I write with more sense and more clarity and wisdom than anybody he knows who doesn't have Alzheimer's.) Thanks, Steve B. I love you, and Pete as well.

How has routine changed your life? Or has it kept it on track? During my lifetime, I've found just being dedicated to work (a task) seemed a bastion for me: a routine. I recall how even during the death of a loved one, I'd often continue working to keep my mind occupied from the obvious stress, the trauma and grief of the loss. Have you found that to be the case?

Can routine be an area we can count on? A place we can run to? Something we look forward to? Is there not something special about that part of our life, maintained, as we would like it – even if it is merely routine? (I believe it is the next thing the 'experts' may come out with. That someone, somewhere, will say that routine enables those with Alzheimer's disease to have quality of life for longer periods of time.)

There is another kind of routine that attracts me more. It is a routine of communication with Creator God, Savior Lamb, Almighty King. One of my routines is to listen to an early morning program which displays nature's scenes and plays grand songs; it is akin to my strolls underneath His awesome canopy, a place where I often talk to Him, walk with Him. These routines: praying, love of music, taking in His nature, studying His Word, all are routines I care little to abandon. They strengthen me, revive me, and give me much to look forward to. Do you realize what else routine has afforded me, can afford you?

†

Thinking of some of those low days that I've endured, long ago and more recently, the devastation that this nation's nineties wars have had upon me (as well as countless other new and old veterans), I have felt that my routine of turning to Him, to the One who first loved us, has enabled even bad days, bad times, to pass more easily. It is His joy that strengthens us! His promises. I cannot help but picture an old friend, Doctor D. Annette Reid.

How she has been under rather stressful times (all of which I will not share), of how through all this pandemonium in her life that would normally cause one to go **c r a z y**, she has at times through her God's smile advised me, "It is time to settle down; I need your patience only a little while longer." This woman of great faith, in our brief moments together, continues to exhibit and affirm the knowledge that God controls all (even our bad days); that He understands it all, that He will yet be, as He always has been, even long after the din of so many battles of mankind, especially the ones we recklessly initiate. *He is after all, Eternal God!*

This woman of caring and fortitude and dog-eared perseverance receives much of her strength, wisdom and love from our loving, living Lord. I am firmly convinced that she seeks Him often and hears His leading voice in order to survive the quagmires not only of healthcare's woes and the bureaucracy that she has to fight, but also the many dilemmas that she faces in her day in and day out often chaotic routine. Indeed, she knows how our hierarchy of authority has affected our society in one very hurtful way: the more things change, the more they stay the same. Yet through these times of trial, my dear friend, D. Annette (as I quietly and reverently call her), works valiantly and tirelessly for each one of her patients, her head held high, her heart touching His, her hands upon each one.

To me, the dear doctor is one of the unsung heroes of today's battle-weary world. Many of them are. Have you not known one?

As I reflect upon Dr. Reid and Dr. Hennessey, and so many countless others that I revere, I cannot help but recall: "THE WIND BLOWS WHERE IT WISHES, AND YOU HEAR THE SOUND OF IT, BUT CANNOT TELL WHERE IT COMES FROM AND WHERE IT GOES. SO IS EVERYONE WHO IS BORN OF THE SPIRIT." —John 3:8

The One Volume Bible Commentary, explains it with plainer words: "As none can trace the source or aim of the wind, yet all can feel and hear it, so it is with those who have experienced the new birth. There is something in the inner life not to be explained, but which reveals itself in its operations, and can be known only by experience."

There's another close friend that I always keep in my prayers: one I also revere abundantly. He lives in Ohio, where I spent many years prior to and post-military career. I call him Mayor Myron Young, although they've never taken a vote, I'd put my money down that most everyone around that neck of the woods would agree that this commander of a small VFW Post (9571), would be voted mayor. Myron and his lovely wife, Elaine, are two humble servant-veterans who have busily served Ellsworth, Ohio, for sixty-plus years!

It is through folks such as Myron, from whom I've learned that it is more blessed to give your life. That it is this love of Christ and family and community that embodies what many of us can only 'shoot for', and if you know me, you know I am not enamored by that term, yet here it seems to fit. Myron has found what Oswald Chambers long ago penned, in one of his many wonderful writings: "When we do something out of a sense of duty, it is easy to explain the reasons for our actions to others. But when we do something out of obedience to the Lord, there can be no other explanation, just obedience. That is why a saint can be so easily ridiculed and misunderstood." (Oswald's February 28th entry in *My Utmost For His Highest,* Discovery House, 1992.)

†

Gracious Master, cause us to not only strive to be as some of these aforementioned, Your servants, but also to be worthy of their emulation because of their steadfast connection and devotion to You. For as they have lived God-centered lives, one senses their love above loves for their fellow beings. Thank You, Teacher, that You enable us to identify You, Lord, in others. It has for me been another one of Your dimly lit mysteries so wonderfully and graciously now and again revealed. Thank You for these selfless ones that continue to touch the hearts and minds of so many people near to them, and sometimes those far away. Thank You, God, for teaching us to live one day at a time; Thank You that bad days do eventually pass.

Another one who has lifted me when I was low: The president of Lambert Book House (which I learned publishes mostly study materials). Thanks, Mr. Garner, for your gracious words: 'I do feel certain that you will find a publisher for your good work.' And thanks to others, unnamed, for you kept me going as well. It is because of folks such as you, and Starling Lawrence (W.W. Norton Publishing), that I have been able to re-cut a path through this work even as I close in upon the veil. Even as I live in fear. Yet I offer this: 'Fear not,' says our glorious Guidebook.

—What We Did With It—

When our lives here are over, do you believe God will be concerned about what we have amassed in real estate or other riches? Do you for a moment believe He will be concerned about where you have traveled or what you were able to accomplish for yourself?

Do you not know that which God has provided you was provided to further His kingdom on earth; that what He provided means the 'gifts' that He freely gave in order that you might be better armed (able) to serve Him? How short sighted we can be, without Him.

Perhaps the most haunting question at Judgment might therefore be: What did you do with it? Whether you were born early and not fully developed, or whether you were one of those units allowed to enter whole and nearly perfectly formed, do you not believe that what you did for God will be what matters most? That not only did you come and go for Him, but that hopefully you also danced and praised Him, even before your expected arrival at His throne?

It is to me scary, when I think about it. I know none are worthy with the exception of the One. I realize that we all begin this race in approximately the same manner; that most of the time we are taught similar basic tenets of our varied cultures, that we nevertheless, practically all of us, sooner or later, hear of One above all. I believe that's His way, rather one of His ways. Although to what extent that introduction is in the beginning (at the onset) may be of greater influence for one than another, sometimes it all seems a puzzle.

Yet I reiterate that in our beginning years and/or some place in time later on, we are certainly given the opportunity to face and more fully either embrace or turn away from His gentle guiding hand. Ever ponder it, friend?

It is about choices. We all have lifetime challenges/choices to do this or that, to go here or there, to love or not to love, to get up from, or remain on the bench.

Do we not also have a choice about what kind of vessel we are to be? I mean, other than the fact that we may have some limitations in the beginning, or later, do we still not sooner or later make choices about our course, or heading? To be a beacon for God, or to pretend He does not exist; to live ever with Him, or to ever remain turned away from Him?

Why of course we do. I am certain of it! We either consciously or subconsciously entertain that it is not simply the winds of life that blow us about, or that there's certain data that we input (that's partly true) during this wondrous adventure which will assist us in an outcome one way or another. Perhaps there will be a situation or two, or a person or two who will influence a choice or many choices; there may be an institution or other influences in our background, yet what do you suppose it is that illuminates us most? What causes the bulb to glow, or not?

Have you ever taken time to consider the meaning of life? Ever stop and wonder why you have been placed where you are, or perhaps why you are (at all)? Do you wonder if it all might be a mere dream? I hope you don't believe that… that this is all merely a happening.

From time to time this very morning, I studied a picture of Nathan and Victor, two of my beloved grandsons. Though the hair coloring is somewhat different, and in this particular photo they seem built a little differently; and as they really had (initially) two different dads, they surely are a happy-looking unit, arms around each other, smiling. They share the same dad now, the same mom. They are now walking similar paths in life. Yet one day they will walk in different directions. There will be certain choices made and different ideas and ideals at stake; and what they have been equipped with and/or exposed to will make a difference in their choices/their lives.

Part of what I will always be haunted by, perhaps, and it's my burden solely, is how I may have influenced family and friends along the way. How did I affect their eternal expanse? By that I mean their greatness, their mightiness, and their enormity. My eyes are again drawn to a photo of these two precious boys, and then my mind's eye zooms in upon me, zooms in close-up upon my very core, so my heart of hearts, my very soul lies exposed, practically transparent. We really are, you know? Have you thought that?

Should I feel downcast by how I have influenced or not influenced these young lives? Should it be a topic that forever works upon my being, or is it a subject easily dismissed? Do we merely walk along this unique jewel of a planet, or do we walk it with spirited purpose? How seriously do we take this undertaking? It is not a question for the faint-hearted is it?

Dear God, I fear I have often failed You, and others. I'm somewhat scarred and scared at the same time. I fully realize that I could have done better with my life. Now, as I center-in on thoughts provoking, thoughts with merit to them, at this same moment, Lord, I come to You once again asking for Your forgiveness, in prayer and praise. Could You enable me to somehow forgive myself? And Lord, if there is one other person feeling much the same, one reading these words, perhaps You could forgive her/him, too?

Precious Eternal Father, thank You for dying for us. Thank You, Lord, for the many times that You thought of me, guided me, prodded me, pulled me ever closer: loved me. Why cannot I be more like You, Father? Why cannot each thought, each deed, each step of my journey be more filled with Your purpose? Now that I am beset upon somewhat akin to Paul, with a thorn or two in my side, is it just a course correction for me? Is it time for that correction, or is it too late, Master? Eternal Maker, I have been blessed to linger near the beds of dying folks who I do not doubt accepted You just in time. There were others who walked not the straightest path – yet I believe they, too, came to live with You, that they now reside with You. Help us Jehovah, to seek Your victory in our daily living. Help us to be Your sure winners, Lord. Enable us to make triumphant decisions during our walk, to make good choices. Is it not possible, One who stilled the winds and waves, if we remain more focused upon Thee, we might be restored, made new, made whole? Fit to more properly serve You? My soul not only seeks after You, Father; it seeks also to be so aligned with You, I might see more of Thee and less of me. For in so doing, I may (we may) do our very best for You, the best for others. It is my prayer, Omnipotent, that You will be spared from asking us 'what we did with it', for if we are centered upon You alone, there will be no need for the question. There is no need for doubt if we live Your way, Your will. We come unto You, Lord, as little children, longing to be guided by Your tender hand. Thank You Lord of Lords, for these words, "THEN LITTLE CHILDREN WERE BROUGHT TO HIM THAT HE MIGHT PUT HIS HANDS ON THEM AND PRAY, BUT THE DISCIPLES REBUKED THEM. BUT JESUS SAID, 'LET THE LITTLE CHILDREN COME TO ME, AND DO NOT FORBID THEM; FOR SUCH IS THE KINGDOM OF HEAVEN.' AND HE LAID HIS HANDS ON THEM AND DEPARTED FROM THERE."—Matthew 19:13-15. Keep your tender hand upon us Lord so we are continually guided to do Your Holy bidding, so there will be no question concerning what we have done with our lives. (Recall Matthew 6:34...) (in part). "THEREFORE, DO NO WORRY ABOUT TOMORROW, FOR TOMORROW WILL WORRY ABOUT ITS OWN THINGS." It surely seems that I sometimes have been unable to do even that, Lord. Might You assist me in the re-opening of this old heart? Might You entwine our hearts. Might You also forgive us for the strange fear that we've often displayed: of being to close to You, or of our fearing failure? For with You there is no failure. With You there is smiling and warmth and grace and success. You so still my soul. Might others also reach out to You, especially those afflicted.

—Family Is Everything!—

Dementia means brain failure. It is not something that I control. Yet, you will find that people forget that from time to time, and it may make life more difficult for you. You may even hear words unkind, that you either don't do enough or you are using your disease as an excuse. I will pray that you might have strength to get through those times, for they will come. Trust me.

Dementia sneaked up on me, yet I still sometimes sense that I am out of my head, or that my mind is no longer right, not fit. But I *do* have the grand blessing of knowing ones around me, knowing that often exhausted family and friends are pulling for me, go to meetings with me, rearrange their schedules for me, and yes, pray for me. When it comes to dementia, family is everything. How blessed I've been. Just study my book's cover. You'll discover a huge portion of family there: friends and family and Christ.

Before I go too far, I'd like to say what Bridget, a program volunteer coordinator for our Greater Richmond Area Alzheimer's Association (and a drop-dead gorgeous young woman by the way) might also say. Dementia can be caused by head injury, strokes, brain tumors and infections of the brain. It is not all AD as such, and yet much of it is AD, or at least these afflictions are placed in that same ballpark, or under the same umbrella.

The *Fam*: Although I laughingly refer to family as 'the *fam*' I must say what is being or about to be realized, AD of a loved one or anyone, is monumental devastation. If you don't see it, you may have failed to focus on it; or are not yet close enough to it. You cannot grasp it… will not yet. That's all right. Perhaps you have not yet dreamed as I, of going through an old evolution, perhaps around an old ship, carrying the old paperwork (totally naked)…

†

Brain cells are damaged or being damaged, messing the patient's brain cell transmissions, or as others have said: AD is an accelerated aging of the brain. It is not a pretty sight. It comes in many different forms. How I wish I had earlier studied neurotransmitters; that I'd learned about serotonin and dopamine ('feel good' neurotransmitters); that I'd earlier realized hard cardio workouts enable the blood flow to get deep within our cortex and enable better blood flow throughout the brain. **That is a great tip, and it's free! It may offer longevity!** Speaking of which, it is what the NEWSFLASH was about (and that's especially good for me) earlier in this work, good that I can recall what I'd typed not that many days ago, er… segments.

Speaking of feeling good, I have realized what a wonderfully compassionate aggressive love (through care giving) there can be for the patient. Those who have loved, cared, and prayed with me, so humble me. Some I have never known or met; yet for me, I know they care. Thank you so very much, especially for your prayers, your warmth, your special love.

I believe one of my earliest signs of a diseased brain was my gut-wrenching feeling as I late in life attempted to become a member of the postal workers world. Normally those little pigeon-hole-type slots are not a big deal. For me they were impossible! Seeking and finding the right location for this letter and that one was very difficult, and I could not figure out why. Now, some years later, I thoroughly understand why I only held that postal employee's badge for such a short period of time. Something had begun taking place within me, I just didn't know what.

Imagine not being able to recall what you just ate, whether you need to be somewhere. Imagine marking your machine tools with arrows showing that this one runs in this position, that that one does not. There are many warning signs, indicators. Yes, you realize that many people do those things, or some of those things, now multiply them by a hundred. Are you getting it now?

As you educate yourself and share and pray and remain hopeful, and as long as you have good support, it's simply put 'One day at a time….' I thank God for people around me willing to help me during this new walk. They are priceless. Their value to me is more than anything I own. To me, they are angels: Caring, cradling, compassionate. They are angel-friends forever!

Sometimes a little heavy on advice, yet still angels. Others seem to forget us, for they seem not to know what to say, do. What a pity. Have you lately forgotten someone?

†

It was not all that long ago that I didn't care that much for looking at pictures. I don't know exactly what it was. Perhaps a throw-back from when I was in uniform and had to shelve so many relationships, for when I thought of those far away, a huge lump would often form in my throat. Part of me now, I guess it's my way of hanging on, part of me finds myself treasuring those sweet faces, those yet remaining memories. Pictures do tell stories all their own. I see something beautiful in each one of them, each is a blessing unto itself. (Thanks, Dave, for the digital photo frame, what a grand present!) What a good friend you've been. You and Glenn are the best brothers a guy could ever hope to have.

As I invite you into my family, reader friend, how blessed and rich and full my life becomes. I also wish to share with you my feelings about writing fast. It's a brain thing, as if each day were my last. You see the troubled brain is a collection of cells, like other organs, neurons containing thousands of branches that carry incoming and outgoing information. But for a moment let me speak more of family (something also with many branches).

Family. Lucy and I recently shared yet another sweet meal with our loving neighbors, Bill and Deb. All four of us understand why God had placed our properties smack up against each other. It was His loving way of saying love one another, and while I'm speaking of caring and love, I must advise you that the disease (AD), has been good for Doll Face and me (at times), good for my Donna, my Lucy, my love. We are now more caring, more tender toward one another, and more sensitive. As I wrote last night, "I wish I had a video tape of this time together."

I recall several great things that had happened that night. Debbie's saying that I am blessed with care partners and also with many others who care. She had been speaking of our beloved church family, as well as our neighbor's love for us, their love. Yet I also recall it as being the first time we'd been together that I had had difficulty.

There had been music and sharing, laughter, and yes: my rambling. Yet suddenly, all of it began to bombard me! Upon reaching for a panic pill, I realized that I had not brought one along with me. I had been sensing bombardment, but had not early enough realized it, and as we discussed portions of a book, *Losing My Mind*, I indeed felt a kinship with its author and I was becoming obviously enraged by something that was going on inside me.

It was that afternoon: the very afternoon of this very long day, that Donna had asked me if I ever saw lights. For me the question seemed as if I'd once again met my uncle's best man, in far away North Africa. (I know it's a completely nonsensical line to you.) But yes, yes I had seen the lights. I was more than a little bit put out. It had been the first time, I later shared with our sweet neighbors, Lucy had been the first person to ever speak to me of the *lights*. It had been one of those dark secrets that I had not shared with anyone (a little like living with post-traumatic stress and stuffing it). I had never read about, or known anything about the lights, until my precious wife had queried, "Do you see lights?" It was a question that had floored me! I had figured I was probably in the middle of a small stroke or a brain tumor, and I'd just keep it to myself. Men can be like that. Never had I told anyone about my lights-show, of the weak, pulsating, battery-dying-like visual sensation. When it happens it's usually after I first awaken early in the mornings, the weak pulsating, life-losing light sensation (again, as if a battery is running low). My battery, right before my eyes!

Although I was with loving friends, my wife, God's music, and was at the same time being bombarded, I did not understand that I had been (partly because of the light revelation) overloaded in the midst of what I now realize had merely been over-stimulation of that day, that moment. (It has something to do with neurons.) Neurons mainly generate an electrical signal (I have read), an action: the signal gets excited by other neurons, stimulates other neurons. (To me it is akin to fission, splitting of an atom.)

My Lucy and I have not only become more caring and concerned one for the other, we are getting back to the basics of living, of loving, part of it is because of our realization that the disease can progress even sooner than predicted. I had to be overtaken and taken hostage and become lost far too quickly, my guess. It makes one feel akin to a horse in its galloping mode, bit in mouth, running along at breakneck speeds.

It is similar for this labor of love: writing, and me. It is a very important spoke: a labor of love, in my Ezekiel's Wheel Vision, more later.

The sweet words of the song jumped out at me. I repeated them practically to myself, our friends nearby, *"no one else can fill my heart like You do..."* Perhaps we were all sharing a religious moment. No, it had been more than that: we that night shared and basked in God's loving, awesome, compassionate Presence. For a moment I had forgotten about the four lobes, sections of the brain. I had briefly risen above it all. So thankful and at peace I had been.

It all comes down to loving God, and loving your neighbor. It all comes down to (the greatest of these is love). For in loving your neighbor as yourself, we are doing what God requires of us. It is the very crux of our faith – is it not? Don't you find it exciting?

†

Family. Earlier in life, living a life within the walls of a United States Embassy at times, I had sensed feelings of family, of abundance. My son, Chuck (We were at the Ambassador's residence one afternoon.), had introduced me to a tall gentleman wearing a patch over one eye: Maxie Anderson, by name. Later I assisted Maxie and his friend in a small way as they were amidst their nonstop flight (attempt) around the globe in their gigantic balloon. (Years later, there would be words in a children's book that spoke to that happening, or at least to someone being sent to a certain location to meet a balloon.)

I'd also given Maxie and his friend a stamped envelope to carry with them, hoping it would one day be mailed from who-knows-where and returned. What a keepsake it would have been, from the men who had first circumnavigated the globe in a hot-air balloon. The very ones to first do it! Yet it was not to be.

Similarly, I had also given Maxie a small container of bleach, as I recall they had had concerns about an anti-bacterial substance for their water supply. The ever-prepared Maxie, the purposeful planner, the amazing adventurer. I still cannot believe Maxie Anderson and his Japanese friend went down in that gigantic balloon, that they crashed in that mighty Black

Forest in Germany. They were killed attempting to set a world record.

For a moment or two, they had become family. And then, like a deteriorated lobe, they were gone, forever lost. Better to have lived and lost, I thought. And yet it was precious little, internally I sobbed, as if I'd always known them.

Family. As you are aware by now, my rich life has involved the meeting of lots of neat folks. Not only were there 30-plus countries represented at our American Embassy School, I was also from time to time honored to meet other famous individuals when in attendance at the Marine House. (Thanks: Bob Creedon, Gunny Keyes! Those were special times!)

One such evening I stood as close to Mohammad Ali as you are to these words. He was young and warm, smiling and suave. What a sense of humor. I had not yet encountered 'my turn' with disease. (I guess in reality I had always had PTSD, but I had tried not to think about it. I knew I hated the sounds choppers and guns and of other certain nearby happenings, I just hadn't realized what had been taking place inside of me. I kept it all bottled up inside. I'd stuffed it.

I could never stop the nightmares, or the pictures that I'd viewed of the atrocities of war. Unfortunately, it often came out in different ways, not always good for others near me.

Then there was Marty Sheen and Ben Kingsley, both in that same country, shooting a famous movie. How about that for a hint? Marty's son, Charlie was about 12 or 14 then.

I had met Gregory Peck in Keflavik, Iceland, and then in another place I met the gal who'd at a Cannes Film Festival recorded _Don't Cry For Me, Argentina_. Later I'd caught her out of her comfort zone, hiding almost timidly behind her huge scarf and equally large sunglasses. So many lovely, interesting people. _Family_: if only for a moment or two. A happening.

But you know what? Anyone can bump into celebrities; meet folks who we seem to place on a pedestal. Do you know Whose face I most long to see? You, too?

On more than one occasion I'd witnessed that huge glistening airplane with the Great Seal of the President of the United States of America proudly painted on its side, often referred to as Air Force One. If your heart doesn't do some kind of *giddy-up* then, I don't know what it will take. On and on the list goes, many countries, many friends, and many faces – *family.*

Did you realize that by 2012, they are projecting the Iraq War is scheduled to produce some 600,000-plus additional VA claims? Another family. Not really, veterans are all part of the same warrior-type family, and I'm proud to be a part of it! (The numbers come from a VFW magazine article, May 2007.) I have tried to keep this topic to a minimum, but as you have read, it is one of my trains, and its noise is very difficult to stifle. We have a huge problem with the numbers of veterans awaiting assistance and/or compensation.

If the numbers for AD are accurate, we are also going to have quite a situation with this disease as well. It too, is growing.

I shared with you in another place, words about Colonel Charlie Beckwith's *Delta Force.* I had been reading it and had been rather impressed by it. At the end of his 18th chapter, I came upon the name of an old friend, a classmate of Colonel Beckwith's, another colonel's colonel: Bob Mountel.

Bob was one of the most daring, dedicated men I have ever had the pleasure to work and serve with. (The Colonel had this tender CWO2 (Navy) who was his Operations Coordinator at this particular embassy.) What fond memories I have of Colonel Bob and his sweet wife, Claire, and their son, Steve.

I quote from Beckwith's *Delta Force,* concerning my old friend and boss, Colonel Bob Mountel, formerly Commander of the 5th Special Forces Group. "Bob Mountel didn't see it that way. He wanted to prove that the Special Forces community could establish an antiterrorist force quicker, better, and cheaper than the Department of the Army. Bob Mountel saw that he had to work very, very hard and he had to put Charlie Beckwith out of business."

I suspect the words above would by now be toned-down a bit on the part of both of those brave officers, after all, we are all on the same team, and the years should have mellowed us somewhat. I will not give an entirely opinionated rendition of what had taken place between the colonels. I had not been there.

(And I would never report in a mean-spirited way for I have a deep respect for both men.)

There was a money situation of sorts, and although Colonel Mountel later realized (according to Colonel Beckwith) that Delta Force could be a good thing for Special Forces, I suspect (through what I've read and heard) that they eventually approached the JFK Center, as the book reads, to get additional funding. (From *Delta Force*): "It was General Rogers, his four stars on each shoulder, who laid it out to everyone. 'The President, Charlie, wants this unit. Delta is important. We cannot afford to mess this up.'"

Not long thereafter, as I understand it, General Meyer clinched the deal this way: General Meyer walked over to an easel and with a black marker he wrote, Department of the Army. 'This is the Chief of Staff and me!' (It was the beginning of a family.) Actually it always had been, it just had never been announced. Below that he drew a box. 'This is the JFK Center for Military Assistance and General Mackmull.' (It goes further, but ends up that General Meyer advises Colonel Beckwith that if he has needs or problems to come directly to him. Not quoted exactly or properly perhaps, but you get the idea.)

Sweet deal... birth of Delta Force, birth of a special family. Colonel Beckwith had to be in Delta Force Heaven. I'd lived that sensation a time or two, albeit in other arenas, but none so lofty perhaps. The exception would be the world of a Face I long to see.

✝

I've often wondered if God, seated at His place of glory, ever ponders, *"I love it when a plan comes together."* I suspect He has a larger agenda in mind than we. Then again, I just don't know. I am comfortable reporting: I just don't know. But I do know this, *we are all meant to be family. We just seem to lose track of that, from time to time.*

"Fam" – We have so often laughed and cried about it, my sweet neighbors, Lucy and me; another sweet deal. I don't believe I've ever in my entire life met such loving, sensitive people. I am sure you can tell. It has been as if I've always known them, miss them when we're apart, and feel great when

we're back together. That's the feeling one gets with family, or should. Can you imagine that last meeting? With God, that one that goes on forever and ever? And you don't mind it...because you're at long last *Home*.

†

Lord God, thanks for family. Thank You for allowing us to be part of the greater family, too, the family of all of Heaven and earth. This is something to celebrate, something to anticipate! Thank You for that sense that as we love our neighbors as ourselves, indeed we may call upon them and not be chided, share with them, laugh and cry, live and die with them. And likewise, it is the same for them. Gracious God, thanks for inviting us into Your loving INCLUSIVE family, the wonderful loving Family of God. That final dining together, forevermore... (Is there not the possibility that this entire planet and its population, of all different backgrounds and cultures could be considered Yours? I believe it is! Might it be so, Lord, as long as they look to You.)

If only it could be...Sometimes I fear for our people.... God really doesn't want to lose one.

Chapter 6

Eyes, Emotions and Stress

—Emotions Run Hot—

I am going to go a little crazy and allow those headings to remain as they are, somewhat different looking. They give editors and publishers ideas about what could be.

"Thank you so much, Lucy, for throwing my Five Wishes (my will form) at me last night", I had begun. *"You did it just when I was settling in for a couple hours of rest."* I went on: *I so enjoyed your tirade, your kind words of: "So! You've listed this one and that one as your health care agent! And what am I?"* (Recall that I had warned you that there would be times when they treat you just the same as everyone else, or perhaps even a little worse?)

It had been readily apparent that Lucy had not studied what the will was about, that they'd recommended sometimes NOT appointing close ones to oversee your wishes and so on. It is an *Aging With Dignity* document. Once filled in, one reads and considers whether a spouse or close loved one may perhaps be too emotionally involved to make certain decisions for the one with dementia. Since Donna (Lucy) had already been involved in such sad passings, I'd figured it might be better for her to be somewhat less involved. (You can find this document online, by the way, or if you prefer as I sometimes do, you can write them at Aging With Dignity, P.O. Box 1661, Tallahassee, Florida 32302-1661.) They are a great group of folks, very kind and cooperative.

It had been a time for Lucy and me that would have been typically easy for me to 'enter the game' and advise 'Doll Face' of the Whys and How's of my decision, yet I have the suspicion that entering that world would have only served to further assist her in her escalation of the, 'What am I?' fury. So I did not play the game. She departed the room.

There are moments of stress involved for caregivers and patients alike, sometimes at the same time. I especially loved it when she used to tell me, "It's all about you, Wayne!" (Such comforting, playful, well-chosen words.) Or how about this one? "Why don't you go back to that place you used to live?" *I guess we should have talked it over*, went through my tired head.

It is true as well: I had not always been the most perfect patient, even under the best of circumstances. As you can see, friend, it is an emotion-filled time (something akin to good drama), the heat has already been turned up twice, now for added viewing pleasure, let's crank it up one more time.

I release and report this drama not with malice, for my love for Lucy will never vanish, never diminish. But when you are living with a roller-coaster-type disease, and the one you are with also exhibits 'roller-coaster-ness' as well, it can become more than a little bit interesting. (Hey, I think the 'roller-coaster-ness' thing might fly!)

I'm sure I've shared how Lucy and I are from different parts of the checkerboard. Can you imagine what it's like being from entirely different planets? I've been there. Yet, if you are so faced with such a situation, remember that I am praying for you, and that I desire you to recall: **Never give up!**

So here's how I assess it. I struggle, as you know, to get word from a governmental agency, for months. There is a sea of bills, including those from an attorney, collection agencies and others, who seem to take pride in calling and even threatening you (even after you've explained and written to them telling them to desist). I am in prayer, attempting to stick to a regimen because of my dementia, when in the mail arrives, a note from a psychiatrist asking me to pay her, so she can close my account! It makes you wonder about the guy who wrote words about a 'wonderful world', doesn't it?

I attempt to sort through it all: the chronic (40-plus years) of post-traumatic stress, the not-that-old diagnosis for AD, the panic attacks. I ache from head to toe, live on oxygen when at rest, and my wife, get this, my Lucy is concerned about paying a cell phone bill! The pastor talks about how we can make ourselves sick, and having just finished talking to my dentist about the tooth I keep busting off, thanks to combat nightmares, I forget about that for a moment and place a call to the Veterans of Foreign Wars hotline.

Two days later, I get *Miss New Person*. She advises me that she cannot speed up my claim, it all depends upon how many other vets are in front of me; more comfort for the weary, I had made a mistake again. I had long ago figured when I had been appointed by the President, with the advice and consent of the U.S. Senate, well, I had just figured it might be a little better than this. (By the way, the VFW later turned out to be one of the outfits that 'saved the day' for me. Sometimes you need a wingman.) Today, you really need one! Maybe a whole flock of 'em. (That, by the way, is a STRONG HINT for any new warrior who happens to be reading a book about Alzheimer's, and needs assistance from Uncle. I am praying for you, daily!)

I had by now contacted doctors and searched files over and again; I had heard from two senators and one gracious Congressional Staff (who probably saved me from suicide); I had walked and prayed and paced, and the great, really good part of it all, I'd been able to relive my entire war history over and over (while being medicated to the nines)! I now have shares in the U.S. Postal System, which is not really government-run any longer, and that may be a good thing. No, that, too, would be a toss up from the looks of the recent lines I've stood in. How about you? A government agency tells us (at what group meetings I can stand to attend) one day all of this will fade into the background. The shrinks hardly ever tell you anything; and your spouse tells you plenty! You've been there, you say?

It all rather reminds me of the mechanic beneath your hood, who begins, "Now describe for me again, that sound it's making." I keep insisting to my children that I'm okay; assure my friends, some who deny my new checks request (at the bank); and I always keep telling myself *It's the best day I've ever had.*

I continue asking the One to enter into this entire bombardment, somehow, sometime. And He has, He does! Thankfully, but then, when I change medicines, my neurologist tells my wife to tell me *Try not to nap.* I'm post-traumatic: *We all nap!* I tell him. (Nobody wants to hear about your PTSD....)

Having mailed and re-mailed documents to various offices and people as the veteran is responsible for 'seeing to it those documents are received by the government agency', one of their famous quotes, it has just been the proverbial barrel of laughs. All the while I'm popping more panic pills in order to survive various maladies, what fun! Not far into it, you no longer care to socialize; in fact, it becomes the last thing you want to think about some days.

Then there's distrust, conniving, your mind's picture of what letters sit where (and which ones you've mailed that have slipped: *'Ooops!'* into someone's trash can, especially if you're one who likes to check on their 'progress'); if there is such a term in the halls of government nowadays.

Should I share or not share any of this with Momma? I mean she's already been through enough in her lifetime for three people. Should I send my brother this **one more bill** (knowing he can't do it all, and knowing that I will feel more and more as if I'm begging from someone who has been so *right there for me*)?

†

I again think to myself: *Does anyone have any idea how many times I have transmitted this **last document** to this government agency, and asked them to please proceed with presenting my months-old application?* Then I always make that fatal mistake of adding: *This is the document that I earlier provided on such and such a date.* **Big mistake.** Trust me. My applications folder, or rather expandable folder by now, ever at hand, conservatively contains 85 to 90 documents, and I keep wondering which ones I have forgotten to make copies of. I often think some arms of our government figure that if they just forget about you, you'll probably go away and/or die. And the problem with most veterans: We're our own worst enemy. We tire, and give up!

(Then I hear a quarter of the homeless are vets!) It's not news: but it hits the six o'clock news now and again. One month after I receive a letter from a congressional person, I am yet chasing down my doctor's helper to get my final papers (medical file) mailed to the local government agency. *One month*! Stand in line, take a number. How it all reverberates in my head. The letter with new (?) information, talks of PTSD, restless leg syndrome, a previous while-in-uniform busted left ankle, hypertension, sleep apnea, skin cancer, memory loss, anxiety/depression, panic attacks (and I pencil in something that will never matter to anyone: bone spurs in my lower neck area). Then there's a paragraph on high cholesterol, and there are side notes: (*Did you know that high blood pressure which takes you years to get, has to be proven within one year of your separation?*) And if you fail to bring it up, guess what: So will they!

And oh yes, what past employers have to say about you gets thrown into the mixture. My guess? I really haven't researched it, but I can tell by some of the questions I've had put to me, something is amiss when it comes to where they get their inside information. Care to take a guess at what part of that listing I was granted assistance for?

Come on... take a shot.... You know what they fail to bank on? They fail to understand that even with dementia, parts of me are still pretty damn good, forgive me, Lord.

I begin to wonder if there's any place within all these statements/forms (opinions), for the veteran to tell about being scammed out of jobs, that there are games played by cliques of people in various work arenas, okay, almost all of them. About the folks who hide the fact that there are no longer any work ethics in today's workplace, but that it's who you know and how you 'kiss up' that really counts. Otherwise, you can be made to look like the kid who's the slacker, or whatever else they can scheme up.

I had vigorously worked my way up to corporate level in a large Richmond outfit, only to find myself being asked eighteen months later to take a five-dollar an hour cut because someone figured I'd been making too much money. I had certainly worked diligently to get into the top 1%, but it seems when you tell anyone how to do their job (even when you've been instructed to), you end up being the one who is 'out in the cold' and what had never been an issue, suddenly becomes an issue! Thanks to the power of the masses, or the fact that I didn't party with the right people. I hadn't partied at all.

†

How many times I've seen workers in nursing homes, leave patients' pills with them (against state regulations in Virginia), and overheard them telling the resident, "Take them when you're ready Sweetie." And yes, just for your information: the local nurse was informed. (And that my friend, is a tip of the iceberg.) On and on I could ramble, but to what end? Do I get a chance to challenge a single employer's opinion, or for that matter anyone who thinks little of conscientious workers?

†

Then there's the document from a government agency that states: *Wayne Terry who resigned from, where was it?* George Mason University, according to their records.

My return letter tells them not only do they have another Terry, but also that this one never went to college. So whatever they have on me (him/her?) they don't have on me. (How's the rest of the paperwork, I wonder.) Yes, I wonder and try to maintain my sanity at the same time through my cloud-infested noggin, which is feeling fried once again.

Not that it has a lot to do with AD, but I contacted the CEO of the outfit that'd offered the reduction in salary. He was gracious enough to tell me that I'd hear from his human resources person. Guess what happens? You guessed it: nada, nothing, zilch! No, I'll take that back. Some real charmer called me and said something about "*if there's anyone you want to thump on…*" What a sweet guy, the Guy that never bothered to ask for my side of the tale. And it was a tale! You just have to be part of the 'gang' don't you? They forget you in the clinches, I guess, after they've put you o u t. Another lady that had just gotten promoted, they decided to 'let go' a week later! Interesting folks….

But back to the 'process', what folks go through when they attempt to get help. I'd say God is the only one who knows exactly how many veterans give up, or get too sick to fight the fight, or who are simply ignored for so long that they eventually get a notice that reads: Did you apply for monetary assistance back in…? *No, that letter never arrives either.*

Your doctor tells you, *"Settle down,"* the agency's voice on the other end of the phone tells you 'If you keep calling, you'll only botch up everything'. In the meantime, you get to re-hear how terribly hard it is to pay bills from the care partner's side of the house. It all puts me in mind of Charlie Beckwith's long ago vantage point: Sea Stallions stirring up huge dust storms at the worst possible time, a stoic warrior becoming somewhat rubber-kneed. <u>Delta Force</u>: It's a good read! That is, if a combat veteran can stand to read it for very long. (I regret how this segment was taken over by ancient problems with an arm of a government that doesn't seem to work for many people, but it all becomes part of emotions so stirred up and steamy that everything is taken to a boiling point; especially when I begin thinking of the brave men (and some women) who died before they were ever granted help from an antiquated system that cannot seem to agree on anything. To me it's as if the *We the people* words no longer matter.)

†

Emotions run a little hot. It's not a time for anyone who finds it too hot in the old kitchen, friend. You may have seen the latest H.R. 327, a Suicide Prevention Bill recently introduced to our congress. The numbers of veteran suicides not just from old wars, but the latest ones, too, would make your head spin, your heart heavy. It is a time to turn to Him, to seek that Light that drives shadows from the room. I end up utilizing how I think of suicide, weekly, in some of my correspondence, *eventually* I receive a letter telling veterans in general who they can contact if they are thinking such things! I don't bother to write to them.... *Why would it matter now?*

Emotions must come out sooner or later; they cannot be overlooked, or stuffed. From time to time I regret my attempts at humor: but honestly, often it's better to laugh than it is to cry, is it not? You, too? How much humor have you read in these lines of late?

†

Creator of the universe, thanks for being and bringing us into being. Although we suffer certain adversity in life, all of it pales in comparison to what You suffered for us. We whine and cry, kick and claw our way along; when all along we have more than we really deserve. In reality, Father, You are better to us than anyone we will ever know. We thank You for the occasional course correction in our lives, the introspection that You daily lead us to.

I come to You humbly, Father, praising You, rejoicing in my tiny problems that often overwhelm me. As we read these words together, we realize that You, God, are in and through it all. I cannot speak for everyone Lord, but this is one time that I am going to say we love You, Lord. Help us to recall the wounded, the dying, families who continue to suffer in silence the atrocities of war. Might You dear God, have something in store that far outshines our nation's Purple Heart Award. For so many of ours have sacrificed their all. We thank You for those who gave their last full measure. They did their duty for the love of neighbors, for the love of country. Thanks, Almighty, for people such as they: our uniformed heroes. We know we must sometimes be willing to fail. If we do not fail from time to time, we may never know what victory tastes like. And it is Your way that brings us to victory! It is a lasting victory and peace. How long will it take many of us to realize that?

"The more you sweat in peace, the less you bleed in war..." —Admiral Hyman G. Rickover

—Stress—

What is it that makes the otherwise achievable unachievable? What is the greatest stumbling block, the albatross that works against every forward step of an AD patient? It is, without a doubt, stress! Not only does stress thwart any patient momentum, it causes caregivers as well as receivers to become unglued, unyielding, and practically worthless at times.

This is more than mere frustration. In a sense the caregiver is also one of the diseased partners, if nothing else, purely by association. And folks outside the circle of those diseased cannot understand it. Often, folks meaning well, will preach to a caregiver or a care receiver as if they were suddenly well, and in need of an instant sermon; what a waste of time and energy and lack of empathy, well intended or not.

Stressors, for example noise bombardment, I early learned sent me running for a panic pill or simply sent me running completely out of the area. Learning also that someone telling me to 'take it easy' or in some other way explaining why I could or should not feel as I was feeling, this too, causes AD persons great stress.

These, though, usually minor challenges in today's fast-paced society for most, often become grave factors for the AD patient because of other inner changes that are taking place. I know I now distrust folks more than ever; that I tire much more easily, and therefore my patience level is often diminished. (See note on brainpower at the end of this segment.)

I just do not handle day-to-day living as well as I used to. This of course is my opinion; it is also symptoms of the disease. It truly disables you in more ways than one. There is a certain amount of depression and anxiety that also accompanies this world called dementia. This is further complicated, moreover, by the fact (which I wish I did not have to include), that I am a victim of PTSD, (previously shared far too often). It is another realm that embodies distrust, and anxiety. (In November of 2007, a full seventeen months after I had begun my application process with a government agency, I was yet awaiting their reply on my 'unemployability status' – this based on the fact that I suffer from AD, PTSD, and panic attacks! **And they wonder why the veteran suicide rate is on the rise!** Seventeen months now! Now here's a real hoot, at the time of this re-write, a full 26 months from my original application with this arm of the government whose name I do not mention, we are yet awaiting the results of a reviewing officer. I hold a copy of a letter mailed to Senator John McCain, who sometimes enters this wonderful world for me, but my friend, John, seems busy of late. (And yes, in a sense I regret that hostile-sounding line, for Senator McCain fights for veterans. He always has, and he always will.) One would think, however, that his people would get word to a vet. (Maybe it slipped off of someone's desk, or they were reading about WMDs. (*I know it's not fair, but I think Lou Dobbs would like it.*)

†

In order to lessen the degree of stress upon the patient's life, a look at the things following is imperative. First and foremost, a routine must be established. The more structured my life, the closer I can adhere to *feeling well,* the better I prepare myself to face the challenges ahead of me. That, by the way is how I cope/live, one day at a time.

Being able to maintain a routine interrupted as little as possible enables me to feel as if I yet have some control over my life, and my ever-changing world. Although I have had to turn in my driver's license (one of the most difficult issues for many of us), after careful introspection I realize the importance of it, that it would happen sooner or later. I also recall words in our Guidebook, about growing old gracefully. And only days ago I signed away any power of attorney and set forth my last will and testament, and that is probably the most difficult thing I have ever had to endure. For none of us enjoys giving up control. I don't care how much head over heels in love, or how close you are to your mate's heart of hearts, when you are signing away control of all your tomorrows, it is a very tough decision. (How I long to receive another editor's letter stating I just didn't get the approval rating necessary to publish this work.)

When someone abruptly enters my routine and asks, "Why did you remove the treadmill to the back porch?" And/or "…how many months will it be there?" You either learn *one*: to not respond, or *two*: to totally ignore the obvious drama, or lastly: just pretend that you are rolling with whatever it is they are muttering (or shouting) about. If you are one who may end up fuming about these outbursts, you may have to grind your internal teeth, as I grind my actual teeth sometimes at night. (Yes, my dentist can verify that, too. Not that anyone will be concerned.)

This example might seem a fair 'let's talk about it and work-it-through issue' for most people, yet it more and more becomes just a plain old stressor for many of us. Or to put my doctor's glib but wise advice to my partner when I was diagnosed, "You're going to have to roll with it." This brings me to my next point.

You may be able to effect much change, if for example your care partner, caregiver, whatever you call him or her, is unable to be flexible during your new, ever-changing life, wherever you are, between who you were and who you now are; it may also be a stressor for you to either engage in and/or ignore that person. Do you remain, or attempt to move on somehow? Sometimes, friend, you are just plain stuck. And perhaps that is not the best way to explain it or look at it, yet sometimes it's true. Or as the old saying goes: *The more things change, the more they stay the same.*

Just as a hostage can be taken and forced to drive his own vehicle in a dangerous manner or into a dangerous environment to evade police, one can easily feel caught betwixt and between two entirely different worlds. If your mate, or caregiver, is unable to carry out his/her duties, perhaps it may be time for yet another of life's changes. This of course depends not only upon what stage you (the patient) are in, it may also be such a delicate operation that you cannot carry it out, or it may dictate whether you can assist in the conversation necessary to enable you to play a role in what is taking place. I yet feel able and blessed to be able to 'play a role' as I am fighting this disease with everything within me, and I'm striving at the same time as well, not to give up my personhood and dignity. (And don't forget my famous words: *Disease can draw you together.*)

At the same time, I fight to remain habilitative. I strive for the best quality of life and longevity that I can possibly have, all things considered. I also desire to keep my marriage intact.

Besides, love is not only a neat thing to be involved in, love is very much what life is all about. What is marriage, or life as far as that goes, without love? Therefore, sometimes, we may have to challenge ourselves! Part of that challenge may well be toughing it out, or being forgiving, or being able to compromise. Yes, I'll be praying. Those of us whose regimen is constantly being bombarded are in a very difficult situation.

—More on Stress—

There are times when the hairnet over my brain and the fog and tiredness that I feel seem simply put, too much to bear. And believe it or not: some of your closest friends will continue to ask again and again: 'What is it you are feeling that is different about yourself?' It is quite possible that you will have to endure their never-ending questioning, even though you've gone through it many times before. Be of good cheer: usually folks are simply trying to support you, but they are unsure (let alone unskilled) about how to do that.

I must acknowledge that I certainly have been blessed to have close friends willing to ask me how I am, or how I feel, and/or what is different. I am also very fortunate to have remembered their asking me previously. Not everyone can do that when fighting AD.

Sometimes though, I am forced to retreat to a place of quiet and/or to my ever thump-thump-thumping oxygen-making machine and CPAP (forced air machine). There are times, too, when simply put, I can no longer hold open my barely opened eyelids. Time my complete system seems as if it is going 'off-line', as if it's saying *buh-bye* now. It is at times such as these that I excuse myself, amidst my 'sun-downing' or I am just plain beat-down tired. Ask Doll Face; she has watched it happen over and over again. God bless her.

Sometimes only a few will understand your disease. Again, often there seem many who fail to recognize it. Sometimes it seems a struggle to get the 'experts' to recognize it. Often a friend with good intentions will attempt to get you to socialize. And that's okay. But I will not normally draw myself away from my routine, unless I feel it is a time that I am able to disrupt it. Often, simply put, it depends upon where I am at a particular time, how I feel. Other times, I seem able to just push through, asking for God's help along the way.

There are also stressors we hardly ever consider. A governmental entity's inability to show any empathy whatsoever for a veteran who has suffered the devastation and re-igniting of unpleasant past experiences of wartime events; the idiotic games-playing of individuals you may have had to 'deal with' throughout your life; the supervisor who thought he knew you when he knew you not at all.

There are also the more subtle distractions as well. The knucklehead who races to get in front of your vehicle before you arrive at the next traffic signal; the neighbor who plays music loudly enough for the entire community to enjoy it (or not); the youngster departing a public school building, exuding expletives that should only be heard on a battlefield or when one is perhaps off alone somewhere. (Oh yes, freedom of speech....)

These circumstances that most 'normal' folks hardly bat an eye at become much more visible, magnified, make me more volatile or withdrawn. I often attempt to ignore such things: yet every once in a while I can act as obnoxious as the best of them. And that may be long after I have encountered just about everything I can think of, and even after I have talked to Father God often and long. Believe it or not, a great deal of this can be diminished with/by the benefits of exercise.

†

Can we do anything at all about these stressors? For me, it is often fleeing to II Corinthians 12:7: "AND LEST I SHOULD BE EXALTED ABOVE MEASURE BY THE ABUNDANCE OF THE REVELATIONS, A THORN IN THE FLESH WAS GIVEN TO ME, A MESSENGER OF SATAN TO BUFFET ME, LEST I BE EXALTED ABOVE MEASURE." Following at verse 8: "CONCERNING THIS THING I PLEADED WITH THE LORD THREE TIMES THAT IT MIGHT DEPART FROM ME." And then the words of our Lord contained within the next portion: "AND HE SAID TO ME, 'MY GRACE IS SUFFICIENT FOR YOU, FOR MY STRENGTH IS MADE PERFECT IN WEAKNESS.'" Paul continues: "THEREFORE MOST GLADLY I WILL RATHER BOAST IN MY INFIRMITIES, THAT THE POWER OF CHRIST MAY REST UPON ME." He completes it in verse 10: "THEREFORE I TAKE PLEASURE IN INFIRMITIES, IN REPROACHES, IN NEEDS, IN PERSECUTIONS, IN DISTRESSES, FOR CHRIST'S SAKE. FOR WHEN I AM WEAK, THEN I AM STRONG."

It almost sounds as if Paul looked forward to stress, does it not? Does it not sound as though Paul could have been as 'messed up' as the rest of us?

Sometimes, friend, do you not feel that you too have been given that thorn? That you were given that something that makes you weak and yet strong at the same time? That something that forces you to go on even in the face of adversity? So we *do* have something in common?

Good environments. Not so good environments. There are folks who listen, but then there are others incapable of hearing anything other than themselves. Are we not all subject to similar stimuli in life? Can you roll with it? Or does it send you reeling? It often depends on where we are in life at that particular moment, does it not?

I easily identify with the apostle. Yet I have suffered only a small portion of what Paul had suffered. Thankfully so. Yet I cannot help but reflect that I, too, have a thorn or two, perhaps they've been there all along. I know this much: Without life's challenges, without a thorn or two, many of us would be rather content to watch life's rivers roll along before us and never be a part of much of anything at all.

We might not even contemplate anything more than our being. We might never leave our comfort zone, or our home. We might become locked away within our own little world. Yes, it's that thorn that keeps some of us striving, dreaming. It sends us forth, propelling us to something we ordinarily might never attempt. And that something might be something very good. If it is of God, it might be something splendid and wonderful, worthwhile. It might even be something life changing for you, for me, for others.

†

"Research suggests (From June, 2007 *Men's Health* magazine) that when you lose testosterone, your memory worsens," says Jeri S. Janowsky, Ph.D., a professor of behavioral neuroscience at Oregon Health and Science University. She explains that a steady supply of T is critical for the neurons in your brain to properly communicate with each other. It sounds quite plausible to me. (I have often read and talked about intimacy….)

†

Father of all, perhaps we will never fully comprehend what to do about stress; I do know however, that we are to turn to You. I am thankful for lives lived before ours, for those who never became conceited or nasty, even when they had a thorn to endure. Father, I am grateful for an un-numbered mass of believers who have been able to identify with Paul's dilemma, whatever it may have been. For in Paul's being able to survive challenges, especially with his debilities, are we not led to yet another great hope: that perhaps we, also, in the face of certain adversity, will be able to prove ourselves more capable? And might we be more able/aware of Your constant love for us? Enable us great God, to lay our stressors at the foot of Your Holy throne, to praise You all the more. Allow us that selfless ongoing that seeks You out, not only when we are being bashed about, but also out of our constant love for You. You, Who created us for more abundant living. For in this way do we not become kindred to the things of Your eternal Kingdom? Are we not praising and worshiping You as we were created to do? Thank You, God, for stress. "SING, O HEAVENS; AND BE JOYFUL, O EARTH; AND BREAK FORTH INTO SINGING, O MOUNTAINS: FOR THE LORD HATH COMFORTED HIS PEOPLE, AND WILL HAVE MERCY UPON HIS INFLICTED."—Isaiah 49:13— *Thank You, mighty Master, for mercy, and for this magnificent life! This life that we should never take for granted, whether the living of it is difficult or sublimely beautiful and filled with peace.*

—Awareness—

I shared with you that early into my early onset (realizing that 'old me' no longer was), I saw things that had always been present, but seldom before noticed. There had developed a certain keen awareness about me: being able to 'see' better.

Is it perhaps not long until I no longer 'take in' as much, no longer realize that I am slipping away, so I am allowed this new sense of awareness? Or is it not that way at all? I am reminded of Ecclesiastes 7:10. "DO NOT SAY, 'WHY WERE THE FORMER DAYS BETTER THAN THESE?' FOR YOU DO NOT INQUIRE WISELY CONCERNING THIS.'" We do not have the material at hand for a just comparison. That last line, it should be noted, also belongs to Reverend J.R. Dummelow, *The One Volume Bible Commentary*, Queen's College, Cambridge. Is the reverend saying we are unable to distinguish between where we were and where we may now be or will be? Is it one of Reverend Dummelow's mysteries? One of God's mysteries? No, there's no comparison here.

Is there not great sensitivity in our time with family and friends? "OH, THE DEPTH OF THE RICHES BOTH OF THE WISDOM AND KNOWLEDGE OF GOD! HOW UNREACHABLE ARE HIS JUDGMENTS AND HIS WAYS PAST FINDING OUT!" — Romans 11:33. We are forced to wonder at His profound love and wisdom, the mystery of His workings. Me? I'm simply in awe of His ways, His grace, His love, the peace that God offers each of us. If we can only be aware and then follow. Yes, sometimes easier said than done. Yet we strive.

I'm not sure this awareness is such a mystery to me, although my heart of hearts believes we will see/discern much more later on, I can't help but believe my keenness, although different, is His way of allowing me one final look. If this brain scrambling or losing of cells means that we are slated to deteriorate, as it appears from the other side (this side), this may well be a gift to us: this gift of keenness and awareness (albeit temporary).

It puts me in mind of cancer patients, and others who sometimes (shortly before death) seem 'back with us', somewhat restored, seemingly wholly aware. It draws us again into the hope for one of His loving miracles. Usually though, the short-lived hope is soon crushed by the inevitable: that slipping away, and then ultimately death, at least, death for a moment. Hold onto that. That *death is only for a moment*! And that there is also loving without the miracle.

There are many things about Him that I cannot understand, may never understand until God shares them further. I have become more aware of how a blind person might feel. (And please excuse me: I know that's a stretch and against every bit of good counseling I've ever learned). But having hundreds of times traversed my home in total darkness has made me more keenly aware of the nature of one no longer sighted. And it's easier for me as I revisit that realm, daily (er... that'd be nightly). In a sense there is sharpness here, too, in knowing, as I study and write and attempt to navigate my living area, by touch, and as I attempt to learn more of this entire realm, it does become easier. It's as if I, too, am able to see in the darkness, though I do not. Do you recall, reader, how they say blind folks have a keener sense of hearing? Can it be that some other diseased folks are also allowed extra awareness in other areas?

I am aware of Lucy's wanderings to my side in the middle of her nights, our nights. This is something new. And it's something I rather like. Her visits make me more aware of the depth of her love, not just her concern for me. Imagine if each of us could be so loved, so cared for, consistently. We **are** you know.

—More Awareness—

Nature is more beautiful than ever before, God's words somehow more splendid. Whether it is the sound of sleet upon the bushes outside my window or warm rain when it splatters against the house, or the thawing-out sounds of the grass in early morning, all seem so much more vivid and vibrant to me. The colors of falling leaves, my deep breathing yoga-type or tai chi breaths. Why am I now allowed this new keenness? Is it because I'm more alert to life itself? No, I believe it is one more of His magnificent gifts to one who has just been given a second Alzheimer's medicine. It is one of His ways of compensating for what He knew would be or not be all along, long before I approached this time of awareness. It is a time that God allows me before I head for my real home. God's Home.

There are times when it seems that I'm slipping away faster than at other times. I have dreams so scary that just the thought of revisiting them makes me not want to sleep. There are dreams of not being able to find my way, dreams of knowing not where I am or whom I am with, knowing not one soul. Dreams that I am locked away within a place without reason, without sanity, just there, stuck. Sometimes, it is as if I'm being held against my will. The worst part: I sometimes know not who I am in these dreams. I'd say they are nightmares, wouldn't you? In some ways they are worse than combat's 'mares. Combat 'mares are cleaner, quicker for me. They are usually the same ones over and again.

But then comes a new day, and God's blessed lucidness, that keenness of consciousness. Or am I lucid during the insane dreams? How thankful I am that we can savor life, each and every moment of it. How thankful am I to be (sometimes) away from nightmares, drug and/or disease-induced, or ones borne from combat. It is akin to the manner in which I am transported to an entirely different realm, my beloved India, or Africa. How I loved those strange new areas of my life, that commonality of life, even when far away. We are all so much alike, even in our cultural diversity. It always amazes me: for even in mystery, the freshness of this new world for me, I sometimes feel so much at ease, it is as if I'd been here before, or as if I'd had AD before. Yet that is absurd.

It was the same (that calm feeling) whether I was visiting or living in Germany, Vietnam or Japan. Naturally England initially seemed more akin to my homeland because of the commonness of the lingo.

Are you, too, aware of life around you, aware of the beauty of His creation, the magnificence of His healing, the awesomeness of God's peace and patience? Are you aware of the unshakable promises of His eternal kingdom? Can you for a moment ponder what lies ahead for those who are at-one-ness with the King? *Fairest Lord Jesus* rings in my ears. What a soothing, mighty magnificence.

How I long to be forever pure, without these albatrosses, without things I should not have to think. Then again, it is also an awareness when I talk of this, and so I share it, if you're trying to be perfect (as a good friend of mine once wrote) please, stay away from me! There is no room for smugness in the righteousness of Him. It all depends upon one's manner, does it not? And that is a tough one for AD folks because our manner and our behavior are often affected. And it isn't always pretty. It's not always pretty to others either.

I can embarrass my sweet Lucy at the drop of a hat: whether it is asking the waitress to place her phone number on the back of the receipt, or that my eyes comb the crowd for that one 'dish' that causes me to say, *Hello*!

†

He has made us a little less than the angels. That is what our Guidebook tells us. Do you believe it? I had another type of awareness, just before awaking recently: It was the most magnificent vision, the most wonderful visit. No, it wasn't anything dealing with victory at sea, or a gunboat, or even a jungle dance, it wasn't about breaking through a glass-topped burial casket that I sometimes envision.

This dream was like none before: There was Grandpa (that's me), and I was staring down into the sweet face of each child: each grandson, each granddaughter. I was telling each one, one at a time through our smiles, "You're my pal, you're my friend." And as each one nodded their tiny head, face aglow, I'd add: "We'll fly kites and go fishing and take long walks, just you and me…." It is all so very real, so very peaceful, each child acknowledging me as if I am the only person in their entire world. "We'll go for ice cream and climb a tree…" … "We'll row a boat and you can run after me." "There are so many things we will do; go swimming again, paddle a canoe."

The *tell-me-more look* in their shining eyes draws me in, as to each one I continue on. We chase the Ganges all the way to the foothills of the highest mountains, there we meet my Shining Star, my Anjuli, (The adopted blessing from India). All of us are there. Each of my little loved ones is there.

Our value is not in our valuables; our value is in our awareness and love one for another. You know the last thing I share with those wee ones? And the ones not so small, "You've made my life so wonderful!" I mean that from my heart of hearts.

†

King of Kings I fully and joyfully praise You for allowing us special times of awareness. The time we are allowed to spend with Your nature, Your animals, family and friends. Forgive us for often 'centering in' upon the reality of today's saber rattling, yet it is difficult ignoring factors that may effect change for this entire planet. If we could only dare to share our similarities. For all any of us really wants is to love and be loved. Forgive our hours and days and years of idle talk, mired in what is less than our very best. Times when the voice of the masses is ignored, or times when they are too often realized, especially when they seem nonsensical or full of selfishness. Almighty One, we pray for our nation, but more importantly we pray for all of mankind. We do not have an edge on the

*marketplace of anything in America, or in any country. In many
ways we are not as advanced as we so often hear and profess,
not in Your ways. Forgive us for our obvious ignorance, our
foolishness, and sometimes-selfish ways. Forgive us for our love
of/for material things that will rust and fade away. Forgive us
in matters of national security and service to country, when it is
typically known that only one percent or even less of our
population is willing to stand up and sacrifice for the rest.*

*But mostly, God, forgive us for so often turning away from
You. The essence of Your heart would lead us more to love, and
less to our warring nature. (Yes, this from a warrior, Lord.) I
praise Thee, Father, and I pray special prayers for that one
percent who do step forward in love and dedication to protect
this yet young Republic. If only we had more folks so committed
to love of country. I often wish I could 'step up and out' again,
instead of dreaming dreams as old men do.*

"O GOD, YOU ARE MY GOD; EARLY WILL I SEEK YOU; MY
SOUL THIRSTS FOR YOU, MY FLESH LONGS FOR YOU IN A DRY
AND THIRSTY LAND WHERE THERE IS NO WATER. SO I HAVE
LOOKED FOR YOU IN THE SANCTUARY, TO SEE YOUR POWER
AND YOUR GLORY. BECAUSE YOUR LOVING KINDNESS IS
BETTER THAN LIFE, MY LIPS SHALL PRAISE YOU."—Psalm 63:1-
3

—The Eyes Have It—

One may not be able to discern whether a person is confused
or normal, not by looking at them. Often dementia-affected
people appear normal, appear to function quite well for a long
while. It is however important to realize, and I early saw it in
myself, to me at least: the eyes have it! It is the eyes that show
something amiss in the vessel, the fortress, the temple. My
neurologist friend had been suspicious as much as nine months
before I'd guess (earlier for me, I mean, I knew something was
amiss). It is the driver who usually senses something's wrong
before the mechanic. Not so surprising.

My eyes (to me), took on a squinty-looking appearance:
after too many long nights, too many sleepless and/or restless
nights. They not only looked rather squinty, they looked as if I
was having difficulty holding my eyelids open; or as I used to
share with the young ones as I watched them slowly and

unmercifully falling asleep: "Your eyes are getting heavy, very heavy."

Mornings are typically the best time of my day, especially after I've had a couple good hours of rest. I say rest, because I don't get into deep REM (rapid eye movement) sleep that much. When you hook up with a sleep cycle of only two or three hours of sleep each night, or at each occasion, it doesn't take long for your eyes to show the tale tell signs of one with dementia: that beat down look. It's as though you've taken up drinking (to excess) all over again.

I had heretofore wondered why most of the patients with AD appeared or were asleep when I'd go to visit them. Now I more easily understand it. It is far easier to understand once you find yourself slipping into a similar pattern, the same element, that inevitable pathway to Who-Knows-Where Land.

†

There are the old aches and pains, too? One is not so prevalent when I first arise, yet it doesn't take long for it to begin, three to five hours into a segment of work, the base of my head used to begin its dull ache. I can only suspect it may be the beginning of my hairnet once again, applying itself either over or somehow into the tangles of my brain, or who knows, perhaps it's my cerebral cortex. Thank the good Lord, I seem to be finished with that now.

Then again, maybe it was a good imagination. Does one's brain simply begin its downward spiral after being gainfully engaged, or did the ache begin as I began working the 'at rest' part of me that had been for a while off-line?

No, I don't suspect the old noggin is ever totally off-line, especially with my now and again recurrent combat 'mares. (And now, after all these months and months since I first applied for help from an unnamed arm of a governmental agency, November, 2007's VFW magazine's cover sort of tells it all: *Current Wars Trigger Haunted Memories of Vietnam.* There are as I'd thought all along, thousands of us!)

What a doubly tough battle, living with dementia and fighting for wartime compensation at the same time. I'll not bore you with the statistics again, but the backlog is unbelievable. Wait 'til the public is brought up to speed on the thousands of applications that are hardly moving. What a horrific, drastic, dastardly shame! Or perhaps even that will not move them.

Fortunately, I hear a song I so revere: *Yes, Jesus Loves Me.* It is as though He is in this very room with me, especially with those sweet words 'they are weak, but He is strong.' I'd often wondered why patients worked so hard at maintaining eye contact during that particular song. It is all clearer to me now. The words are so strong and effective and believable.

It is important to use this organ, this controller of so many processes. I will continue striving to work my brain regardless of whether the eyes indicate my disease or not. Remaining busy, learning and reading, all are recommendations of various health books. There is much you can read about that you'll not hear from doctors. Then again, what doctor have you talked to that volunteers much of anything, but once again, in fairness, so many of them are swamped: sitting with and striving to ascertain and/or diagnose and record that which they may already suspect, or soon will know. And there are so many of 'us' affected and afflicted with/by this and that, and only one doctor to see the 'so many'. You may ask them questions.

(Did you see that lady who slid off of her chair in a New York waiting room, see the people walking by as if she were nothing? Does it cause you to sense that we have all gone absolutely crazy, especially when you ponder how hospitals are to be safe havens, places concerned with the lives of our beloved brothers and sisters?) I believe it was back in July, 2008.

I've found most doctors when they have time to respond, will respond, even if you're not face-to-face with them. They are akin to good nurses. They really care, most of them. Keeping the brain busy, some suggest, seems to slow the progression of the disease, so naturally I'd recommend you keep the dust blown off the old gears of your noggin, keep her in motion. That's a challenge! But again, sometimes doctors do get a bad rap.

I've found, as other brain-impaired people: colors blend for me, especially if they are similar hues such as blues and greens and yellows, they seem to blend more easily. I have noted that my eyes favor the brighter colors now, especially anything red or with a shade of red therein. No, I don't suspect that this infraction between eye and brain has anything to do with my droopy-eyed condition. Yet I wanted to mention the vivid colors, how they at first STOOD OUT so, when I had first noted it.

These little tidbits that one discovers along the way are part of the revelation of the whole. It is one reason I love reporting this, for those who have also shared have meant a great deal to this writer. I so appreciate their selfless efforts to the cause of others. Our sharing is a sign of our caring, and our love one for the other.

✝

Then there's the *gaze*. I may have hit on it some. It is different from my squinty-looking eyes look, my eyelids that need the proverbial toothpicks to keep them held open. Folks with the gaze, I can spot from twenty-five feet across the room. They also seem to mostly sit facing one particular direction, often reminding me in their stillness and stiffness of a doll-like manifestation of their former selves.

Squinty-eyed or glazed over, what is taking place is a partial disconnection or cell deterioration (I suspect). It is a brain hosting a tangled network that is disrupting the natural healthy flow of blood. (Throw in the words this layman can't pull out, doesn't know, or just cannot figure out). The eyes have it. While I'm on the eyes: Did you realize that a lack of exercise can affect your eyes so very much that it could possibly lead to blindness? I know, more good news.

Seriously, I read it in Men's Health, (March, 2007); page forty, under a topic entitled: *A Bad Case of Lazy Eye*. It speaks of blood vessels expanding and contracting, how exercise improves endothelia function, according to Dr. Michael Knudtson, M.S. He recommends a good workout at least three times a week to insure your eyes. Yours truly recommends you work out every day, as you may already have gathered.

✝

There are so many of us affected by this 'interrupter', this disease that slowly changes the course of a man or woman's life. I always pray that the change is for the better, after all, there's sometimes not a whole bunch we can do about it. Yet I do know Someone Who can!

Stay in touch with Him: That's another challenge! He *is* One more beautiful than diamonds: God.

†

Living God, thanks for AD. For me this thorn in the side has been a leading back to You! "YOU ARE THE FATHER OF ALL WHO BELIEVE. (Romans 4:11 paraphrased): *What comfort it has been to me, coming home again. You are that touch that we often long for, that healing balm that we often seek. You know our longings and needs before they are ever uttered. You come when invited, and You are always here if we'll simply accept that fuller, more constant Connection. Whether we go to a secret prayer place, talk to You as we walk along, or throughout our day and night, You are never far from us! That is a praise item. We praise You, Healer of Healers! I long to be more at-one-ness, whatever my lot, Lord, and I know that You know that. It so soothes me.*

Chapter 7

Depression's Best

—Distrust—

Although this is a portion also prayed about, I did not sense much excitement about scribing it. Yet eventually I felt led and somewhat compelled to address it: *Distrust.* There seems today to be such a perverse attitude of distrust within our society and that of other cultures as well. It is very sad. Some of it I can readily understand when I read and see and hear about the mess some folks have made of their lives, how almost instantaneously we're notified when someone has 'gone astray,' if you will. It's as if some enjoy sharing the dirty details with everyone, as long as it doesn't harm them themselves.

If you are one fortunate enough to be in today's work-force, and therefore paying into benefits and programs that somehow assist those less fortunate, I say God bless you! I don't question those less fortunate than myself, as if I distrust them, nor do I sit in judgment of them. Later on my words may make me out to be a liar. (I also sense that I may have written about this matter somewhat earlier. If I have, please be kind enough to forgive me.)

Another example of people not trusting others nowadays is readily available to me. I'll always remember when one of my first works was published, the questions from a good percentage of people (and some were friends): How much did you pay to have it printed? Who helped you write it? Aren't children's books so much easier to write? Once in a while this kind of curiousness is not too bothersome, but it would have been so much more refreshing to have heard, "Well done," or some laudatory form of exchange once in a while. I'm attempting to explain this in love, as many have loved me, and many have as well been very gracious to me.

Maybe it's part of our frailty, or being unable to accept someone else's success, the product of just plain old hard work. It puzzles me, for we all have been blessed with one talent or another. It's in our Guidebook as well. Why? is my question, why are we so unwilling to say *"Wow!* I'm certainly glad you were able to do that, I'm so proud of you."

Do you yet sense why I did not wish to write this portion? It so demonstrates how selfish and conniving and misled we can be. Momma, long ago taught me this: She had worked a food bank; in fact, she was the organizer of a large food bank, which involved many different churches working together.

Late one afternoon, I had asked her about the number of clean, sometimes expensive-looking vehicles parked outside the church (driven by those coming for food). How, I'd inquired. How do you determine who is really in need? Well, it later on did evolve into a little checking out of this one's income and that one as well, but at that particular time (the time of my question), Momma turned to me and simply replied, "He sorts it all out. There are no secrets kept from God."

I've always admired Momma for that, that and her gracious service to literally thousands of families that came into that church building year after year for assistance. Thanks Momma, you did well! *And thank you, God. You provided so much, often when people wondered where the help and food would come from. You are so gracious, Lord.* (Mother's volunteer workers were gracious and dedicated, too. And some of them continue on today.)

Surely the not-so-trusting folks have every right to their opinions and emotions, don't we all? But isn't it time to be more than looking out for number one? It goes on yet today: I recently caught a segment on CSPAN, where the generals were answering questions put to them about warriors recently returning from combat zones. It is a little more than interesting to me, as you know, I am one of those returned combat-exposed veterans from a previous war.

What makes me crazy yet, is that too many of my returning combat type men and women (I am hearing) are being told more or less to suck it up, pull yourself up by your own bootstraps. Although I hear the generals saying each case is handled separately, and that this is monitored and that is monitored, I am also keenly aware that getting a troop to return to full duty, and perhaps combat again, is a large money saver for Uncle. So yes, I, too, distrust. I warned you that I'd become a liar. But I tell you, I have reasons to distrust today. And I have many reasons to stand up for returning veterans!

There's an eternal flame burning in Arlington, Virginia. Not many of us, let's say fifty years of age or older, would not be able to recite what that particular man once shared with us,… *about asking not what our country can do for us.* That's wonderful stuff, yet sometimes a country owes more than it can repay, and why is it that the ruling class, the bank owners, the mortgage companies have ripped off so many? And what is this reverse mortgage stuff, where now we're saving our citizens by selling their homes little by little, until nothing is left? I believe that is nothing short of shameful.

On the other hand, it has for sometime been shameful: the numbers of folks who figure the country owes them a living. But isn't it sadder still, when combat veterans (or any veteran for that matter of any war) return home and must once again fight, sometimes years later, to prove they are eligible for aid?

They must fight bureaucrats, caseworkers and psychologists, folks that hold out long enough that the person in need eventually gives up, or simply tires because they begin to feel that they are *begging for help.* It is indeed a sign that too many of us have our sights on the visible world, and we've forgotten things invisible.

Had our Lord decided ahead of time: *Hmmmmm, shall I sweat droplets of blood in the garden, and be beaten and spat upon and pierced and degraded for a single soul? Or should I turn My back on a world of lost sinners?* Do you believe for a New York minute that things would've turned out better than they are? Do you believe so many would have come to realize they should do what is right for others, out of love? Or would they have told debilitated soldiers to *suck it up*? Compassion doesn't take a shuttle scientist! Nor should a vote in the House or Senate!

It's awesome to me, how God can turn despair into joy, a broken life into abundant living, a thief into someone who shall proudly walk into God's eternal kingdom! Yet I suppose some of us need to place our hand inside that gaping hole in Christ's precious side. We are so distrustful. I'd guess part of it's due to the fall of man. And yes, that includes ladies, too.

Another injustice taking place: folks that have nothing better to do than rally around the rumor room: So small their world has become, they spend a great part of their days sharing stories about someone else, anyone else, in this way they take any attention away from their own sorrowful lives. They trust no one. Not even themselves.

I do not relish these mean-sounding syllables. Yet I don't believe they are mean sounding when they ring true. I figure sometimes I just don't think too highly of myself either. I, too, am a sinner, and often I have been distrustful, have become hardened. But then I recall God's words about forgiveness, and how we must.

I'm certain there are those who are asking: 'What has all this to do with Alzheimer's disease?' Actually, anything detrimental, aids in the deterioration of folks. I am not saying that I have figured out that the world's environment, or our particular stress factors cause AD, but I am saying that we would be better off if we learned to live in harmony one with another.

Would it not be better if we could learn to understand another's point of view instead of involving ourselves in this daily worthless calypso of being callous? It drives me nuts! At this writing, the approximately 7 to 900,000 veterans waiting to hear about an application for assistance are waiting on a government that is so bogged down in *nothingness,* it will be literally years before these once uniformed men (and women) are assisted, if ever.

And sometimes it is the little things, such as a new Speaker of the House coming into office and complaining about the size of her airplane. No, they shut that story down real quickly didn't they?

What on earth is going on? When I begin to think of the literally thousands of homeless, lost and maladjusted folks in our Republic alone, as we continue to give money to countries that continue to bank it or simply misappropriate it, I must stop, grab a panic pill, or do both.

Not long ago, I read where four or five 'distinguished' psychologists/psychiatrists (Notice I didn't use shrink.) got together and decided they were (and are) going to house young returning warriors in units where they will be rehabilitated, and that thereafter some 90% of them will be fit for return to full duty! *Right!* Please tell that to the thousands upon thousands of Vietnam and Korean veterans who are exhibiting symptoms of PTSD that for some had been stilled in the background, or their train was as mine, on the tracks: waiting to be stoked, only so it could later get back up to speed once again; back to full-swing, full-blown PTSD.

Do you know what it sounds like to this distrusting soul? It sounds to me as though they are trying to figure out a new way to not get bogged down any further in paperwork, let's just call PTSD something curable. Well, I hope it is curable, folks, but I think they are a hundred and eighty out! What if the 'experts' find out 30 or 40 years from now that they (the warriors) were not cleansed, never made ready for return to war? What if these new warriors start encountering what many older Vietnam veterans are facing right now?

—Agendas—

We see it in the chambers of our U.S. House and Senate: everyone seems to have an agenda. Sometimes that's okay; yet too often they seem to spout off with such golden tones, words so easy upon the ear, spoon-fed words as some of them are, carefully crafted, doing what for us?

Why are we unable to get bills passed that are clearly written or at least have a table of contents showing exactly what is contained within these voluminous documents that are being blessed, when all along no one is able to read them (as JFK is gone), therefore they are just passed with the wave of a special wand, the wand of an undivided house!

That is, if they can settle down and quit talking 'at each other' long enough to agree on anything. To me, they have seemed so much like children in the schoolyard, and what they have been showing this Republic of late is deplorable, inexcusable and not defendable.

And behind these words, these bills, is your distrust, my distrust. It reminds me of Thomas Paine, not that long ago. When will our nation, if ever, truly return to one governed by the people and for the people; or as Senator Coburn spoke of not long ago, transparent, understandable, acceptable?

How long until we will not have to entertain hearings regarding the apparent ignorance of *leaders(?)* as they daily turn their collective backs on soldiers at Walter Reed Army Medical Center? Yet I echo partly, words of VFW's Gary Kurpius, its Commander-in-Chief then: "What occurred was disgraceful, but it was an aberration that should not be allowed to taint the dedicated service of thousands of military and civilian employees who provide outstanding care to our wounded at Walter Reed and elsewhere around the country." (See Ohio Veterans of Foreign Wars News, Volume 68, No. 2 of March, 2007.) I'm sure the story was carried elsewhere as well. There is always good work.

Yet I am suspicious. Somewhere within this work there are words about how long our representatives spent talking about Walter Reed Hospital.

Yes, this is the portion that I never wanted to write. It shows us at our worst; then again, maybe it shows that we're still thinking. God help us all. I know HE CARES AND I AM THANKFUL HE CARES; I know He lives, and I do: *I trust in Him*!

†

Thank you, Elijah, for these words: "I WILL INSTRUCT YOU TO TEACH YOU IN THE WAYS YOU SHOULD GO; I WILL COUNSEL YOU WITH MY EYE. BE NOT LIKE THE HORSE OR THE MULE, WHICH LACK UNDERSTANDING, WHICH MUST HAVE THEIR MOUTHS HELD FIRM WITH BIT AND BRIDLE, OR ELSE THEY WILL NOT COME WITH YOU." —Psalm 32:8-9. *We can trust in you Father, because you know our rising up and our lying down. So gracious and understanding and loving are Your ways, Father, so far from ours. Assist us gracious God, to live together in harmony and peace and with a sense of dignity and trust. Help us to somehow become more transparent, more caring, and yet at the same time remain vigilant. Assist us to reach out to others in love, to concentrate on winning souls for You!*

(Lest we forget, a portion from 2nd John): "THIS IS LOVE, THAT WE WALK ACCORDING TO HIS COMMANDMENTS. THIS

IS THE COMMANDMENT, THAT AS YOU HAVE HEARD FROM THE BEGINNING, YOU SHOULD WALK IN IT."

When we walk according to His commandments, we are able to discern mediocrity; we become more able to look beyond our selfness, there is borne the possibility of mightiness. Then we are no longer fixed upon a hierarchy of authority, and at last His authority, an authority with a difference, a transparency, becomes our authority!

—Growing Old And Dying—

Sometimes I think my combat nightmares assist my writings about life. It's true: no one gets out of this life alive. It is more troublesome for some than others, drawn out for one, over in the blink of an eye for another. There's a list that comes out when you are in the Armed Forces. I am not going to tell you what it is called, yet it always brings up the question: 'How did this guy make it, how did that one get promoted?' It caused me earlier to think something not very nice to say: 'That the one who got killed, or died in the blink of an eye may have been the lucky one.' Of course that's not true either; it's just that most of us fear death. And many of us think we'd rather die than fail. It's not true. At least, I don't feel it's true for me.

Naturally, you know I'd like to be the **Never Give Up (guy), who tells you he doesn't fear death.** But I can't say that. And I realize that we obviously die a little each day; something akin to the new car that depreciates the moment it leaves the showroom floor. And then there's the daily wear and tear, and how environment/conditions, or our own ignorance affects any and all of the original value. For me: it's striving to get the old jalopy back to pristine condition, where possible. The **Never Give Up!** profession serves as my daily reminder to do my best for God, as opposed to thinking that someone who died was more fortunate.

Should we simply forget to look within? Are we to be able to consider how we might be of assistance to others without introspection? Does it not enhance our entire being, our world, perhaps a legacy? I am not crazy about the word, legacy: to me it smacks too much of thoughts I don't care to induce, thoughts of me. I do, however, enjoy portions that define 'What sort of

guy was he?' or 'How did he influence the lives of others?'
'How was he to strangers?'

Suffice it for me to share, as we make ourselves open to
God, to His constant Presence, we soon learn not only that He
does affect everything we do; He also effects change, often
great change in our personal lives. Are you open to such an
invasion? Open to realize that change may 'take over' your very
life? No matter where you are in life, no matter what your
burdens - are you willing to become an open vessel, God's
vessel? Are you willing to become that person who realizes that
the story is no longer about you? Never was about you.

Know you not that regardless of wars and rumors of wars,
regardless of how close we may or may not be to 'end times',
do you realize that God is our only way to eternity? That's right.
It is why I am fond of calling Him my life's Savior.

Have you ever thought as we trudge along or bravely
approach the paths to our own end, that without being centered
on Christ, we cannot possibly glimpse perhaps the best part of
what our lives could be; what our life was destined to be? It
frightens me. Yet at the same time as I see my words coming
easier before me, as I sense His sweet companionship with me, I
KNOW, deep within my very core, anything is possible with
God – at any time!

So whether we die a little each day, or look forward with
vigor to each remaining morning, I am keenly aware of His 'He
leadeth me' words, aware that we are citizens of another place.
And that place is not here.

It makes life for me more palatable as I think of God's
constant guidance and what it does for me, how He energizes
my entire being. I sense no downward trend whatsoever, not
even what is considered scary to some: death, for example. For
are we not promised eternal life through God's grace? Because
of His loving sacrifice: *Why yes, we are!*

Should growing old frighten us? It does, I know, but I don't
think it should. I believe growing old is merely more and more
of our placing ourselves in His hands, more of trusting
thoroughly in Him. "BOTH RICHES AND HONOR COME FROM
YOU, AND YOU REIGN OVER ALL. IN YOUR HAND IS POWER
AND MIGHT; IN YOUR HAND IT IS TO MAKE GREAT, AND TO
GIVE STRENGTH TO ALL. NOW THEREFORE, OUR GOD, WE

THANK YOU AND PRAISE YOUR GLORIOUS NAME."—I
Chronicles 29:12-13.

I would not dare elaborate or attempt to change a word in
any way. But I gladly share them with you. You see, growing
old and even dying are not that scary when you consider His
power and might; and that God has had plans for you, even so
very long ago. Before your beginning.

†

*We daily, some of us, Father, intensely realize that we are
nearer dying, yet we are also closer to our rising: thanks to
You! Thanks to the empty tomb! Citizens of another world are
we indeed. Yet while we are here, Savior, assist us to be
servants and not selfish, seeking to be more of what You would
have us be.*

—'Mares And Meds—

This area is where two of my particular dilemmas meet. The
nightmares or 'mares, emerge from wartime experiences, yet
sometimes I am certain that they come from dementia
medicines or dementia itself. The sleeplessness I suffer, that is,
the light-to-restless sleep, is indeed shared by both these worlds.
But again, 'mares and sleep problems overlap, and therefore it
would seem (to me) difficult to determine from whence they
originate.

It was quite obvious after the fairly recent death of a
uniformed nephew, I had placed myself in his situation, or at
least my inner self had so imagined it. For a long while I
pictured myself crashing into the water in a chopper, being
found dead, floating. There are other more recurrent nightmares
for me. One is from when I embarked on my famous gunboat
patrol. You may already have tired of hearing of it, but it plays
an integral role here.

These vivid, sometimes recurring nightmares are most
traumatizing and in all likelihood will continue with me as long
as I have breath within this broken vessel. I must confess as of
this writing, I regret having 'stuffed it' (the not sharing of the
nightmares) for so long. My war wounds of the mind I later
realized would loom larger, sooner or later. I did my best to
conceal any suffering, and I did a pretty good job of it. I did

- 157 -

however, 'get off once'. I had turned myself into a psychiatric unit in 1982, but even then, I spoke little of my war trauma.

There is a strong caution here, however, and it is why I wish I could give every returning young warrior a copy of this work. (Maybe some entrepreneur, reading this, will take that on as a project.) Though this is generally about AD, I believe, deep inside, if we harbor guilt and trauma and deny the haunting within, from combat for example, sooner or later these ghosts will come out and vibrantly reappear, regardless of how and/or how long we've kept them 'genie-like' all bottled up inside.

My soundest and soberest wisdom for any returning war veteran, especially for those who were exposed to combat, would be to get yourself somewhere where you can openly talk about your experiences. Do not attempt to accomplish what so many literally thousands of other returning veterans have successfully accomplished (we thought). Do not keep your emotions, your pictures of the mind, and your innermost secrets of atrocity – do not allow them to rest within your vessel!

On the other hand, I am not thoroughly convinced that this rehabilitation they speak of today will mean an end to your 'mares. Sorry, I do not necessarily agree with many of our current 'experts'. I do not believe they can predict your future, or how you will react to certain stimuli/triggers down the road, especially when conflicts arise and your recurring and/or new thoughts come into play. Your past is not that easily erasable, trust me.

The first time I swallowed their (our) modern-day cure for AD, (and by the way, there's no such thing yet); but the first occasion when I took the number one-named drug for dementia, my dreams and/or nightmares took on such an ugly turn, not only did I have more and very troubling dreams, but also as I had shared with my neurologist friend, I had decided pronto, I could not live with the obvious side affects of that particular medicine. Therefore, I am now plodding along on another medication, which although it also gave me some initial weirdness (dream-wise), it was eventually conquerable, that is, I have been able to get to the place to where I can live with it. *Hallelujah!*

—An Interesting Area—

This area I have found to be of interest: as there are times when I am uncertain what it was that encouraged my internal computer to play it before my mind's eyes, that is, what had caused me to have a combat nightmare and/or caused me to suffer another weird and/or brand-spanking-new dream territory. In other words, I am uncertain whether some visions are combat-originated or medically induced, and/or disease induced, allowing this sometimes-new seduction of the mind. I know I would not talk of my recurring burial dream (being buried alive) as if it were a medically affected 'mare. Besides, friend, it is one of my hauntings, one I've lived with for many years since my 'games' in country, Vietnam.

I also continue to wonder if it's simply that the clock that's supposed to monitor my inner timings has somehow become eaten away and/or simply rusted so it is beyond repair. Dementia and/or dementia medicines sometimes make me seem even more restless than ever before. But if that is part and parcel of what one has to endure to slow the progression of disease, so be it.

Although I would love nothing more than to continue this rambling, and often that's what my reporting seems to me, about the various possibilities of/from 'mares and medicines, I will not. I am instead going to 'cap this well off' for now. There is plenty of room for research and schools of thought for the more scholarly. Thoughts I have offered again are merely my observations of what has/is-taking place within me. It is my prayer, reader friend that you are and will have more gentle nights, more restful moments within that sometimes-quiet realm known as sleep. At least, it is a world I look forward to, one I may get now and again, when I am dog-tired or cobweb-ensconced when I hit the hay.

†

Father God, thanks for life. Thanks for experiences and sensations that we relish. Thanks, too, for the scary times, ones caused from our scarred lives. Your Omnipresence, Lord, is a grand comfort to us. Thank You Savior, for words from Proverbs 16:9 – "A MAN'S HEART PLANS HIS WAY, BUT THE

LORD DIRECTS HIS STEPS." *I will never feel 'puppet-tized', Creator, yet I do feel Your loving and gently guiding hand upon my very soul. You have become my all at last. As is also written in our Guidebook:* "TRUE WORSHIPPERS SHALL WORSHIP THE FATHER IN SPIRIT AND IN TRUTH: FOR THE FATHER SEEKETH SUCH TO WORSHIP HIM."—John 4:23.

Friend, we are to worship Him genuinely, sincerely, and often.

—Tired Of Being Tired—

It is easy to understand that sleeping for only short periods of time without deep REM sleep makes one tired, enables us to realize why our 'awake ness' in daylight hours may sometimes seem utterly long. It is good for my writing process, however, and communion with God. These words say it better: "ONE THING HAVE I DESIRED OF THE LORD, THAT WILL I SEEK AFTER; THAT I MAY DWELL IN THE HOUSE OF THE LORD ALL THE DAYS OF MY LIFE, TO BEHOLD THE BEAUTY OF THE LORD, AND TO INQUIRE IN HIS TEMPLE."—Psalm 27:4

Long days are easy for me to identify with as my worlds of chronic PTSD and AD and an occasional panic attack often merge: making sleep a luxury, or at the very least a tertiary category. When I'm not writing or reading, I can usually be found exercising. That includes walks (day and night) as well as an occasional meeting. All in all it makes for not much rest at all. I often feel as I'd once professed at one of my former group meetings with other wartime veterans: *We are the walking dead,* and I am tired of being tired. I had been diagnosed with PTSD and long awaited a government agency's final determination (due in part to our *leaders* in Washington, and their record-breaking speed at making decisions). Sometimes I wonder if they figure veterans will die, and that will be the end of that. Sometimes, I wonder if they know we are 'out here' at all. I fear that we have too few veterans representing us. Too many silver-spoon-fed folks who are out of touch with the masses.

Those are not words I enjoy regurgitating with an already burdened family and/or close friends, but the truth is: sometimes it's as if we're simply waiting for the other shoe to drop. You know yourself, if you occasionally have a sleepless or rather restless night, and then a grueling day thereafter, how quickly you can become rundown, devoid of energy, rather lifeless. Now multiply that for the person who lives with dementia. Do it once again. It causes my brain to feel entangled and abuzz. Yet I must now admit, since the recent receipt of the patch (where one wears his medicine all day long instead of getting jolted by so many milligrams at once, the entanglement and feeling abuzz or 'fried' may be on the way out). And what a blessing that will be. I am almost prepared to say 'is', or at least to confess that it is at least more manageable.

—Awaiting—

There are times when I attempt to identify with our Lord's beatings, His being dragged to the cross and then having to drag it, little strength remaining within Him. I'm striving to be very cautious and to remain far from any blasphemy, for NO ONE, not one other than the One, will ever know what or how much our Loving Incarnate One suffered for you, for me. Yet I often feel deeply depressed and beat down when I think of it.

On the other hand, it can be a time when I also remain fairly optimistic, hopeful, or just plain 'pumped' thanks to Him. Thanks to God's free and abundant renewing power that we gained at the foot of the cross. After all, His death means life! Can you imagine that? Do you realize that it sets us apart from all the others? "THOU SHALT BRING DOWN THE NOISE OF STRANGERS, AS THE HEAT IN A DRY PLACE; EVEN THE HEAT WITH THE SHADOW OF A CLOUD: THE BRANCH OF THE TERRIBLE ONES SHALL BE BROUGHT LOW. AND IN THIS MOUNTAIN SHALL THE LORD OF HOSTS MAKE UNTO ALL PEOPLE A FEAST OF FAT THINGS, A FEAST OF WINES ON THE LEES, OF FAT THINGS FULL OF MARROW, OF WINES ON THE LEES WELL REFINED."—Isaiah 25:5-6 - (KJV).

I am thoroughly convinced that I have been led to share those words. My every moment is now more golden and cherished. I feel akin to the galloping horse, bit in mouth, the wind in my mane! Part of me knows it's the writer's disease, this love of writing I suffer from. It makes one seem totally driven and committed. It is an energizing labor.

Yet another part of me senses the urgency that I more acutely sense as more than ever I realize that time is 'running out' for me, okay, for each one of us. This is not to assume the worst. It is not a declaration of giving up; rather it is the gateway to those old words above, about that sweet wine. I continue to fight and am a soul winner/warrior. The combination of these emotions, commitments, and the 'driven' part I am not sure are good for one's longevity. But most of it is good. Sometimes it feels as if I'm on a kind of collision course, because of the 'driven' sense of it all. Sometimes it is simply said: too urgent. Yet in the end, it leads to the gate, that grand gate and the bringing down of the bombardment of life's noise.

I revel therefore, in each moment, as I've shared with you before. I eat of life. I love life. I love God's grand nature displayed in so many ways, and above all I love His committed people. It's just: sometimes we do some pretty stupid stuff, don't we? That's where forgiveness must come in. And we are forgiven, and He's alive! Even YOU are forgiven. Ask God.

—Renewal—

This love and action and sense of urgency combine to cause one to feel in need of an overall physical more often than might be necessary. It is important to maintain ourselves spiritually, physically, and emotionally. Senior citizen words concerning what is first lost would be easy here: parts of me have already flown the coop. Nevertheless we march on, knowing that life is rather short and that it is also very fragile. It is indeed a priceless gift, a fleeting gift. Do not take her for granted.

No matter how much we love life, laugh at life, or fear the inevitable, once again, we are fragile creatures. How much we affect ourselves physiologically, psychologically and overall by our attitudes, well, it's all bound to be studied somewhere by someone or by groups of someone's, even as I write these words. I'm certain it has and will be again and again. Thank God for a brain, for thinkers and shakers, for those who renew and revive us. I especially thank Him for constant revitalization and renewal. Not long ago I read a draft of a page of one of my segments to one of my daughters over the telephone. I recall hearing her become more and more quiet, and then I sensed that she had begun to cry. Crying some four hundred miles away. That would go for Momma, too, only differently, as I've heard her say, "I need positive things now," or in other words, her sweet way of saying she, too, is tired, and in need of not being beaten upon (by life) any longer. Such is life, as even loving families and recollections, both good and not so good, surround us, affect us.

—A Challenge—

Through tired eyes I see a good deal of history on my picture mirror: memories of ones I've loved and hopefully influenced in some good way. It's a family memorial/portrait, and it contains a few of my (our) beloved friends as well. So blessed have we been with friends. What you see upon the jacket cover of this book is itself a story. No one will fathom what it has meant to me during my deteriorating phase, with the exception perhaps of Him. No, Lucy would get it, too, when she can bring herself to look at it. Where He leads me, I will follow.

(Miss Lucy is growing old with me, and I am so thankful for that.) You, too, 'Doll Face', have made my life incredibly wonderful. I would do it all again, and it would seem fresh and new and wonderful all over again.

Even if you, my friend, are fortunate enough to be one who rests throughout your entire night, perhaps you can understand part of this if I share that it is now five minutes before two in the a.m.! That causes one to become tired real fast, when you begin your day so early. To me, however, it has been a mission, an energizing challenge. The steady rain outside my window, the flowing music inside, it's the perfect writing environment even for one so very weary.

Part of this comfort is because I long ago invited Him into my space – not that God ever needs an invitation. But I do feel His blessed, loving Presence with me. There are prayer warriors such as my devoted neighbors: Bill and Debbie; and I must mention Reverend Mike and Linda. (Between you and me, I call him Uncle Mike.) There are so many folks praying for this work, and this patient. Actually, I have asked the entire church family to pray for this work! What a privilege being surrounded by prayer warriors. There are other prayer people close to me as well, and there are many prayer warriors farther away, so I thank Momma and siblings, and so many old acquaintances as well. I am thankful for each and every prayer, each and every warrior. *Thanks so much. I love you all.*

I believe from the top of my normally aching noggin to the bottom of my formerly heel-spurred feet, God is in and through everything. Anyone who has not felt His awesome brilliant Presence, who has not found a loving church family, is quite possibly missing out on the very best part of life, for without Jesus, we cannot 'make it' to God, and we cannot worship in spirit and in truth.

One of the paths that He has set millions upon millions of people on is the study of His marvelous Guidebook. Herein my friend, you learn of the most magnificent way to live an abundant life, for you learn of Him. It is where you meet Jesus; and it is Jesus that leads us to the Father. "COME AND SEE THE WORKS OF GOD; HE IS AWESOME IN HIS DOING TOWARD THE SONS OF MEN."—Psalm 66:5

—A Real Fear—

In my tiredness I fear for our God-founded society. I fear too many have traded the things of this world for things so far removed from His expectations. We have only prospered these many years because God has allowed us by grace, to prosper. I believe He may have favored us somewhat because we were willing and able to call upon Him, to praise Him, to live and give our all for Him.

Yet it seems now, so many are more concerned about a different kind of prospering. Indeed, I am in fear for our beloved Republic. I fear that we are being swallowed up; that we are too much within ourselves today. As are agnostics: noncommittal. How can anyone alive see all God's beauty surrounding them and be noncommittal? His created wonders alone ignite passion!

As perverse as life has become due in part to this eroding distrust, the eroding of our values and traditions, our very hope and faith, as well as our being washed away as we seek the taste of a life similar to the cave dwellers near the Dead Sea, we are at the same time being tempted to be so much less than that we were created to be. There seems little health in us.

On Another Front. Mike and Linda, I sense your prayers. No, I wholly feel them! And by the way: I no longer assume the worst. I have several friends whose mother or father has

Alzheimer's. Right now I am thinking of Carolyn, and I am so thankful for her prayers as well, as I know her mother is suffering from the pangs of dementia. Debbie and Bill and Momma, and Mary and Gale, and Dave and Glenn and my children and grandchildren, I so love your tender prayers for Lucy and me. There are so many others: Jessie and Levi and John and Lori, Jim and Amy, Chuck and Debbie, my Anjuli, and of course my sweet Lucy. And there are the wives of brothers and sister's husbands, and I can never forget the brother and sisterhood of my wonderful New Hope Fellowship. You're all tender care partners. I love you so very much.

I would not doubt that Mary Ann Johnson and Nancy and Sherry and Alyssa and Bridget and so many others involved in guiding and running our great Alzheimer's association (in Richmond) are in prayer as well. So many wonderful people who have been so very gracious to Lucy and me. It all reminds me of words from our precious Guidebook: *"See how they love one another."*

I am sure as well, there will be names I have missed or cannot recall, but each one is special. Then there are my writing buddies, Ken and Steve and Pete, folks who have sent music and letters and words of encouragement, sometimes a book or two. Thanks, so very much.

†

The second time I awoke from a combat 'mare, 0345 (military time), I should have been weary and wrung out, but you know what else God does? He revives us! It causes me to turn my mind's eye once again to Doctor Doris and others similar. Even as beat-down-tired as she sometimes gets, having given her all to her patients, she knows in her heart that His living waters will refresh her; His tender 'follow me' words will sustain D. Annette and others for yet another day's battle. Whether it is the battle at the doctor's office, or your personal battle, even mine.

People who live with Christ beside them cause me to recall a melody, and I am ever aware of its sweet lyrics: *Because He lives, I can face tomorrow*! Now I know sufficient is the day unto itself, yet how invigorating it is with Him, to march into the possibility of tomorrow! It's not a question. It is indeed a declaration.

—The Invitation—

I often see faces of visitors caring for lost souls. I see faces of other prayer warriors and soul warriors. I am blessed that many of those faces have been very close to me. I ask the God of everything in the universe to enable me not to ever be without the vision of those sweet faces – even in my almost constant state of exhaustion. They are faces of those who know God, faces of those yet to come into being. If you are one of those, yet to come to Him, do not be afraid of these words unless you're simply dismissing Him altogether. All are invited. Yes! That includes you!

God's invitation is a loving invitation. A standing invitation. No need to ring up ahead of time. It is a humble prayer and a touch from eternity. God longs for you to come and visit Him, even if you enter His chambers for only a few moments. Do not be afraid. Perhaps that's what He meant by the words, "FEAR OF THE LORD IS THE BEGINNING OF WISDOM." I tell you this: Do not fear God, even as awesome and powerful and as all knowing as He is; for He will invite you into His loving Presence, for none compare with Him. Just ask God if you can come in. Just ask. This, my friend, is get-serious time! He will not let you down.

There is a place in our Guidebook that speaks of fear of our Lord, and I know that's in Isaiah, and that it says the fear of the Lord is the beginning of wisdom, but that, friend, is a different kind of fear, and a different passage. Do not fear the One Who has so powerfully and mightily created you to be the best you can be, One Who simply wants to hear from you again and again. He so looks forward to your seriously genuine inner longings and praises.

He will allow you to sit with Him, quietly if you wish. He will simply allow you to come into His magnificent, holy, selfless, infinite and loving Presence. Here, His mighty wings will enfold you, and you will feel a warmth and comfort and completeness otherwise not felt before, otherwise unobtainable. His love Spirit is akin to none other. He alone is worthy. He is your Teacher, your Master, your Redeemer, your Savior, indeed God is your all! He is King of Kings and Lord of Lords!

So bend your knee now, or bend it later. It's your decision. But I tell you for certain, as our Guidebook says: "EVERY KNEE SHALL BOW..." Were I you, if you have not already, I would hasten to follow Him now, to seek God out, for no one, literally no one knows when Christ is to come again. Do you not want to be ready, filled with Him, even as He shall surely look deeply into your confused and tired eyes? You may be whole or with illness, but the time to come to God is now! Put it off no longer! Whether you are reading these words or having them read to you: put it off no longer!

Behold His grace, His unending love, and His forgiveness beyond compare. Praise God and love Him and keep Him ever near. He will cause you to pray for places and people and situations that you've never thought about praying for, or would ever pray for. Believe me, He will enable you to go wherever He needs you to go. And you will be powerless to think twice about it. You may have kept God at arm's length for most of your life, friend, but as one of my brothers wrote not that long ago: *He cannot be kept in a neat, tidy little package.* If you go to Him, life will no longer be neat and tidy. Yes, it can be scary; but the changes for you and your life will be so drastically elating that they will invade every part of your being. You will never, ever be the same again! Just ask.

Heavenly Creator, Friend to all who come, some will encounter bumpy roads, difficult trails and rain-filled skies even after accepting Your loving invitation, even after they have promised themselves wholly to You. Lord, might You allow them to have that patience that You are; might we be readily able to learn Your ways, to learn that You will be with us even unto the end of the world. (See the last part of Matthew). And new friends, Lord, let them know that they are part of this huge, warm, loving family, that although they may have never sat in a church pew, or one of the many places that they could have contemplated You, it will be acceptable because You are a powerful, loving and forgiving God. You are the essence of love; the Great I Am. Lord, there are a number of us who have lost friends and family, jobs, all kinds of things have taken place to us and around us, especially with relationships. Yet Father, You know so very many hunger for you. So very many are just tired of being tired. And you, Father, are the very One who revives us. You have saved us! If nations are a drop in the bucket (Isaiah 40:15), how small we must be, and yet You continue to seek us out. What more can we say than 'Thank You', thank You for being such a wonderful Encourager, the only One to ever arise from the grave!

Chapter 8

—Roller-Coaster Ride—

Before I once again attempt the beginning of this portion about this 'ride' and about an adventure, I wanted to say perhaps you may be wondering why, at this juncture, at the halfway point of the work, yours truly is speaking of other things besides Alzheimer's (or at least has been, and will continue to speak of other things as well as Alzheimer's). It is because I am speaking of things happening in and around the patient, as is the case with each person (diseased or not). It is also here, because the work is not solely about Alzheimer's, and as you will learn in a later chapter, chapter 13, I unveil that which makes one more familiar with my paradigm, my model. And I do not explain the word paradigm as if I am talking down to anyone, I simply want the work to be understood by a vast audience.

Therefore, in chapter 13 you will note that my regimen is contained upon/within the spokes of my wheel vision, the wheel, which surrounds the center of this AD-enshrouded life, that life which is centered on God. And the spokes of course are a necessary part of the wheel. They are (the spokes) those essential areas, which I believe will assist Alzheimer's patients in the living of their lives in as optimal a manner as they can. I take time to explain this which may appear as minutia now, as we are again approximately halfway through our journey together, or as others might say, at the middle of the work.

—An Adventure—

Reading about AD is sometimes akin to using fog lights when you can't see your hand in front of your face, not always that good. But this adventure will cause you to reach for whatever straw you can find, whether it's short or long. You continue to hope that something will provide the answer you seek, some kind of cure. If I had the money, I'd fly off to Switzerland or some other location that has a cutting edge breakthrough years ahead of anything we can imagine. There I would find an experimental drug or a procedure unknown to us.

I'd even be willing to use a medicine not yet approved. When you're in trouble, dangerous studies or attempting to grasp a cure not quite thought through don't seem to cause lots of heartburn. We reach for the straw. It is very similar to the person who has never before considered God, yet easily reaches out to Him in their time of desperation and need; when they have bottomed-out so to speak.

Now, somewhat older, a little wiser, further into the *real thing,* I'm comforted in knowing not only that am I going somewhere, but it's also possible that I'll learn valuable data along the way. The adventure I'm talking of is exhilarating and yet confounding at the same time. Often I've asked, *Why Lord, why have I been chosen to do this work, to walk this particular pathway?*

Were I one to share with you that God talked to me just now, I'd reply after you'd looked curiously at me, that He countered with a question to my question, and then I'd continue His dialogue: *Why not you?* Scary? No, not at all. When I think of what He endured for you and me: how God The Infant, appeared to mankind to die for us, it's too much a puzzle for me, too much to take in at once. And the more I think of *going somewhere,* the more I realize who isn't? We all run out of grains of sand. Yet we must always remember God's gracious and awesome sacrifice, and that His blood has washed away all our sins, and we are His!

I may have shared with you before. Dementia-affected folks are informed (sometimes) that puzzle working and other brain-working games are well worthwhile. Believe me! No. *Believe God!* Learning new things: studying something that you may never have studied before, all these can be helpful for the brain.

—Life Happens—

I wish I could explain (to you) what I am going through in order to re-write and re-ponder things that I had said and studied before, as well as what I am enduring at this keyboard, and what an extraordinary hardship it has been for me this time through. It has indeed been an adventure.

Why is this an adventure? Simply put, I believe it is because we more vividly realize not only that are we slated to be in transit, but also that we always were: always have been. So, is it not an adventure for one and all? Yes, life is. (But this one, as you sense the cogs and gears, whatever you wish to utilize to describe the apparatus, the 'stuff' that is slowly being changed within you, is a very frightening dilemma. I need to go ahead and say it. Sometimes I live in fear.)

It is strange how life is what happens as we strive to plan our way. It seems that even those of us who talk about other controlling people, even we admire being able to control, do we not? Perhaps the adventure is one of God's ways of saying you cannot control Me, no matter how diligently you work at it. Maybe you can control your wife, your kids, your boss, but not Me.

Twelve hours after writing those words, I again witnessed that life is what happens as we plan a book, too, or as we're in the midst of planning one.

Our little dog (a Yorkie), had been acting rather strangely for a couple days. Unfortunately for me, Doll Face was out of town (as is usually the case when one of the animals gets sick). She'd been away watching grandchildren, while I'd kept the home fires stoked. Around 1300 (one in the afternoon, civilian time), Cleopatra started to whimper and whine. It had been an unusual time for that. Although I'd taken her outside, being gentle as I did, when I sat her down in the grass, I noticed that she could not walk, in fact, it appeared that she could not even bring herself upright again. It was as if she were hyperventilating as well. Something was definitely amiss. Off we flew to the veterinarian's (fortunately I still had an operator's license back then).

We soon learned that all the body fluid in her little stomach was a sign that her heart was no longer working properly. Me? The one with chronic post-traumatic stress, panic attacks and dementia, I'm told I'll have to wait for the doctor. He's currently performing surgery on another pet. It was one of the longest hours I've ever spent. My mind revisited one of my worst combat 'mares, only this was a first for me, during the daytime.

I'll bet I was a sight as I remember being curled up on one of the animal hospital's long benches, knees pulled up to my chest, one hand upon our dear Cleo. The daytime nightmare was highly unusual, but finally it was over and Cleo, as we affectionately called her, was finished, too, both of us at peace. Relatively. Her for sure.

Later on I was surprised to learn that dogs sometimes become stressed when their closest friend is away from them. They are much like people, are they not? I had earlier wondered why she had been whining so, scooting ever nearer the back door: her idea of where Mommy comes from. It had all caused me to contemplate whether I whine too much myself, whether I sometimes wallow in my weaknesses. I do. I admit it.

—An Adventure-Continued—

We used to say it in the Navy: *It's not just a job, it's an adventure*. Not only for the Navy, that's something that can be said of life, and it's true of AD as well. This adventure is similar to others: were I merely to sit in a pew each week longing for pastor's sweet words to enable me to feel better, instead of realizing that I am to be a soul warrior (even though I am first a sinner), well, you can decipher the difference. It is similar to this disease. One can sit idly by and wait and not plan any habilitative measures, just try to survive, or the patient and care partner can work at exercising, reading, word games, and never assuming the worst. Remember that: things can always be worse. Perhaps it's why the **Never Give Up!** words continue to ring in my ears.

Thankfully, they are deep within me; then again, it may make departing this realm more difficult. Who knows? (You know that answer.) For me, it's as familiar as *Yes, Jesus Loves Me*, or *Happy Birthday*, or even that twinkle-twinkle song that I share with other diseased folks. Part of me keeps wondering what makes the songs stick to us, like plaque to our vessels: that plaque that interrupts our bodily processes. It's akin to the adventure topic somewhat. I believe that being in the Armed Forces today is yet an adventure. Who could call it anything less during wartime, when you're young and sense that you are yet brave? *Some call it HELL!* They have my vote.

Do you relish adventure? I do. I've also sensed a possible problem because of adventure within my personality. It is being too quickly drawn to not previously known females, especially if they are cute little packages as one was this very morning, at the same place I met my pastor-friend, Reverend Mike. It is a listening and watching so intently that I could easily be drawn as the moth to the candle's fire; not always a good thing. But thank You, Lord, I'm learning that whenever I begin to sense this being drawn in, I attempt to focus on making that person a friend instead of a find. What a deal breaker it has become for the guy with the horns and pitchfork. Every now and again this chink in my normally shining armor is revealed. Strange how (this situation) shows up at the same time as my pastor. I love you, Brother Mike.

†

So, instead of popping the pretty lady's phone number into my cell's computer, I very cautiously, intently, strive to understand not only how futile it would be to once again make an idiot of myself, I also work toward making the focus more of a joke. Yet this, too, can be of some danger. It's a challenge, an adventure, Right? What I'm attempting to share and risk tarnishing my perfect-appearing image while so doing, is we either transform the quagmires of our lives or we become drawn too close to the flame. We get near danger so perverse that it can get us into serious trouble. Perhaps destruction. At the very least, it will draw a not-so-friendly glance from your spouse if she happens to be along with you.

Not long after these words were put to paper, I discovered the increased sexual thoughts and awareness that I'd addressed in chapter three. I also learned that AD patients are sometimes quite verbal about sexuality, lucky me! And all of this was only once again verified when I went with my family on a 'fun cruise' to Freeport and then on to Nassau.

I had the time of my life, but I had not come away totally happy, for my spouse, my Lucy, had suffered a huge amount of anguish. I had only done what my neurologist had suggested, and I had loved being so young-at-heart again! **Big caution here: It's not seen quite the same way by your caregiver. (If you get to go on a cruise, be very discreet!) Take her with you, as I did, and hopefully you can communicate with her.**

And now, in the silence of my room, and during this time of this rewrite, I must confess: This is honesty time. Although it seemed that I was not quite as capable of controlling myself onboard the 'fun cruise', I **did** realize exactly what I was doing at the same time.

†

Can you, patient, or caregiver, think of a way to turn the chinks of your armor into highly polished areas of your life, areas that will enable you to buffet incoming adversity? Can you during this adventure called life enlist the aid of One who can assist in protecting you from further harm? I have every confidence you can! (I am not too proud of wearing out my eyeballs, yet I did enjoy dancing the night away.)

—From Crazy Fun To Mourning—

As a soul warrior, I am usually deeply committed to honing-in on the chinks in my armor, to finding ways to smooth them out and get them polished so they will later work toward my advantage, God's advantage. I care not just to be soothed and made to feel warm and fuzzy in His temple. Would you not rather be challenged where you worship? An adventure? No, it is much more.

It is knowledge about the disease, or when you're serving/reporting the disease and its affects upon us: even if it is just crazy fun. But this is much more than an eye opener, my friend. Refer to Ephesians, chapter five. (Yes, the entire chapter.)

Breaks are often allowed during my writing process. I had turned to a scene on the tube this morning, this day smack up against a rather emotion-packed day that I'd earlier endured. Although to me it was all part of the same day, that aside, I must share that as I spotted the televised man walking his little dog, I broke down and cried. I briefly mourned the passing of our beloved Cleopatra. My mind flashed back to the wrapping of her lifeless little body, the later breaking of fresh soil.

Yet in this brokenness, during this time of sadness, I thought, good Lord, I haven't told Lucy what's happened! In my current condition, I often forget things I've done almost immediately, that is, I cannot recall having done them, or whether I did not do them. This time I hadn't forgotten, not altogether. This day, too, would prove to be a tough one. Then, recalling Lucy, the woman with the toughest job, I wondered how she would react. It was at that moment that these words came:

Father, I dedicate another day to You. As I praise You, I ask You to assist me in becoming gentle, more caring, assist me in becoming the perfect deliverer of some burdensome news: The passing of a very close friend.

After all, Cleo had been our baby. After I'd paused and thought about what I'd just prayed, I felt rather foolish, for I realized that God knows all, even before it takes place, and it is all rather a replay for Him.

Well, we had at least talked about Cleo's passing possibility, (Lucy and I had). Later still, I wondered about our Cleo and my Lucy. I wondered how it would go upon Lucy's arrival home. I knew she'd be looking for various signs: I knew there'd be no high-pitched tiny bark, no little tail wag to greet her, no little dance. Next, Lucy would immediately note the absence of the little mat, that tiny bowl, all those little observances that no others would immediately seek.

Fortunately, Donna had earlier talked to a veterinarian who had shared, *"Perhaps it's time* to put her down." Fortunately she'd had time to process the possibility that I was now anxiously internalizing. I knew this would be another of life's adventures. I pictured holding Lucy tightly, attempting to console her in her initial moment of sorrow. This after her long and very tiresome days with the noisy, jumping-beaned grandchildren. (Actually Jessie and Levi's kids are the highly unusual 4 children that folks gravitate towards when we are in a restaurant, where people often say they have never seen such well-behaved children. And that is sincere truth.)

On that final call, the evening of the last day before her return home, I asked God to assist me in keeping her mind occupied. Thankfully, with what's left of my noggin and through His grace, all went well. The call, that is. What an adventure life! And later still, as I'd earlier envisioned, I did wrap Donna in my arms, my Lucy. Perhaps our time together, mourning the loss of a close friend would make the earlier memories a little easier.

Okay, now that I've mentioned Jacob and Rebecca and David and Abigail, kids' names above, I feel compelled to add this. And it is a free one, especially for anyone yet well enough in mind and heart to understand and utilize it. I have noted that not only does Jessica have the uncanny ability to get eye to eye with her children, when they have a particular situational problem (I'm going to call it), but also I must advise you that she has always done it in a loving and tender manner, without shouting, and ensuring that the children have gotten the message. It is simply a matter of clear and direct, yet calm communication, yes, so unlike our folks who some people call our leadership (?) in Washington, D.C. I have also noted how Daddy Levi takes the children by the hand often, whenever he is painting or working, and what wondrous things he teaches them in a loving way. Lastly, these children are allowed to view television one time each week, on Friday night, often to watch an old favorite movie or and animal show or the likes of.

An adventure? Yes. It is all of a piece (an old editor had once shared with me), all an adventure. Might all your adventures have peaceful endings, or at least endings you might endure without too much discomfort; or, if there is discomfort, might it be with God's grace.

†

Eternal God, Your Holy territory extends beyond the infinite. You were, You are, You always will be. It is my prayer, Soul Receiver, as each of us lives our adventures, that You might be pleased with their outcomes – pleased when we search for You, praise You. Help us, God, to realize that there is an unseen realm awaiting us that will never fade, that this, too, belongs to a new adventure. (Read I Peter 1:3-7. It addresses various trials.) Could it be our animal friends share in man's homecoming? I pondered that as I read these words:
"REMEMBER NOW YOUR CREATOR IN THE DAYS OF YOUR YOUTH, BEFORE THE DIFFICULT DAYS COME, AND THE YEARS DRAW NEAR WHEN YOU SAY, 'I HAVE NO PLEASURE IN THEM': WHILE THE SUN AND THE LIGHT, THE MOON AND THE STARS ARE NOT DARKENED, AND THE CLOUDS DO NOT RETURN AFTER THE RAIN; IN THE DAY WHEN THE KEEPERS OF THE

HOUSE TREMBLE, AND THE STRONG MEN BOW DOWN; WHEN
THE GRINDERS CEASE BECAUSE THEY ARE FEW, AND THOSE
THAT LOOK THROUGH THE WINDOWS GROW DIM; WHEN
THE DOORS ARE SHUT IN THE STREETS, AND THE SOUND OF
GRINDING IS LOW; WHEN ONE RISES UP AT THE SOUND OF A
BIRD, AND ALL THE DAUGHTERS OF MUSIC ARE BROUGHT
LOW. ALSO THEY ARE AFRAID OF HEIGHT, AND OF TERRORS
IN THE WAY; WHEN THE ALMOND TREE BLOSSOMS, THE
GRASSHOPPER IS A BURDEN AND DESIRE FAILS. FOR MAN
GOES TO HIS ETERNAL HOME..."
—Ecclesiastes 12:1-5 (in part). Sometimes I so long for that
eternal home. Do you not also?

—After A While—

God's healing grace always sends me into a tailspin! It is
important for AD patients to learn/know that after a while you
begin to realize that you can (or some will not be able to)
comfortably live with this disease. It is different for each one,
again there is no model. It may not be pretty, yet sometimes
there is a breakthrough. For me it hit as lightning the morning
of my oldest daughter, Amy's, birthday, one day in February.

Unique happening? No, I guess it is not especially unique,
then again, perhaps it is. It is simply that we are bound together
within and without of our different worlds, times and places.
The bond between us very strong and I am happy to report that
it is the same with all my children, and our extended family as
well. Often you can sense that something is taking place, even
before you hear about it.

You may have recalled that Amy and I had awaited the
arrival, rather the pick up day of another daughter, Anjuli. I
laugh as I think of Angie and her brother, Chuck; all three of
them are characters, but then again who of us is not? All three
have assisted me in this breakthrough, the realization that I can
yet move on, *keep on.* They daily bless me to move ahead with
their love and their confidence. It so enables me to abide in and
be flooded by God's gentle spirit, His awesome love, and their
love. And it is the same with my Lucy and others ever close to
me.

This is not nonchalance. After a while we really surrender
all. After a while there is comfort not only in knowing of your
diagnosis and prognosis, but also in realizing that you can
continue to live even amidst this deteriorating dilemma. To be

quite matter of fact, I'm not all that certain where the line is. That is, I am not totally sure that between the time that we are sensing that we are in the 'here and now' and that time that we can no longer think and/or reason in the here and now is surely so definable. That is, there's a time when we cross over an imaginary line of sorts, or for the lack of better words: There comes a time when we finally begin the lengthier journey, the out-of-our-body-lost-in-earthly-space journey to Who-Knows-Where Land. We are no longer cognizant of the here and now because we are no longer in the here and now. Simply put: I do not know. Yet I know that time approaches, for I have often seen it.

Sweet Carolyn, a good friend, recently lost her mother to the disease, I can only imagine that her nights are rather turbulent and without rest at this point, yet I continue in prayer for her, as I always have. And God continue to bless your dear mother.

I can sense that my love, my Lucy, sometimes fishes for it: attempting to decipher if I have yet boarded the train. It is her, *Can you count backwards by sevens, from a hundred?* Right out of the psychologist's/neurologist's, someone's, textbook.

Well, Lucy, sometime it's easier than others. Sometimes it seems that I do it easily, then there are other times that I just don't care to focus, or perhaps cannot. And yes, Sweetie, I know you're not being mean, as you would say. I will love you to the end and beyond!

Is it the compromising of my **Never Give Up!** attitude for one of submission? No, I do not for a moment believe that. Is it reaching the realization that we are close enough to that line, or is it that the line no longer matters? No again, is my reply. It only matters as long as it matters to you, brothers and sisters of dementia, as we await the grand crossing.

"FEAR NOT, FOR I AM WITH THEE." It is very appropriate for me right now. And these words as well: "THE LORD WILL GUIDE YOU CONTINUALLY, AND SATISFY YOUR SOUL IN DROUGHT, AND STRENGTHEN YOUR BONES; YOU SHALL BE LIKE A WATERED GARDEN, AND LIKE A SPRING OF WATER, WHOSE WATERS DO NOT FAIL." —Isaiah 58:11.

Do we all fear failing? I believe we do. I know I sometimes do/have. Even with God's love and assurance, the comfort of His strong hand at the helm, even with the tender caring and loving friends that surround me, even after we've decided that we can live with this disease, is it not yet a natural part of us to fear it? Though it sounds rhetorical, I am going to answer: Yes!

I may have shared it before: If you've met a combat veteran who claims he was never afraid in battle, be very careful of the next words that exude from that misled lad's mouth. Is it not much the same with the world of dementia? Yes. Some of us sound so tough, when in reality we are as in fear and thankful at the same time, as if we were a wet puppy being let back indoors and are met by a warm dry towel and loving hands and arms. Perhaps an excited face to lick.

Speaking of troops, I cannot get them out of my mind, and heart. Keep them and their families ever in your prayers. I guess we'll always be in wars from now on. Yet after a while....

So, although you are 'living with it' and although you may be afraid of it, you need to know that I continue to pray for you, friend, just as automatically as I breathe, until God allows otherwise. As I breathe daily, I also pray for you and yours daily! Is our best Friend not also in prayer? You bet He is!

Even after a while, He knows your getting up and when you 'give up' for the day, God is aware of it all, at all times. He hears your every breath, your every whisper and whimper. He knows when you shift your weight, which may cause pain simply by the moving around of your body. He is keenly aware of your agitations, your dreams, and God goes with you *always*. Believe it! He is the One who believes when others cannot or do not. He is ever mindful of you! Ever watchful and faithful. Ever wonderful.

—Over Stimulation—

It takes little effort to recall how I felt as I sensed this very real part of AD: over-stimulation. Early on it mostly occurred when in the company of others, or when in new surroundings; now I know I sometimes over-stimulate myself when I am not even aware of it. Even the changing of my routine can cause me to go somewhat haywire.

One of the most recent encounters with being over-stimulated was when my wife and I one evening spent precious time with out loving neighbors, Bill and Debbie. I have that sometimes-helpful ability to be able to speak and listen at the same time. It can also, however, be a hindrance in that it can cause one to become agitated and confused more quickly, more easily.

Sometimes I also speak quickly in order to keep from forgetting what I need to get out. I used to do it out of pure ignorance. Now I sometimes do it because of the disease.

As the four of us, seated closely to one another shared a kitchen island, barstools on either side, as we shared our lives and good food, I had attempted not only to pick up on as much as I could, but also to tell my story at the same time. Listening to praise music in the background, I soon sensed myself shifting in my chair, that feeling of uneasiness coming over me, that brink of **bombardment**. Some refer to it as noise overload or noise bombardment. Part of this bombardment was from music turned up too loudly. It was something I had not noticed immediately, and one of those things we are taught not to mention, especially when we are visitors (although by this time we had become much more than mere visitors).

Fortunately our neighbors are understanding, flexible and compassionate folks. These friends, once sensing my 'dis-ease' (interestingly appropriate), took steps to assist me in becoming less stimulated, and they did so with great dispatch and out of love. How often I have thanked Father for placing us near this bastion of love and strength – these loving Christian friends. Or as once said in a movie, to us it had all been MTB (meant to be). It only reverberates a long-held belief: *There are no accidents, especially with God.*

Although that particular evening was somewhat curtailed, mostly my choice, I sensed immediate relief as Lucy and I wandered through the stirring pines between their home and ours. The urgency of my adrenaline or active misfiring of neurotransmitters or whatever those 'in the know' would call it began to settle. Thankfully.

—Caregiver's Burden—

There have been other similar events. More and more I did not feel ready to enter that arena of over stimulation, especially when I felt that a routine or particular mission would be curtailed or interrupted. I at the same time realized how vital it is for one's caregiver as well, to be able to *get away* to make/take time for herself/himself. The caregiver's task is much more challenging/burdensome than most patients will ever be able to comprehend or appreciate.

Somewhere betwixt and between stages three and four, I felt in touch with my former and future self at the same time. I cannot imagine what the caregiver is enduring, other than the thoughts of what is unyieldingly clear and scary indeed.

But back to that evening and my temporary uneasiness about going next door, something not often felt, thankfully. That is, as friends, the four of us share a *mi casa es su casa* attitude. We would do anything for one another. We are devoted, loving friends. When they feel down, we are right with them; and the opposite is true of course. It doesn't get much better down here.

I think now of the time of this next ensuing sensation. I had failed to consciously take into account that I had unfinished work to do. Naturally it was this text, this labor of love that consumes me, turns me into a machine of sorts, a galloper if you will, in search of that illusive ending to the tale, I suspect. (It indeed seems a more difficult and illusive task the more I go through it. Sorry. I guess advice from long ago always sticks with me when writing. Be dissatisfied.)

This particular evening, how gracious Lucy and our neighbors were as they rallied around a roaring fire, not pressing me to join them. How relieved I'd felt, as I had not been pressured and was able to have some quiet, precious time, time to think and not feel as though I had to immediately appear. What a continued blessing, a considerate, loving, caring relationship: Sometimes sensing that we are not being prompted to socialize can be beneficial. After all, there is less and less that an AD patient is in control of, so it seems any control at all is of utmost importance.

I continued for a time to work at whatever topic I'd had in mind for the evening, and as my uneasiness eased up, I began feeling forward momentum on this work that was/is always calling me. Not much later, I felt drawn to comradeship as well. Having not been pressed, not pursued, I felt much more willing to transport myself into that caring, sharing realm. Soon I trudged next door to be with my Lucy and friends.

The sensation derived from over stimulation is somewhat easy to explain, as it is very similar to the strong sensation that I used to get from hypertension, before I was medicated for it. It is another enemy that threatens these old bones. Before I was properly medicated for high blood pressure, something brought about by living in a combat-minded attitude for many years, I often felt much like a grenade, ready to blow into tiny little pieces. What an uneasy sensation. Then there is Restless Leg Syndrome. This one can seem even worse at times, at least until it's treated. That governmental arm I never mention by name, I believe, they would not wish to hear about RLS either: it might mean that they have to relinquish another five bucks! It seems that it is much easier saving that money for the ones currently being shot at. (Thanks Generals! You guys knuckled under, again.) I take nothing from the active duty folks fighting, but you guys should know better than to forget those, many of whom fought for you and alongside of you.

—Then There's Panic—

This one took a little longer for me to understand. Normally I take medication, what lay people call a 'panic pill' before I attempt a nap or before bedtime, (Yes, I'm aware that's not what they were intended for….), and almost daily now, I take one or two when I feel distressed. And there may be one needed depending upon my mind's eye and/or combat remembrances/'mares. Often I take one as I prepare to be in a crowd, or before I must enter unfamiliar environments. The pills have been a boon to me, habit-forming or not.

Sometimes, however, I sensed that I might have been weak enough and faithless and hopeless enough to do something really unfair to loved ones and family, that is to disappear early, on purpose. Should you, reader friend, ever feel similar to the above written words, I plead with you to enter into serious prayer, and/or to quickly seek immediate help. Maybe an emergency room, or someone you can talk to who will listen to you (I am also sensing that I may have addressed this before, rather briefly.). ***Do not pick a waiting room in New York,***

*however, how sad was that atrocity; people walking beyond
and away from a dying woman? Disgraceful!*

What has worked for me? Imagine what damage you can
cause loved ones, what a terribly dismal, nasty outgoing that
could be. Please heed these words of caution not only for
yourself, but also for the sake of the loved souls around you.

There are also other over stimulations, I call them, caused
by not following your doctor's advice; or not taking medicines
as they are prescribed, directed, or failing to take them at all.
There are unnecessary addictions that very well may cloud an
already less-than-perfect visibility. When we seek 'an out' on
occasion, we often learn that it is only a temporary out, and
we'll simply suffer a re-entry into this same cycle later on. Ask
any drunk.

—Simple, Yet Sound Advice—

Over the years I've learned it is best to attempt to get proper
sleep and exercise and to eat a well-balanced diet, to be
moderate in most everything. Years ago I ministered to a man
ninety-plus years of age, I may have shared this with you
before. One of his favorite repetitions when I visited was:
*"When I'm hungry, I eat; when I'm tired, I lay down. I don't
figure that's too far from wrong."* His wise words have led me
to a few good habits. (I've often said you receive much more
from ministering to people than you can ever give them.
Besides, we're not the Giver, are we?)

'De-cluttering' mentioned elsewhere herein, has worked
wonders for me, and now I find myself picking up more and
more around my area. It is a blessing my wife rather enjoys. It is
a change worthy of some celebration, at least at this point in
time. (Beware though, not all of us can pick up after ourselves,
that's the bad news.)

As for celebration, I believe it is very good to pamper
yourself now and again, time for introspection, or simply time
to take a break. If it's at all possible, no matter whether you feel
that you can do this, writing can be both a mental and a spiritual
blessing. How often I have felt God's gracious, amazing sweet
Presence when writing in the middle of my nights. I have noted
also, when I cannot be out underneath His magnificent blazing

canopy, I sometimes imagine myself there, in His open vastness, His overabundance, His awesome creation. (He has named each star, you know.) Sometimes these moments are solemn; they are also often so euphoric, the entire remainder of my day is as if He's yet by my side. And He is!

It is a grand feeling. Of course God always is beside us, we just don't always sense it, can't get it. It's too much for us. I wonder if it's because we feel unworthy, or have clouded our minds with something else of lesser importance. And of course we are not worthy; only One is worthy, and yes, we cloud our minds even when they are healthy.

—Do Not Fear Closeness—

If out of all the lines within this work I would want you to remember one, this would be near the top of the list: **Never fear being drawn too closely to Him**. I know many of us seem afraid to encounter God; some of us are afraid to relinquish control. We strive to maintain distance. There are always those who know of His mighty power and grace and illumination, though, thank goodness. Why do you suppose that no one could ever look directly upon Him? Yet might I share a secret? If you have seen Me, says our Jesus, then you have seen God. If you have found the Almighty within the pages of our Guidebook, you have in effect had a God encounter.

Listen to these words of Jesus: "...I AM THE WAY, THE TRUTH, AND THE LIFE: NO MAN COMETH UNTO THE FATHER, BUT BY ME. IF YE HAD KNOWN ME, YE SHOULD HAVE KNOWN MY FATHER ALSO; AND FROM HENCEFORTH YE KNOW HIM, AND HAVE SEEN HIM..." —John 14: 6 & 7.

†

Gracious God, thankfully we are able to call upon You, even in our over stimulated times. We can count on You and know You will be with us always. And, Father, thanks for dentists, for in another recent combat 'mare, I've busted a tooth to pieces. It seems You allow these different circumstances to enable us to carry on against all odds. Teacher and Friend, cause us to learn to lean on You alone, even as we seek You out, perhaps for the very first time. We know You are all, and in all, and

*through all. Thank You, Jesus. Hallelujah! All praise to the
Mighty One, for no one is above Him! Not one.*

Do you think perhaps that some of the money I have finally
been awarded from Uncle might come in handy when buying a
new gold crown to hold a tooth together? Only at a cost of two
thousand dollars today.

—Disease Can Draw You Together—

The devastation of this disease is drastic and preys upon
cultures and backgrounds and folks both rich and poor, young
and old. It means trauma for millions, and more are on the way.
It has no aversion to singling out any particular section of a
society, or any particular person. Sometimes though, there have
been suggestions: One is that those well read and/or more
steeply inclined to higher education are more likely to be spared
this suffrage. I would refute that any time, especially when I am
aware that persons the likes of Shakespeare, Emerson and even
Erasmus (the scholar) were not skipped over by dementia. Even
as I reflect upon those of my now close-up group, it is easy to
find chemists, journalists, bookkeepers and even doctors among
them – no one is overlooked. None are immune to this
deteriorating disease.

My beloved Lucy and I have strolled, walked rapidly, and
even skipped childlike down a few paths in our life together.
She has been able, more than any woman I have heretofore
known, to touch the very deepest recesses of my soul. She has
raised me to the very top of the highest mountain, and comforts
me when I plunge to the deepest depths known to this same
soul.

Naturally part of me, and the way I have evolved and am yet
changing, plays a part in the aforementioned. Lucy can be as
soothing as a violin or sometimes as the rest of us, harsh and
cold as a rocky strait being crashed upon by even colder
seawater. *That is cold!*

Yet though our ways have been sweet and smooth or
furiously harsh, I have learned throughout it all, disease can
draw people together. I am unsure whether my finger is on the
pulse of it, but there is something in it, about it, when two souls
who often hunger for one another become exposed to this roller-

coaster-like ride that turns them at times into devil-take-care units, separate units; units that can deflect, and that is understandable; units that can stand afar off from one another. I have learned that it is important to stand together as far as is humanly possible. Make it your goal to be together, undivided by outside forces as much as possible. It will do wonders for your relationship, especially now.

We even sustain a rather distant air at times. We may indeed become units that choose to completely ignore one another for a time. I believe it may be caused by the intensity of the disease, as it can push and pull upon every emotion within us (you).

Often it causes even the stoic, compassionate, committed and rational partner to seek out (to learn again) the nuances of the dating game (at least in the mind if nothing else). (See chapter on sexuality.) Then there are other times when God calls *me* back, reminding me of His grand intentions for my life, for Lucy and me. So, I gradually settle back down, and sometimes in prayer I scream at Him. Yes, you can do that. I don't know that I'd recommend a lot of it, but you can do it. You can kick and scream because God understands; He's been here, and He still is!

I recall one particularly restless night, (not long ago as of this last rewrite) after the signing of our wills and my turning over power of attorney. Serious stuff, scary stuff. Not only was I uptight about 'stuff' that I swore would never shake me, I was upset as well because I had once again pushed the wrong buttons on my computer, and at the 220-plus page mark had managed to 'screw up' the works.

All of a sudden I found dots in between words, headings with new boldness that I would swear I had not placed there, and when I approached Lucy with it, she did what she could do.

At least she ensured that it was all 'saved', but she could not get it back to what it was, so once again I was left with: *I don't know what you did*, and was again on my own (to begin anew).

It is not a real great feeling for one with Alzheimer's, attempting yet again to get his work out to another house for consideration. So I ended up taking a midnight, okay, way past midnight, stroll. It is not something I highly recommend. But as I felt very stressed, I put on my shoes and socks and a long bright ribbon that reads Alzheimer's association. It practically glows in the dark. And, as I probably have mentioned before, I have my tracking bracelet that you would mostly see worn by perverts, that is if they were made to wear them where you can see them, most of them have them placed on their ankles. (I believe they should be bright red and placed in other parts of their bodies.) Sorry, Lord.

I found the walk to be good for me. I got a chance to talk with God again, to look now and again toward Heaven and that be-speckled canopy filled with a myriad of bright shards so beautifully shining as if each one were a diamond in God's sky. And when I returned home, quietly entering, I did feel somewhat calmer, more relaxed, prepared to 'slog on' with my labor of love.

The *Why me,* that I've often written about concerning the caregiver also applies to the patient. Ignore it not, for if you do, she will persist and become an even greater burden to you. She will threaten to overpower you, just as PTSD can and will. But you know the fighter in me, reader friend. May there exist a fighter in YOU as well! And may you have that God-connection which is so vitally important during the rocky times. Oh, recall this, too, we need God even when times seem smooth and calm. Be with Him always. This is a bond that must be kept strong and secure.

This dilemma, this threatening, these changes are akin to the disturbing feelings I sometimes conjure up when I contemplate our nation's (leaders'--?) current ploys: the gamesmanship and politics of our time, the general malaise. Often it seems that our blessed Republic is being tossed to and fro as if it were some bit of flotsam and jetsam upon an unruly international ocean. My very soul seeks the words from *Sweet Hour of Prayer*, or some other lovely hymn with lyrics and sway equally soothing. That today is sometimes difficult to find. (Often, it is found, thanks to close friends who have supplied me with ample Godly-filled Heavenly music. Thank you all, so much.) Especially Chuck, Debbie, Steve and Pete, my Angie.

And I must never forget my Emmy-winning friend, Roberta, whose magnificent, <u>No Way Back</u> DVD is part and parcel of this work. At least I have mentioned it.

—A Matter of Communicating—

It seems that we are so concerned about being first in line, quick and bold, loud and impressive, instead of listening and attentive. The quiet and soothing songs assist me in centering-in on what I know to be more akin to God's tenderness, for is it not also written: BE STILL AND KNOW THAT I AM GOD? –Psalm 46:10

We are to celebrate life, but my, does it have to be so fiercely and noisily done? I suspect that the distaste for this upheaval originates within me because of my disease. I am the one who has to take his earplugs with him to go to any dance floor or other noise-bombarded location. Sometimes more often than not; again and again I attempt to do without, but I'm normally driven back to the bombardment stage that is very distressing.

The quieter, soothing hymns almost lull me to sleep. They so refresh me. That sometimes can be much to Lucy's chagrin though; she might give me the old elbow, especially if we are in church.

Yet back to the *Why me?* It seems that our age and lifetime experiences *do* offer us certain wisdom and solace and a spark that ignites an idea so profound that we are forced to run headlong with it, regardless of its results. Oftentimes it is simply a matter of communicating. And I yet believe this might be the case with communicating. 90% of what we worry about never happens. Yet sadly, I must report that that is not yet the case with this disease. Not yet at least.

†

Father God, thank you for coming to join me once again.
(And as you'll hear more than once, God is always with us, but it's okay to ask Him to come into your presence, but please hear me when I say: God's always in your presence.)

So if for some reason you are feeling as if you need to call upon Him, or as if He's far away, you might want to check and see who's moved! (I always liked that line, Rusty.)

In the wee hours, where much of my life is spent, I unfortunately began again to ponder some of the afflictions I've endured. The ruthlessness of PTSD continuing to show the momentous rise of the dragon's everlasting head once again, as it is with thousands of other new and older warriors; the loss of a nephew in a special operation in East Africa; another nephew now in a war zone; the recent diagnosis and prognosis of this new challenge; the aches and pains and general malaise that accompany it all; skin cancers; Restless Leg Syndrome as well as terrible leg cramps if I forget my meds; that eerie hairnet feeling that often pervades my skull (although the patch that has recently come out seems to be dampening that some); the unfortunate evil one's taunting me to contemplate suicide, well, it all serves to make you a little less than the 'glitter and be gay' type of guy you'd like to be. (Don't even go there, Gunnery Sergeant!) And then there's the loss and passing and/or removal of so many wonderful friends, associates and family members – signs of (the inevitable) growing older.

Does it not pull all of us down? No! Okay, not too much. Not with God's help.

Speaking of topics that bring us down, I have worked diligently to keep from naming an arm of our government. An agency that cannot keep up with the amount of applications for assistance coming their way; (Get your hands on a *Veterans of Foreign Wars*, magazine, November, 2007 – it addresses the literally thousands of men (and some women) coping with PTSD. One of the lines in a subheading reads: "The link to the ongoing wars is indisputable.")

Ponder that one for a while, shrink friends. Alright, you may think that highly unfair, but I so tire of small bands of folks who believe they can twist and turn years ago decided upon topics to their current advantage—or to the advantage of a few (who seem to be attempting to once again treat military folks as if they are third-class citizens). My opinion? We need more psychiatrists and psychologists who have bravely and honorably served in uniform.

—Being Ignored, or Forgotten? —

I was sick to my stomach when I heard of the Walter Reed Committee, and of how quickly certain parts of our government attempted to quiet that mess. I couldn't help but wonder what has happened to those who used to keep an eye on the ball? Or why is it that we have so many 'Yes' men, and everyone too busy to follow up or find a way through the impasse on situations that need attention? Why do our *leaders (?)* continue this bickering back and forth as if they, too, are racing to the next traffic signal and pretending not to know what they have done?

I had a whole different work begun. It contains 80-plus documents between a government agency and myself, and yet they still have been unable to complete the issue at hand! This after a full 26 months ago, that is if this work were placed into print and distributed today it would be twenty-six months!

(You can of course scrap all those words: that was quite some time ago.) You can't help but wonder whether you'll be as tens of thousands of other veterans who either gave up, or simply died before they received any help. Are we being ignored, or simply forgotten?

This segment actually began as a letter to another department of the government, or a regional office at least, fortunately it has been revised and 'toned down' so you will not see the copy to addees, or hear all the *nice words* that rolled off this crusty old military man's tongue.

Thankfully, God has led me to revise it, and it will naturally make it far easier for a publisher/editor to place into print. Not only do I feel God's leading as I share these words, I also sense His prompting me to be more open about some of my disgust/distrust. Therefore, some of what has taken place heretofore I now share:

I could not believe it when I yesterday (This was a portion of a letter, before the time of this actual writing you are now reading), when I called a government office (location and name intentionally left out), to learn that another group of applicants had to be 'rushed through this week', so apparently my application was not really yet at the Board level. Is it? Was it? (I had wondered and written at the time.)

You see, I had been advised a fortnight previously that my application had finally been hand-carried to the illustrious Board. I also surmised that I had hounded this office so much, so often, that it was a minor miracle that my 'stuff' had not been lost. Prime example: as of this writing, on this very day, (back then) I am working paperwork that goes back to my local hospital (imagine that), where it all had begun. I have advised them that it's rather strange that they denied my application for PTSD, as they were part of those who diagnosed me with PTSD, some number of months I can no longer calculate before! (At that time.) Simply amazing.

And in April of 2007, a full ten months later, I had sent notes to the Board of Corrections of Naval Records concerning this department's apparent disinterest in my PTSD situation.

What kind of craziness is it when veterans and/or patients of any particular illness are forced to run pillar to post and back again with that old 'hurry up and wait' attitude that had been prevalent half a century ago, yet still persists to this very day? Years ago it only seemed to be at the 'grunt' level. Now it seems to be inherent to almost every level, in many different institutions. (Those of you, who have been grunts, please realize what an endearing term that is coming from an old mustang that was a grunt himself far longer than a 'leader of men' in uniform.)

In fact, I had been one of those grunts who had said I felt they should invert everything and appoint the grunts to run the outfit, and allow the officers to do the work for a change. Later on I learned that officers really work, too, and just as long and hard, hindsight and all that.

—Other Agencies—

Not only has the 'herding' of military men and women become commonplace, it has somehow come to the halls, walls, and insides of other institutions as well. What fun! What for so many caregivers was a 'given', almost an instant granting of assistance for their AD partner had for this veteran become another total nightmare all its own.

As of this writing, (Again, many moons ago) my file, which had been red-flagged for 'expedite', had not even shown my neurologist's diagnosis until a full nine months after I'd first talked of the disease's affect upon me. How is it that such data gets 'overlooked' or misplaced? How does very personal pertinent data simply disintegrate?

Is that what we're saying today: *lots of luck?* It makes a person feel as if he/she should walk around with a little pocket recorder and keep repeating, "Hello, today is the 18th day of June and I am here to talk about a condition I have..." all the while making sure your machine is not out of tape. "You are not scheduled to retire soon are you..."? (Sorry, I was yet recording.)

As for the one part of the story,... my only saving grace this day, weeks and weeks after a U.S. Congressman's letter to an agency (back then), is that my Lucy, the wearer of another *Safe Return* ID bracelet, had taken me in person to that office to insist that we get a look at my medical file! (You talk about a hyper-vigilant post-traumatic veteran trying to keep from going to general quarters! Any grunt past or present would have been proud of the rage boiling up inside this old warrant!) I only hope God appreciates that I didn't let go with all those crazed feelings. To give you the shorter rendition: We were eventually approved! I have actually received *some* assistance from Uncle. So, miracles still do happen.

†

It is unreal that couples are drawn together by agencies with about as much empathy as a mushroom. I believe this devastation, not only of living and suffering with various maladies, but as I think of what various agencies and arms of our Republic are getting away with, with older citizens, it is one horrendous, antiquated, unprofessional attempt at keeping compensation from folks who will surely often die before it is received! I only pray that I am incorrect about much of this. When I am finished with this work, I may be forced to write one solely on the inability of our government to properly care for the hurting people of our society. It is absolutely unreal! Or as Lou Dobbs might say: *It is an atrocity!*

†

Father God, I ask Your forgiveness for my troubled, tortured, trembling and sometimes-whining ways. I ask for Your patience and guidance. I am also asking that You might enable me not to feel ill feelings for those seated in offices and agencies who seem to enjoy taking their time and T-ing off people. I am sometimes so confused at/by our inhumanity to one another, our inability to care for folks in a timely fashion, I so tire of their picture games and questions and endless prodding of us, as they continue to strive to make us feel 'very intelligent' when in fact we are just very troubled and very enraged, and so very tired of it all. Thank You, Savior, for the love and devotion of partners willing to sacrifice and fight for us, just as Christ will one day sit as our Advocate.

Thanks, Father, for prayer partners, who are also concerned about/for us. Bless each and every one of them. Loving Lord, be in those thousands upon thousands of waiting rooms where folks sit shaking their tired and often hurting heads, wondering why they are being so 'kicked around' by a cadre of 'leaders' who seem to give with one hand even as they scheme to take away with the other. Indeed, Awesome Creator, it is a complex and perplexing subject with passionate warriors on every side, with a leadership that always manages to 'get by' more than quite well.

Why does that part of the equation never seem to change? Are the great slave owners yet within the walls and halls of the country's seat of government I have for so long loved and fought for? Or has it always been so? No, I prefer to call them the ruling class. And that, too, is a topic for an entirely different work.

Lord, I sometimes wonder if I have been allowed to make this journey so I can more closely identify with brothers and sisters in need. Will this prayer be the portion that causes a publisher to throw the entire manuscript across the room? O Devoted Divine Deity, thanks for a disease that draws Lucy and me and others closer together. Be with the thousands upon thousands who are feeling these same feelings. I can't get over the fact that You knew each of these situations before we were even formed! That this piece 'popped up' for reworking on this particular day, the day I sat with yet another doctor. How I love

Your tender ways. They are incomprehensible even to my 'very intelligent' scrambled brain. Draw us together as a nation once again. "TURN AWAY MY EYES FROM LOOKING AT WORTHLESS THINGS, AND REVIVE ME IN YOUR WAY."—Psalm 119:37

Chapter 9

Love Or Loss?

—Where Is My Friend?—

This one was easy. It gushed out like tears from a new bride, like blood from Christ's side; a mere forty-eight hours before I had buried our lap dog, rather Lucy's all-of-four-pounds lap dog.

One of the songs Helen Reddy often performs is the subtitle of this segment. When I listened to the lyrics again today (back then), I admit to a tear or two for Lucy's little dog, for others and myself as well. That's hard for some of us to admit, especially guys. That's just the way it is.

Some of the words go like this: "Where is my friend? The friend that I lost, at a fork in the road…" Having sat in on support group meetings as if I were a caregiver has assisted me immeasurably in deciphering and gathering a huge amount of empathy for the caregiver, as well as the receiver.

In the caregiver's effort to discuss his/her burden, to focus on their lot in all of this, it is natural during times of momentary detachment from the one that they are detached from, that they feel that they really are not detached at all. It's a momentary change of environment. The patient is moved, has moved. It sounds fairly easy, but it is not. It's not simple for anyone within or even near the Alzheimer's circle. This said, a change of environment is now and again of great import. Just as mates sometimes need time apart in order to more properly enjoy serious introspection, it's important for caregivers to make time, take time, to be alone, to give themselves a break from this topsy-turvy diseased world.

To me, the job of the caregiver, as I've shared before, is a much more demanding and difficult task than being the patient. It is a job even tougher than the 'going someplace else' that the patient must eventually endure. (Perhaps God will let me come back and report on it. I really think otherwise.)

First off, we don't know where it is we're going. Nor is it possible for us to visit where we are to go until we get there.

But as the onlooker, we sit, we visit, we occasionally sense that they (Now I'm speaking as if I'm not involved) are lucid for a fleeting moment or even part of a day, yet we have no real idea what they are internally encountering, contemplating.

From having sat with literally hundreds of patients over the years, (at one time I ministered to three different nursing homes simultaneously), I noted the largest portion of patients with dementia to be quite docile, rather friendly. They are seemingly *at home* in their new environments, and after a time they seem to fit in. Most of them.

You can catch them in conversation with their neighbor through gibberish, with words or without. It is as if they have been lifelong friends, and sometimes they practically are. It is truly amazing to me, at this point. How thankful I am for having had the opportunity to witness it – that I got a sense of it before I myself get to fully experience it, before I myself make the complete journey. *God's plan perhaps.* At least I sense that.

This reporting seems more and more difficult for me to write. Do I write it as though 'they' are physically present, or as though 'we' are physically present? I've done it before, have I not? For now, I'll continue as though it's all happening outside of me, to someone else.

Though they are physically present, you easily and rather quickly discern that parts of them are not present any longer. And so comes the inevitable sadness, the loneliness. So enters the *Where is my friend?* articulation, an emotion so strong that it envelopes caregivers and/or family. It can take over our world, whether we think we can or cannot allow it.

Though we have not or may we ever enter their world, it now becomes very much a part of us, having seen a glimpse of it. It is a person losing his/her loved one, and spending the rest of his life fighting that battle for the one lost over and over again. Talk about turmoil, my friend! It is turmoil and stress and loss, all at the same time.

Our Lord's words in John 8:12, speak volumes to me as I write concerning this aloneness, this darkness: "...I AM THE LIGHT OF THE WORLD: HE THAT FOLLOWETH ME SHALL NOT WALK IN DARKNESS, BUT SHALL HAVE THE LIGHT OF LIFE." And later, in verse 14: "...FOR I KNOW WHEN I CAME, AND

It sounds much akin to what the patient is facing, does it not? It just is not for us, friend, not possible to know the *Where is my friend?* part of it, nor where it is they go. I like to think as many of us become more childlike (see that chapter), we are surely in a friendlier place, I mean: they are in a friendly place.

It often becomes a particularly difficult time for the one who remains behind, after all, the one who remains often feels abandoned, forgotten, so very much alone. Is it this aloneness that the patient senses? I am yet unsure that I totally believe that, although sometimes I do feel alone (as the patient). Yet being in touch and out of touch at the same time puts me in a situation sometimes almost unbearable. Sometimes we see it, too. Sometimes we witness the great frustration of the patient. We see someone very distressed as they attempt to make those final efforts to communicate, as their cobwebbed brain becomes more confused and distressed. After this period passes, this particular stage, the patient finally seems more at ease in the aloneness, their 'away-ness' if you will, somewhat settled.

—Visiting—

There is a lot to be said for your visits, friend, whether to those with dementia or not. There is much that can be accomplished by touch, through song, by a now and again recollection for them. Just as I sensed and long ago learned when visiting folks in hospital beds, not done so much by me any longer; it was another time of aloneness, and yet enlightenment.

I always spoke and/or prayed as if that person (being visited) was yet present, whether conscious or not. And the stories from families and friends of what they'd overheard (people who had been in surgery for instance, supposedly under), well, once you've heard one or more of their tales, believe you me you'll NEVER treat a patient as if they are unable to hear you, (or you: doctors), not ever again!

"...I'll never, no never, no never forsake." They are a portion of God's most tender words. Words for ones who have departed, or even before we are allowed to go on. I often pray that the patient has had a permanent, solid relationship with our

Lord throughout her/his life; a relationship that accompanies them wherever/whenever they go. It is my deepest hope that for them it has been as a portion of the 63rd Psalm (from vs. 2): "...I HAVE SEEN THEE IN THE SANCTUARY," (and 3) "BECAUSE THY LOVING KINDNESS IS BETTER THAN LIFE, MY LIPS SHALL PRAISE THEE."

I have often sensed it when I knelt next to patients and softly sang, "Leaning, leaning, leaning on the everlasting arms," and as they sometimes joined in. I had sensed that they indeed had at one time, had that relationship, and whether they have had it or not, I yet worked as though it were my most important task: imparting God's precious love; bringing them home to Him. You see, dear friend, God wants not one excluded. Did you realize that?

Again, there is aloneness in this devastating feeling of separation. (This is me, the patient speaking now.) This is such a lonely journey, devastating, often seeming devoid of any warmth and kindness. It is scary when we ponder losing our way, no longer having much control over our lives. Even as you run back and forth between this doctor and that one, and then other agencies and offices and doctors (who somehow have the 'final word' on whether you receive assistance), you wonder, *What else can they possibly need from me?* Does anyone get this? It is something I've often muttered to myself. (At the very time I had typed these words, you would not believe how many months into my particular process for assistance I was, and I'd hate to tell you how many inquiries my wife and I had had to make up to that date.) Closer to a full year out, we finally made it!, at least with our Alzheimer's request. (Sorry again, if this is repetition for you.)

Next to my pool cover going into place in the fall of the year, one of the saddest moments in life is Helen's song's lyrics referred to earlier:

"Where is my friend?
The friend that I lost, at a fork in the road,
that led me to the life I've lived?
Where is my friend, who knew me when,
I'd love to meet her again.
Where is my friend?"

"The friend that I lost at the fork in the road,
and never, ever, found again?
Well, I wonder what she'd say,
if we met today,
has she lost her way, and does she need a friend?
Does she feel the same, when she hears my name,
does she wish we were together once again?
The road to the talking, we keep living again.
Ah, but it gets lonely, ooh so lonely, now and then.
Where is my friend,
the friend that I lost at the fork in the road,
and never, never-ever found again...?"

I cannot help but think of my lovely, lonely Lucy, my children and precious grandchildren, the family doctors I so revere, Momma. Then there are sweet siblings who have so supported us during my transit, our transit, as well as nephews and nieces and on and on, my close friends, Billy and Debbie (next door), a far-off and far out Gunnery Sergeant I sometimes refer to as 'Lenny', though he'll try to find the exact coordinates of where I live when he reads that. The neat thing: David is now a soul warrior and prayer warrior, as is his sweet wife Barbara. We call her Saint Barb. (A whole 'nother story there.)

When you ask, *Where is my friend?,* you automatically think of your church and it's warm envelopment of you, at least I do. The church, as Christ, wraps you in everlasting arms. These dear friends are constant loving mentors, brothers and sisters; witnesses to so many lost sinners, other sinners such as you and me. It is home to our Savior, our Friend. Church is that place where you share sadness and joy, new life and death. *The very real knowledge of your Tomorrows Forever.*

I pray for you that it will be the place where you feel so very much at home in, you won't want to leave it when you have to head back to the home you live in. I also pray that you sense God's Presence there, now, later, most of your life.

Naturally I also think of those many folks mentioned in my acknowledgments. And as therein was said, get on my knees for anyone not intentionally left out or forgotten. What a cold lonely devastating subject, being left out, somewhat akin to departing early without any 'good-bye'. Fortunately, I've had time to say 'so long' or see you later.

Then there's Luis, the nephew who honorably gave his life for our beloved country, of the profound impact his living and death has had upon others, as well as me. *Thanks, Luis!*

And I think of new life that has blessed our families over and over again, all these new beginnings. The threads that will weave tomorrow's Forever blanket of joy, honor, glory, praising, dancing, singing, so much more.

I am praying such a new beginning for you as well, Michelle. *Really*.

—Another Not Knowing When—

There are other favorites: with a story behind each face. I have fondness for each one, how they have directly affected my life, this person somewhere between where I am and where I will be. Is it not true of each of us? Is it not true that each of us will evolve in one-way or another? This or that?

We either become more gracious, wiser perhaps, or at least hope to, or we may become combative and nasty and yelling at everyone as people sometimes do from medication and/or when becoming further along in their disease, or simply put, older, or stubborn. Sometimes we are allowed these choices; sometimes we are not.

Part of me is aware of something else, too. There are, in the midst of my remembrances and fondness even for the din of life, these words: "BEHOLD, I COME AS A THIEF. BLESSED IS HE THAT WATCHETH, AND KEEPETH HIS GARMENTS, LEST HE WALK NAKED, AND THEY SEE HIS SHAME." —Revelation 16:15. I could traverse such vast territory with those words, but I especially focus upon the I COME AS A THIEF portion of the words. I have always been haunted by words of Christ's return, that no one knows when. We should be comforted by those words, never in fear of them.

†

Anticipation. Is it not that realm that causes wonder as we walk so many pathways during our short-lived lives? New places can be looked forward to with great anticipation or with feelings of anxiety and loss, and anything and everything in between.

So why hold on? Why fear aloneness? If you have been watching for His return, I suspect that your life has been a special life, probably a serving life, a loving life. Should you therefore ever feel alone? Yet sometimes we do. That's the humanity in us.

For me, too, it is a big **Yes!** How often I've felt totally alone, whether on a ship at sea or in the midst of war. Something clicks inside. One can be with many brothers and sisters in various times and places and stages of life, and then suddenly, or at the same time, feel so alone, utterly, relentlessly, terribly alone. It is scary. *Where is my friend?* Think about it. You know the answer.

†

Almighty Father, as I watched yet another space-walk on a chilly November evening, and now morning (long before this rewrite) - it only reassures me of Your graciousness to each and every one of us. And to me there is something almost sacred about an International Space Station. The working together of people from various nations and backgrounds makes life so rich and wonderful. My prayer now, Lord, is for sinners thinking or knowing where they are, or for those not so certain, the prayer that exudes from within me reminds me of these first few lines: "O GOD, THOU ART MY GOD; EARLY WILL I SEEK THEE, MY FLESH LONGETH FOR THEE IN A DRY AND THIRSTY LAND, WHERE NO WATER IS; TO SEE THY POWER AND THY GLORY, SO AS I HAVE SEEN THEE IN THE SANCTUARY. BECAUSE THY LOVING KINDNESS IS BETTER THAN LIFE, MY LIPS SHALL PRAISE THEE. THUS WILL I BLESS YOU WHILE I LIVE: I WILL LIFT UP MY HANDS IN THY NAME." —from the 63rd Psalm

How unfathomable Your ways, the vastness of Your love and grace, Lord. You seek us out. Even when we attempt to run from You, You draw us back under Your remarkably mighty wondrous wings. You protect us; You care for us; You long for us.

And so it is with this prayer, gracious God: For it is at this very moment, in this stillness of the middle of one of my dementia-laden nights, I again turn to You in silence rather than aloneness. I have been privileged to know and feel Your

Holy Presence and power, Your eternal patience. At this moment, God, I pray that You'll continue to bless brothers and sisters fighting their assigned causes; that You'll comfort the bereaved, and visit one's alone in prison cells. Be with any contemplating suicide; spark that previously dull life back into a new revitalization and wholeness. Perhaps You might allow love to come into other lives again, so some may look beyond themselves, toward You, to service for You.

And then there are the hungry, dear Lord, how my soul cries out for ones without enough to eat; and ones dying, or worse yet, ones lost who hunger for Your special way. They seem forsaken, even as You for a short while felt forsaken. I pray that we do not ever forsake You, we never forget where our Friend is. For we do know where You are, Everywhere! (I recall having written an *Upper Room* piece about that, many years ago.)

—Joy!—

Some may color me **c r a z y**, instead of a guy with AD. Yet I now share with you that it is of utmost importance: caregivers and receivers alike must focus upon joy where possible. Joy is strength and vitality, the hope for what is yet up ahead!

"O, Lord my God, when I in awesome wonder, consider all the worlds Thy hands have made."

What grandeur. What soul-stirring lyrics to a song and proclamation I so love. There are these words also: "THE PEOPLE WHO WALKED IN DARKNESS HAVE SEEN A GREAT LIGHT; THOSE WHO DWELT IN THE LAND OF THE SHADOW OF DEATH, UPON THEM A LIGHT HAS SHINED." —Isaiah 9:2.

The light this prophet looked forward to made his vision assured so he addressed it as having already happened, as if it had already dawned. Joy is like that. Our hope is instantly made whole and in faith our souls grasp that which is no less than the greatest satisfaction on this earth. Joy enables us to die with delight ahead of us, with the knowledge that we are sailing toward our eternal home.

—It Cannot Be Contained—

Joy puts me in mind of a fishing remembrance, a picture of my oldest grandson, Victor (who just happens to be here on vacation, right now, in the other room). He is looking to his right, pretty much pleased. Yet he seems a tiny bit envious as Grandpa (that's me), holds up the first catch of the day. Only moments later, as he holds his fishing pole in another captured picture, as he proudly displays his catch, what obvious joy is splashed across this nine-year-old face. (Actually Victor is eleven years-young now, and by the time this work hits the street, he may be twelve!) At any rate, his look in that picture can only be described as joy—joy, and perhaps a shade of pride as well.

Joy is an entity that must emerge from your being. It is that awe-inspiring and invigorating feeling that one can never hide, never contain. I've often told the story of a vision that could only have come from God, when I was much younger; of how our pastor then, Pastor Bill, in a Zion, Illinois church, allowed me that next Sunday the privilege of using his pulpit. Okay, you know I mean Christ's pulpit. In this way, I could share that fabulous, soul-stirring event with the entire congregation. It had been a vision I'll never forget, as was the sharing of it.

Because of that day, and that *telling*, I later did progressively more leading of worship services; I kept getting more and more involved in God's wonderful work. And let me tell you before I forget it: It's not always an easy plea, getting a pastor to relinquish that pulpit. But sometimes, especially if he's Spirit-led, it is easier to get yourself into it. And in that particular case – way back then, the invitation was extended. Thanks, so much Bill. God's continued blessings. (Yes, I, too, still miss Mary.)

The early beginnings of what would years later become my involvement in ministry, of my finally surrendering to God's call, that stranglehold around my throat, I totally realized that balloon-filled emotion inside me. It is the *I-cannot-contain-this-only-unto-myself* sensation and truth. It is akin to a pastor anointed of God.

For this fullness, this anointing, causes one to invite every living creature into God's Holy Presence. He invites them to partake of this divine splendor that he (the one anointed) cannot himself contain inside. That is joy. And I have been blessed to feel it often, and strongly.

God and a pastor, or other loyal, loving leaders invite one and all to come *home*. If you are a pastor, and have not sensed that feeling of late, you might consider selling shoes, or some other field of work. (No, that's much too harsh. It can be righted, my friend. And you, with God's assistance can carry on as He longs for you to do. Trust Him. Seek the joy again! And allow no one to let you look back! Not one!) He is, as a friend of mine has written: *A God of second chances.*

If you, reader friend, have not felt this buoyancy, my very soul cries out for you at this moment. It is not a joy that is reserved solely for ones who wear the collar. If you have failed to ask God to join you in this walk of life, or have slipped and taken a few backward steps, know that you can enter this dance of life right now! I encourage you to let Him know that you confess you are a sinner (even if you've done it before), ask Him, after having asked for forgiveness, to enter your heart again, right now! Now there are those who will write and tell me that I am crazy, that once the invitation has been extended, you don't need to do this again. Let them have their say. Whether or not you feel that God has entirely disappeared from you, trust me for a moment. Trust God, as well! (And always trust Him first.)

For those of you who would say that I have an agenda, it is nothing less than true. I know within the deepest core of my being, if you have failed to sense God in all these years of your life, you, too, have missed out on the greatest, most joy-filled life that you were meant to live. How sad is that? How it afflicts me: It is worse than my most vivid nightmare; worse than this hairnet-like feeling that comes upon me, especially when I have been awake far too long; or whenever I have managed to go at full steam ahead for far too long. Sometimes, I can go for quite a stretch.

—The Works Go On—

You see, friend, when I sensed His Presence again, in the midst of this writing, I also sensed the urgency and joy that culminate at nearly the same instant. Had it been much the same with the Babe, I have sometimes wondered. The One, I am hopeful you have (if necessary) just re-invited into you heart and soul. Know you not God's eyes were and are steadfast upon the cross, as He knew He had been commissioned, was sent to earth as a Child only to be crucified on a tree for your sins, my sins? He sensed this self-destructive, yet soul-winning urgency during God's entire thirty-plus years on earth. He was fully aware that He was about His Father's work.

When He walked into those temples on Saturday, what we now celebrate on Sunday, He walked in with great authority and power and blessing from the One above; with confidence and zeal and Power, filled with love, the Lord, (Who actually was God Incarnate, come here in the form of man). For in knowing that His death, this divine sacrifice, was to be atonement for all mankind, how could God not also have been so joy-filled that He could never contain the works: the sampling that Father had sent Him to show at the very same time that Father had sent Him (our Savior) to die.

Indeed, again, God had sent Himself! Therefore, the works displayed were far more than a mere sampling. They were and are a sure sign that they are to go on even today and forevermore (regardless of location, personhood or form).

This *at-one-ment*, this making right or good, is it not the Omnipotent's way of leading us also to a life of purity? For in purity we find joy, and in joy we find peace and strength; a new calming and reinvigorating assurance.

So, if you are reading these words and have somehow missed this divine initiative prepared for you, I right this moment beseech you to fly to Him! I don't mean go in a strolling manner. *I mean fly to God!* Find a place where you can be alone, or grab hold of a loved one you already know to be one of His – but seek God out! Or speak to one who needs to be His as well.

Speak gently and calmly and lovingly, yet fully knowing what is happening to you. For it will be the beginnings of *j o y*. Not containable, exhausting and exhilarating, filled with God's Spirit, we call it *j o y*.

Grasp this new feeling that will change your entire attitude, your future, your life, your entire world. Go to that quiet place right now! Humble yourself before God and attempt to empty yourself of the entire world's clutter and chatter. Empty yourself of all those voices that have kept God away for far too long. Center in upon His wonder and awe, place your head to His loving bosom. Stay with Him; talk with Him. Tell God exactly what it is that He already knows, but share it with Him, for this is important. Share where you have been, tell Him where you think you are now. It will be an amazing new beginning again.

—Do Not Run Away—

Surely in this meeting, in this time of *at-one-ment*, as you humbly and honestly seek God, He *will* invite you to come in. *He will!* You might not feel an immediate jolt or sudden change right then and there on the spot, or you may. But whenever it comes, you will not mistake the change that is taking place within your very soul. You will not mistake how wonderful you feel as your burdens melt away, as your mind and heart and very spirit realize that there is another way to live your life; that you really don't have to work so very hard at it, nor do you have to run from Him any longer. *Do not run away from the very One who has so powerfully made you.* You will learn what an awesome, wondrous, forgiving, loving and Holy God He is. You will once again, or for the very first time, learn of joy! *His* joy!

The knocking. Those of us in the faith, the family of God: we call it knocking on the door. And actually, it is Jesus knocking upon YOUR heart's door. Ask Him to enter in. What do you suppose will take place? Do you for a moment doubt that you would not answer Him? I am in special prayer for you, for you and your answer, and your entirely new life!

—Not The Sunrise—

One of my closest friends on this entire planet happens to be a U.S Marine. He is quite possibly my very closest friend. David has often shared the story of one of his awakenings, his sensing the day's warming sunlight in his eyes. David was actually *coming to* in the bright beam of a State Trooper's flashlight. David had lost control of his motorcycle, the way he'd lost control of his entire life. He has often shared with me through laughter now, "It wasn't the sun that I saw, it wasn't sunrise, it was the beginning of a miracle that led me to His Son."

David knew if he did not abandon this kind of foolishness, of himself being thrown in the opposite direction of his bike, if he did not abandon the course he had begun, his life would simply become less and less of a 'living' (if he survived), and more and more of a dying, as he himself had been dying inside all along. What a tragic thought. What a wasted life it could have been.

Thanks to Father, I years ago stood alongside my friend at a *Promise Keeper's* meeting in Pittsburgh, Pennsylvania. Here, I had observed this heretofore-awakened-by-a-Trooper's-flashlight person, witnessed tears rolling freely down his chiseled face, that face between huge shoulders that were one of the signs of a proud, slightly-used, U.S. Marine. As I looked over at my friend, I recall asking this hulk of a machine, this combat-hardened warrior, "What's wrong, Dave?" only to hear an almost inaudible yet committed, simple, sincere statement: *I think I just gave my heart to Jesus!*

How many times we have revisited that very scene. That new beginning for David, that instant for David had become his new beginning. It was a moment that enabled my friend's life to be touched and his course to be forever transformed! It was and is yet today **joy**!

†

We never really lose those memories, those moments with God, those sincere commitments. Sometimes we slide back a little, or strive to go it alone for a while, but thankfully our loving God always calls us back home. So joy-filled am I when I recall how many wonderful Christ-filled people I've been fortunate to share my life with. This walk.

Certainly Momma comes to mind early on. She could have been as David, and so many others. She could have become booze-induced and led astray; she certainly had that proclivity. Many of her siblings and her father suffered from it: that *play all night, sleep all day* realm of some musicians which sometimes leads folks to certain mischief, and later utter loneliness, and sometimes brokenness. Defeat. (No meanness intended: it's often factual.) Instead, however, Momma came to know 3 wonderfully exciting, God-fearing men, who she has outlived. But what a life it has been for her, for us! What a witness she has been for God!

—Intervention—

My car broke down when I had first arrived on the tiny island of Guam, back in the seventies. One of its essential belts had dried out and snapped with a resounding '*buh-bye* now' sound. Suddenly there appeared this tall, rather stately looking man, even in his weekend gardening clothing he somehow looked differently, friendly, no wrinkle lines on this brow, self-assured, confident, and there was something else.

Soon he was underneath our hood, calmly talking of this and that as he removed the brokenness and later reappeared and repaired the vehicle. Repaired what had been so very frustrating for any newcomers to an island out in the middle of nowhere. The Western Pacific is way out, this part is beyond Hawaii.

Only days later, was I to learn as I looked upon him again, now in a crisp white summer uniform with four broad stripes over each shoulder, that we had been rescued that day of our utter frustration by the senior chaplain on that tiny island in the middle of the Western Pacific.

To me it had been nothing less than an intervention of joy. To our family he quickly became a fast friend. One day he would be assigned to the Navy's Office of the Chief of Chaplains, this mechanic!, this man of God, this down-to-earth, tall and gentle stranger who had become for me a good friend and advisor. Do you not find great joy in people similar? I can yet remember his favorite hymn: "*O For a Thousand Tongues to Sing…*" it begins.

Has it ever impressed you how God took the tax collector, the drunken Marine, the mechanic and some common fisherman to become examples? How is it that He draws each of them to His unequivocal side? Why the common people? Why that commonality?

I believe it is for each and every one of us to sense, no matter where we find ourselves in life, that God sooner or later reaches out to each one. No matter how many times we try and do not succeed; no matter how often we have failed Him. All of this, this mess of a life we may have been living far too long, cannot all of it be reversed? Reversed, revived and made new and whole, forever? Certainly you know we can be made to feel whole and new and justified perhaps for the very first time, or all over again? We can realize that we are one of God's, first thing upon awaking, because we ARE! Christians call it being sanctified, set apart.

When I think of my lovely Lucy, and how her dad spent most of his married life with a sickly wife (until her passing), of how he would come home and nastily take it out on Donna, I cannot help but find myself yet hurting inside for her. She was one slapped about and screamed at, and often hidden away; and yet, she was one who honored her dad even to his end. She had made that right decision not to allow those terrible picture-memories to take over her spirit. She would not allow the degradation to accompany her into eternity. She had loved the seemingly unlovable. She had endured the unbearable. How I respect my loving bride for that. How I admire such fortitude. It is baffling to me, the strength, often times, of the human spirit. I do not know if I could have forgiven someone who had treated me as Lucy had been treated; much less ever forget it.

Yet that, friend, is what we are called to do, even you and me. You see it is one way God allows our burdens to be lightened.

—More Joy—

It is a simple matter for me to speak of the cover picture of this book, of what joy it brings me. Look at those faces, enter that portion of my life so enriched by family and friends, by faith. Why is it these loved ones mean so much to me? It is because they are not small tokens; they are the lives of the ones I have so dearly loved, been surrounded by, will never forget. And yes, they are who have mattered most to me.

Can you not understand why it is that God wants us surrounded by friends, by like fellows? Those who are like-minded? And should they not be like-minded, don't you believe he wants us to gently attend to each one until they find the courage to ask for that, what I had referred to earlier: to realize that it has been God's knocking upon their heart's door?

Life works out easier if you simply pursue the real longing for joy. That one Relationship many of us cannot seem to speak of, let alone pursue. There was a time when I had ministered to a woman who had cared for her mother for years on end. Only shortly after her mom's death, she was to learn of her own particular battle: a type of blood cancer. A cancer that eventually placed her in a wheelchair, and debilitated her more and more for the remainder of her years.

As I would now and again wheel her out to my car during our preparations to depart for a nearby worship service, I long never to forget this hope-filled woman's repetitive words: "What a beautiful day it will be." The cold winter wind might be biting at her already rosy cheeks, but always the same response came from within her: "What a beautiful day it will be."

Those words that came from beneath those white locks of hair; hair that sometimes almost hid her ice-blue eyes, were to me words filled with nothing less than pure joy! Even as 'beat up' as she most certainly must have felt from time to time, she had managed to learn one of Paul's secrets: to be content no matter what her lot.

†

Omnipotent Father, You see into and through each soul. I hear Your sweet words, "...Ye who are weary come home." To me they, too, are words of joy. Thank You, Savior, for knowing us so well, for caring for each of us, and thank You for this wisdom from Romans 8:26 (NKJV): "...THE SPIRIT ITSELF MAKETH INTERCESSION FOR US WITH GROANINGS WHICH CANNOT BE UTTERED." *Dear Father and Friend, thank You for Your promises, Your peace, Your declaration later in Romans 8:38-39,* "FOR I AM PERSUADED, THAT NEITHER DEATH, NOR LIFE, NOR ANGELS, NOR PRINCIPALITIES, NOR POWERS, NOR THINGS PRESENT, NOR THINGS TO COME, NOR HEIGHT, NOR DEPTH, NOR ANY OTHER CREATURE, SHALL BE ABLE TO SEPARATE US FROM THE LOVE OF GOD, WHICH IS IN CHRIST JESUS OUR LORD." *You so seek us out to give us Your joy, Father. We so love You for those great and wonderful promises!*

(Read Psalm 63:1-4, and then read in Psalm 145:3-4, how we pass these wisdoms on to the next generation.)

Chapter 10

—'Sun downing' Or 'Sun-Upping'—

A time of being unusually tired, or feeling as if I am in a fog, is what I refer to as sun downing. I am in it as I prepare myself for bed at night, as I do all those little things in preparation for sleep. Therefore, what is sun downing for you and sun downing for me might be quite different. I do seem to sense a more pervasive confusion late in the day or when I have pushed myself further than I think I should have. But then again, pushing is what a *Never Give Up* guy does.

As you know, I don't get much rest, at least not a lot at once. Part of that is the posttraumatic syndrome, the other part the AD. Sometimes I only get an hour or two of rest and then *Bang!* I'm right back at it. And it may be I have brought some of this about myself as I push to complete this work before I cross that line into a different kind of reality. I look for help from God, and from my regimentation. I seek change for the better, and I believe my paradigm will work and prove eventually, to be very beneficial!

The frustration I refer to as *sun downing* is sometimes caused (for me) by too much sound, or activity, such as music played too loudly, and or television, or just being over-stimulated: that is, too many things going on at once. And this area is different than/from noise bombardment. Again, it is caused by my body preparing itself for that blessed relief known as rest, and/or sleep, especially when I am tired; so it is I may be getting prepared for rest at that time *sun downing* seems so prevalent. And yet, whatever it is or however it is brought about, I will not allow it to beat me.

—Patients And Treatment Ideas—

Those I have been heretofore blessed to visit, who sat rather quietly, almost motionless and/or half asleep, looking glassy-eyed, it is my belief were in the later stages of the disease. Although it would not surprise me that some had been sedated (on purpose).

I have read, and now more readily understand that it is often beneficial to remove the patient from the din and clatter of mealtime preparations, as explained in Dr. Mace and Rabin's *The 36-Hour Day*. It is an excellent read about Alzheimer's disease.

The doctors explain therein how the patient is taken to the park, while people are arriving home and things are being readied for mealtime, let's say the table is being set and so on. Great idea!

My loving wife has even sensed this about me, and knows there is less agitation for me if I am *out of the picture* so to speak. Since there is confusion, moving the patient or separating her/him from this agitation is found to be beneficial, then later, when preparations are completed and things in place, the patient is then returned to sit down and eat with the rest of the family.

It is my belief that it would also be a good thing for the elderly, whether or not they are diseased in this way. (After all, they have had their years of business and engagement and 'going nuts' along with the rest of us.) The craziness we seem to continue to allow because we do not seek a still, calm center. And what a shame that is.

As previously described, I suffer mild agitation as I prepare my writing room before I lie down to rest. I make little trips back and forth: readying my CPAP machine, ensuring that my coffee maker has water in it, seeing to it that I have an apple or something to nibble on in my workspace for later on. It is during this time that I usually feel my hairnet-like fog feeling coming down over my brain, and/or my aching brain syndrome I used to call it.

Yet I must confess that since I wear the 24-hour patch now, and also have another medication as well, I am not feeling those hairnet sensations as much, or at least as vividly. The patch has been a definite improvement for me.

Exhaustion definitely exacerbates confusion, therefore, I would recommend attempting to ensure that the patient is kept rested, and not forced to go too much longer than they normally go (without sleep) unless it is necessary, for example, when traveling. As of this writing, it is much the same as it was last year at this time: that is, I seem to run a cycle of a couple hours of rest and then I'm up again. At the end of three or four days of this, I am so 'wiped out' that I usually get a longer stretch that seems to somewhat revitalize me. And of course this not only depends upon my weird AD dreams, but also whether or not I get one of my combat 'mares. (So once again, what happens to me may be different than it is for you.)

Much of this can be changed and challenged as I attempt habilitating myself as much as possible. That again includes exercise, a positive outlook, having a labor of love (some kind of hobby), a proper diet, enjoying music, good support, and where possible, attempting to keep my life somewhat 'de-cluttered' and simple. *For me a good prayer life is also essential.* There will be more details about this paradigm of which I speak, in chapter twelve.

—On Socializing, Again—

Usually I have a problem attending meetings; sometimes I just do not want to bring myself to them. In fact, I would rather isolate than socialize. So sometimes I do not make the effort. (One exception has always been my good attendance at Alzheimer's meetings.) I am told that others with dementia suffer a similar type of longing: to be left alone.

I do know that once I am at the meeting, such as an Alzheimer's meeting, and am involved, it becomes easier for me. At times, depending upon the hour of a meeting and/or where I am in my day, I have a tendency to want to sleep instead. And this, too, changes as we enter different stages of the disease. So sometimes a patient will have to fight it, or rest up in advance if that will help.

These concerns sometimes bring about unnecessary guilt, and/or you might get *the look* from someone close to you if she/he is in the same room. (You guys know about the look, right?)

Thankfully, I am more concerned with *upping* than I am with *sun downing,* that is, to me 'upping' is my clear concise and consistent effort to remain focused on current goals in this early onset patient's mind. Of course my wife will disagree and tell you I am no longer in 'early' onset. Then again, she may now and again agree that I'm doing pretty well. *Either way, I love you!*

A good attitude, family, the One, the struggle to remain 'on track' seem most important to me now. In this way I challenge myself more than I would if I simply allowed sun downing to take place. I do suspect, however, that this type of regimen may be possible for some folks with early onset and much more difficult for others.

For some, this 'working' to become more regimented will be looked upon as a rather rigorous element that they will not wish to pursue. But if it is followed, there are certain benefits from a regimen, and working to keep one's self active and engaged. At the very least, it will prolong quality of living and can effect great attitudinal change, or we could say a great attitude is what makes it possible for one to prolong quality living and longevity of living as well.

It is the fighter within me that opts for 'upping' as it is my way of staving off this giant that will one day no doubt overtake me. That is, unless I am granted the miracle, never rule that out.

(Speaking of fighters: it was this very day, as I later worked this final rewrite, that I pondered one named Tiffany, who is on to more training and then to an assignment to Iraq, as so many before her. Our church body prayed for her and her mother and for so many others involved in serving this Republic for the rest of us. I am proud to hear and learn of some yet willing to go that extra mile for the ones who remain behind today. Tiffany and others remain in our daily prayers. And how thankful I am for you, and your service to your beloved country.)

The illusive, rather obscure, somewhat sneaky progression that gradually spreads and causes more and more deterioration until it simply 'takes over' is part of this life with AD, this path that you may now be set upon. Yet it's natural for me to hope and pray that you can keep this deterioration at bay for as long as possible, that you might remain lucid and vital. I pray it often, tenderly, in earnest. And I pray that you might be able to ward off those folks who mean well, and tell you: *You can remember,* or *You could live this way for 20 years.* Though that is sometimes the case, their words of encouragement sometimes lack empathy, and you are therefore not allowed to feel sorry for yourself. ***You are entitled to your emotions.***

So, reader friend, whether I am a participant in perceived sun downing or am actually involved in this slosh that I call 'hairnet time', matters little to me. I will not be one in denial. I'm simply stating for me, the preferred goal is the 'upside' of it all! I therefore encourage you, as well to focus not on the 'poor me' aspects of the disease (although again you may), but am hopeful that you will find much that is cathartic about working to keep yourself as upbeat as possible. Even if you are sightless, or on the way to it, and therefore cannot read these words, is it not wonderful to have someone read them to you? It is surely one of God's ways of showing you how very much He cares for you.

Might I use a little joke here? I call Jesus' returning to the Father, ***Son-upping!***

†

Lover of our very souls, thank You for enabling us to have the 'sunny side' of our vessel exposed more than our cloud-filled side. O God, as surely as You said, "It is done," upon the cross, You have done/and yet do such wondrous works for Your praise people. Thank You, Teacher, for allowing us to sense Your loving Presence wherever we are. We know we need not even ask You to come and be with us, for You are Omnipresent. We cannot always sense that, it seems. Thank You, Lord, Savior, Friend, for the awareness: that it would serve us little to be different at various times and places, for You know our actions, You know every tiny detail of our lives. Assist us in becoming transparent people, as You would have us be. Therefore, transparency in living is our striving to live for You. It allows each of us to know that You are always near, and that can be a marvelous comfort. Assist us in this grand walk with You. And assist us in recalling that when Christ said 'It is finished.,' He meant that evil had been conquered, and that God's mighty foot had been placed right smack in the middle of the evil one's chest!

Read Hebrews 9:14. It is offered here from the New King James Version, ... "HOW MUCH MORE SHALL THE BLOOD OF CHRIST, WHO THROUGH THE ETERNAL SPIRIT OFFERED

HIMSELF WITHOUT SPOT TO GOD, CLEANSE YOUR CONSCIENCE FROM DEAD WORKS TO SERVE THE LIVING GOD?"

TIME ZONES (Slipping away…)
Wayne Glenn TERRY

Chapter 11

Giving Up and Looking Up
—Relinquishing—

It is difficult for one to give up what he'd figured was his duty: home security. But when I turned my handgun over to a friend, it was quite a feeling of freedom. It is also difficult coming to terms with what most of us know to be reality: that we control very little in this life, and indeed, we are rather fragile creatures; that we rely upon God for most of (and should say all) our protection.

Near or in stage four, (my perception), I read and share this very appropriate poem I love:

I am not here anymore.
Somewhere else is where I am.
A place so hard to find,
you cannot see me here
or visit me there,
or wish me out of this anywhere.
If this is where I'm supposed to be,
why can't I find me?

(Poem from *Learning To Speak Alzheimer's,* Joanne Koenig Coste's work, Houghton-Mifflin Co.)

Though these words may seem somewhat sad, I realize how true they ring. They have some time ago assisted me in turning my disease over to God's care, I have indeed relinquished control. I only wish I had accomplished this much sooner. Really. It's made a transition easier, me thinks.

Several things take place when one surrenders control. And I do not wish to give you the idea that it's just 'giving up', for in a way I will never give up. In another way, I have. When one relinquishes control, life becomes instantly simpler, easier, clearer. It seems the more we strive to control, the more we learn that we actually control very little, or as the words of a song that I have sung declare, "What I'd often longed for has been here all along."

Further knowledge gained upon relinquishing is that we begin to learn how important is trust, and for many of us, that's no easy lesson. For others, it may never happen. Relinquishing allows us freedom; it allows us to go to a place we may never have been or could not have gone before, not on our own at least.

You know the man, the one who has attended your church for thirty or forty years? Finally one Sunday he gets up out of his seat and walks right up front and humbly confesses to the pastor, before God and all, that he'd never gotten it, all those years, until this very moment! That is relinquishing.

As patients, we turn control over not only to our Lord, but we turn control over to a friend, a mate, a relative, perhaps a facility later on. I might even go so far as to relay that control is overrated. Did you ever watch the tough guy that runs and shoots and acts invincible until he's finally stopped and cuffed and in a prone position whimpering, "Please, please don't hurt me!"

I sometimes find that scene humorous, as I'm thinking: *This is the same fellow that just shot at law enforcement officials without regard for anyone else's life – and now he's begging for graciousness?*

Relinquishing often has much to do with admitting that sometimes we are just plain wrong. That is often a tough one. Even though we are changing, in transit, losing parts of us – we, too, can be wrong. We can make mistakes, too. For me, I would say: *Attempt to go humbly where possible, and that's difficult for a combat veteran to share.* Yet I am reminded of ancient words written by one sixteen years of age: "…Approach thy grave like one who wraps the drapery of his couch about him, and lies down to pleasant dreams."

It may well be a blessing for us to think we are dying before we're actually dying. The positive offshoot: It makes each day sweeter, each moment more important. I've heard it said before, as each day is marked off, we are one day closer to paradise! That's not such a bad thought. Actually, IT'S A WONDERFULLY JOYOUS THOUGHT!

Relinquishing also enables us to allow others to more easily assist us. I used to hate it when Lucy would drag me through crowds, her hand squeezing mine, my arm all twisted in an awkward way. Now, her sweet firm hand is a comfort to me. I daily, as do others, seek God out. Lucy's hand reminds me of that. It is her gently guiding me nowadays, as if God is closer through her. And believe you me, He feels closer now.

How I used to hate her words: "Don't smoke that cigar in the house!" I have since learned that they were blessed words, that that listening, may well have allowed our home to stand another day, and there are other real personal benefits of course. What used to seem painful to me now seems more worthwhile, perhaps I might proffer: wiser.

Yet with all this said: relinquishing may be the one thing seeming almost impossible to the patient/receiver/diseased one. In my layman's opinion, that's because it diametrically opposes other words that I've shared herein. Do you recall those, friend? *Never give up!* You know what I have discovered? Relinquishing is NOT giving up, it is merely turning over control and trust to our Creator God, the One Who knew all before you even were begun.

—Praying for Others—

I often am in prayer for veterans older than myself. Without someone's **immediate assistance**, the older combat veteran is slated to be forgotten and sometimes never assisted. Lost!

It is similar with working a regimen, as I am suggesting for AD folks. If it is not worked, there will be no gain recognized, no good changes made. And again, if we are unable to relinquish, we will never know why trusting our tender God can assist us in living. *His eye is on the sparrow, and I know he watches over me....*

I used to regret having merged these two worlds: of the veteran and dementia, but I am beginning to think it may be quite helpful. Have you noticed nowadays how much air we are finding in our bags of 'stuff' at the store? Too many bags filled with a lot of air, and less and less product. What I am getting at is that what was, and what is supposed to be, are two different things. And we, the consumer, all I can say is they must think we're all out to lunch!

Are you, or the one reading this to you aware that some 1200 World War II veterans are dying daily now? That means, unless someone prompts that senator or congressman, the 7 to 900,0000 veterans (And you can't even get an accurate number anymore) whose applications seem suspended somewhere, well, they may as well be out to lunch, too. I don't relish saying this, but it seems it may well end up that many of our older veterans are in the same boat as a good friend of mine, rather a recent Vietnam-era friend, Steve; God's continued blessings, Steve. No more asking for help with your T-shirt.

Steve recently died before he heard anything from a government agency. (I dearly miss ya, Pal.) What do you suppose they will do for Steve's wife or his mother or father? *Bingo*! You guessed it! *Nada, almost zippo—zilch....* (Oh, let me not be remiss, there are a couple hundred bucks for burial fees, I hope we don't break the bank.)

What has happened to initiative, fair play, taking care of those who have served this country so bravely? I would be terribly remiss here if I did not mention my Congressman J. Randy Forbes and the marvelous support and assistance I've had from him and his great staff in Virginia's 4th district. What they have meant to Lucy and others and myself! I placed a hand written note on his desk in D.C., telling him that. And I mean it, Randy.

Perhaps, by the time this work is published, an arm of the government may have decided that a guy with Alzheimer's and PTSD, who suffers panic attacks as well will no longer be employable, in their eyes. So far though, no soap. NEWSFLASH: I have to take that back as of this final rewrite, in August, 2008, I have been notified that I will be on Medicare effective in December. *Thank you, Father. It **IS** a praise item....*

I continue to wonder why this great paper mill that only cripples any forward momentum continues to exist. What would be wrong with some agencies using a few of those fax numbers everyone is aware of? So typical of today's malaise. You think I find myself in a fog? Watch the U.S. House or the Senate for a few weeks! That's an eye opener, especially watch the programs in the middle of the night! It is truly frightening to sit there awestruck, at what they fail to accomplish. (I am sorry,

Lord. I do not understand why our Republic seems crippled to honest and forthright communication. Transparency. (Why and how does the gamesmanship go on?)

—And Then There's Denial—

I really wish I could report that all will be well if you choose to begin a regimen and fight your debilitations. Yet here is a single line that you may wish to place upon your bathroom mirror or refrigerator, or somewhere prominent: If you are willing to fight to be as good as you can for as long as you can, there will always be those who figure that you are not in a 'funk' that you indeed are not sick, and therefore I don't know exactly what they will think of you. All I am saying is: for some it will be classic denial, and for others, they will remain skeptics until your body is lowered into the ground once and for all. That's just the way it is!

Yet you know what else I've learned, dear friend? I've learned that it just doesn't matter. After all, those of us who know God, are sincerely interested in knowing that not only is He alive and in charge, but also that He knows all, sees all, and that things are going just as He had planned all along, regardless of how you and I sense it or feel about it.

I'm sure you've heard it said, sometimes your best is not good enough. What I am saying is a little different. Sometimes your best will be too good for them to believe.

But as I am one of the *Never give up!* Guys, I'd say go for it! Do your best, for as long as you possibly can. Live, love, dance and laugh. Enjoy every fiber of it, and keep recalling that each day you are one day closer to eternity and God! (Thanks, Leroy, I loved that sermon!) I can hear pastor's wife laughing it up now (since I called him Leroy).

—Memories—

Never let go of your precious memories, even as you relinquish control. As far as possible, hang on to every single one. I pray that for you. Somehow, I realize, God's grace again, that when one part of the noggin's not stroking correctly, another part remembers old times quite well. And that's nothing new, not really. It depends of course on what part of the brain is being attacked, does it not? There are times (the doctors say), the patient is simply confused, that we really can recall a person even though we (the patient) are confused about who that person is.

Don't ask me, this part gets a little tough for my brain. I figure if we act as if we don't recognize someone, perhaps there's a good possibility that we just do not recognize him or her. Then again, I'm not the brain man. And much of what I am offering is what I am sensing or have learned through some study.

I wish I had been the one who founded the *Stephen Ministry program*; Reverend/Doctor Stephen Haugk and some of his wonderful associates, however, accomplished that. This ministry has sent literally thousands of ministers to retirement facilities and nursing homes and to those living alone. There, the ministers listen intently and often pray and sometimes read Scripture with their visited one. It is a grand calling, and a program that I would recommend to anyone, on any continent. They are also found in churches, prisons, in the middle of persons suffering divorce, or the death of a loved one, and so many other situations.

—Fear Again—

I honestly am in fear for the future of our Republic, whether we will gain or lose our desire to be a compassionate people. Right now it seems a toss up, but then again, it may be my fried brain talking. I surely hope I am wrong. Compassion seems far removed at times.

Remember, if you do visit senior citizens, many of them, the more they are visited, will remember you and look forward to your visit, your reappearance. They may not recall what you had to say – especially as you are to mostly be a listener, but they will remember that you cared enough to come and be with them. Often being there says more than what is said. Amen?

BUT BACK TO relinquishing: Imagine if all of us relinquished, so that somehow, in some small way, we would work to make just one person's life a little sweeter? Maybe just reach out to help one person have better quality of living. Can we not work to assist someone in becoming a citizen of another place? Why certainly!

The best part of relinquishing (before I put the subject to rest): it allows one to walk where he/she might have never walked before. I've known friends near death, knowing cancer would soon overtake them. I've watched them work and visit, and do for others, until they could no longer get up and out. This work, visiting others better or worse off than they themselves, so much of this reminds me of a song about surrendering all. What a blessed thought and God-filled song. But for me, the remembrance of that last courageous struggle of those folks is such a moving, wonderful inspiration, I only pray that Father would allow us to recall such memories forever. I sense His loving touch as I say that; *I am sensing God is very near.*

✝

All praise to the Majestic One. The One Who first surrendered all for you and me. The One Who has set us free! Savior, Friend, thank You for this grand knowledge: "FOR OUR CITIZENSHIP IS IN HEAVEN, FROM WHICH WE ALSO EAGERLY WAIT FOR THE SAVIOR, THE LORD JESUS CHRIST, WHO WILL TRANSFORM OUR LOWLY BODY THAT IT MAY BE CONFORMED TO HIS GLORIOUS BODY, ACCORDING TO THE WORKING BY WHICH HE IS ABLE EVEN TO SUBDUE ALL THINGS TO HIMSELF." —Philippians 3:20-21.

Every knee shall bow… Believe it!

—Exercise—

Although this topic comes up now and again throughout these pages, its value can never be overstressed. I am certain that you read the first NEWSFLASH earlier on in the work. I have been excited about arriving at this juncture.

Exercise, which quickly became a regular part of my routine, is a Godsend in so many ways. Whether it is in the form of simply warming up and stretching exercises, or a light form of aerobics, or a form of yoga or tai chi, I am totally convinced of exercise's grand influence not only upon our bodies, but also on our spirit and especially our minds.

I have read briefly about chemical changes that take place within the brain that has an exercised body. I also recall reading that even our eyesight is affected by exercising. I am beginning to wonder what systems/processes are not affected by the moving of our bodies. (No wonder so many of God's creatures have four legs, so they can get around more easily and be better off.)

This is another area I am certain of: I have felt the definitive release of stressors through an exercise regimen. And anyone who has studied AD realizes how devastating a stress-filled life and environment can be upon this already tension-filled progressive disease. Knowing of this benefit alone: that it keeps our stress levels down is enough to keep me diligently working on my physical well being. It is an attempt to keep the old machine well oiled, my dad would have said. At least he would have said it.

A warning here: It is important to remember that sometimes folks with dementia withdraw from participation in events. It is one of the ways they (we) continue to exist on their own level, to 'deal with' a particular situation. Do not force these folks. Simply love them and listen to them. Most of the time that is what matters most. Safety and reengaging them are other matters. And of course, I would encourage reengaging them and getting them started 'moving it' later on, if possible. It is vastly important. It can be life changing.

—Better Blood Flow—

Not only is exercise vital to the patient, I'm sure Lucy would not mind my telling you how much better she feels. That she sleeps better, has greater stamina because she moves it, and she has the sense that it is moving her as well: to better health! I do know it's a wonderful bi-product seeing her smile again. She is perkier after she has exercised. Indeed, she becomes more alive and vital. And a good cardio workout, as has been stated elsewhere herein, has proven to be one of those wonderful mysteries. It allows our brain's cortex to receive better blood flow, and therefore so does the rest of the brain as well!

Hand in hand with exercise is a well-balanced diet. I have chosen not to address diet too much, not only because I do it later on, but also because I believe this line stands out on its own: *Our bodies, as any other living thing, are not only in need of fuel, they also need good fuel.* And fuel is what gives us energy! I do know that foliates and anti-oxidants and certain vitamins DO have a positive sway on our bodies, especially those living with AD. (As a matter of fact, you want to see a good example of what fuel can do for you? Research what Michael Phelps, our recent Gold Medal Winner in China takes in for fuel as he works hard in the Olympics!)

Further, I encourage you to keep studying. I believe there are words following soon which contain a similar line of thinking.

—Not Fuel Foods—

I had a friend who used to stop for something, (something you can eat while you drink coffee) every morning of his young fifty years of life. Note I said 'used to' stop. I had mentioned it to him, but apparently my words went unheeded, or I was too late with them. (No nasty notes from treat lovers.) Everyone knows how some of them are prepared and what they are heavily saturated with/in. I believe his daily habit was the culprit to this man's early demise. (Yes: anyone can sue for anything, but it doesn't mean you'll win....)

On the other hand, I do wish to offer great hope that's been recently released – well, I read it in April of 2007. *Best Life*, April 2007, page 48 contained words from a study in the Archives of Neurology. The article speaks of foliates, and relates that green leafy vegetables, beans, peas and citrus fruits can reduce the risk of developing Alzheimer's by 50%! That's worth reading a second time.

—Repetitious, But: Work It! —

Exercising our bodies, even if it's simply for muscle toning/stretching, aided in addition by a good breathing technique, will cause you to feel so much better and less challenged when it comes to moving the old bones around. You'll love it! Stretch it! Use it! Breathe deeply, slowly at first. Work it!

Cardio work is something I wish my dad had used after he'd departed the Army Air Corps. This man of only forty-three years of age at his death, used to share with me how he could jump as high as he was tall. He also had talked of performing the Canadian Shuffle (an arm and leg coordinated exercise that I have yet to investigate). Unfortunately, I can hardly recall seeing Dad run and I hardly ever saw him exercise. The sedentary lifestyle will take your life quicker than it should be taken. In fairness to Dad though, part of that was due to heart difficulty and being seated in front of a linotype machine for many years after service. *I miss you Dad, every day. Thanks for your service to our country!*

The recharging of our batteries takes place when we manage a good cardio workout. As a young worship leader and minister to folks, I recall another, older leader advising me to be careful of my tongue when the old battery is run down. It is so easy for us to be human.

Of course we are, what I mean to say is: we do not have to be nasty-tongued humans as well. Take this important time for yourself and for others you love. Stay rested as far as possible. And then, move it! Rest and exercise go hand in hand.

It is not difficult to chart your exercise progress, once you've talked with your doctor concerning your plans. When doing a task that causes your breathing and heart rate to increase, something **strongly** recommended, you can easily tell how far you've come by paying attention to how long it takes you during your 'cool down', that is, how long until you get back to your normal breathing cycle. If it is taking too long, you are in need of more work, perhaps you may need to move it a little faster. See your doctor first!

I have failed to study yoga much, but I offer this: The stretching of muscles and tendons, the quietness of it all – the 'centering in' really carries a new dynamic with it. The relaxation of the workout, and the stress-reducing pace of it all seem well worth researching - again, if you are physically able. (And again, I dearly love the free flowing and easy movements (for the most part) of tai chi. Investigate it.)

The inhalation, exhalation, and different body positions have an almost trance-like affect upon me. It causes me to wish myself back in an Asian country, or another place where I might befriend a good follower or teacher of yoga. I have also noted from what I've seen and read, a kinship with dogs, cats and swans, different body positions. *Prepare for pigeon.* This might be a good time for me to check my humor at the door.

These worlds mesh splendidly: yoga or a relaxing, thorough warm-up, followed by a strong cardio workout. These enable the main organs to operate at their peak performance. Here again, I've noted that some of my fellow patients become not so comfortable with regimens; so go slowly, remember that just as no two humans have the same fingerprints, we are all at different levels when it comes to dementia and exercise as well. Yet a good writer must challenge without saying: *You are challenged!*

While I'm visiting the world of exercise, I want to once more emphasize my new fascination and following of Tai Chi. Goldhil has produced a tai chi workout DVD for beginners. I like it a lot. It is narrated, and David Carradine demonstrates the introductory movements. This tai chi workout for the mind not only has an introduction, but also a portion on stretches, stances, Tai Chi Ball, 8 Moves of Chi Kung and Dan Tien Ball Rotation. I recommend it to anyone, diseased or not. It is refreshing and calming and cleansing (to me). (The DVD is designed by Anthem Digital, and again is entitled: *Tai Chi Workout for Beginners.*)

As the decision to begin this new regimen, if it's a new one for you, involves a positive attitude that may very well lead to certain longevity and perhaps a healthier you, I cannot once again overstress its importance. You'll also note, men, if you seek out a trainer or a club, this is no longer a 'girls only' realm. The facilities are much nicer now, better organized, better equipped, and the social aspect alone can be a boon to your day-to-day living.

—Challenge Yourself More?—Certainly! —

Whether you are a boy or girl, man or woman, picture the one who is unable or just doesn't choose to move, then picture the person who moves easily and can walk longer, and by God's grace at a greater level of maximum performance. And keep this in mind as well, if you find a person who is serious about good conditioning, you most likely will find someone with better overall lifestyle habits, that is, how many hung over people have you met at the Y early in the morning? (PS. Do not forget to rest; even Father rested on the seventh day, it is meant for us as well.) And one more while I'm on exercise. I prefer challenging myself a little more.

Sometimes I also utilize *Tae Kwon Do* movements. (It translates into the art of kicking and punching, but if you're up to it, it is an excellent heart-starter and workout guaranteed to keep you fit. I was fortunate to have my first exposure to it with the Korean Tiger Battalion when I served in Vietnam. A good friend, Benjamin Franklin Mercer, and I used to try our hand(s) and feet at it early in the mornings. It is well worth the extra effort.)

†

Awesome One, we come to You fully realizing that You mean our lives to be lived at their fullest potential. We wonder, as You walked all those dusty roads so long ago and climbed those hills for us, if You were not even then giving us certain guidance. You sometimes mention the slothful in your Guidebook. It is not the way You want us to be.

Read God's beautifully picturesque and descriptive 104th psalm! Linger over it. It is well worth your time. It will be a relaxing time, a time of worship and praise, a time to spend with Him. You won't find a better use for your time.

—Quality Of Life – Individuality – Striving Not To Drive Your Caregiver Nuts!—

During this time of the Beijing Olympics and a moon in the north/northwestern sky as I re-entered my home, I recall (at the time of this final rewrite), that striving not to drive someone crazy can be a challenge beyond anything the heretofore-diseased person has ever experienced. That is, even though we strive to live in/as what we have already become, it is necessary for us to strive to maintain forward momentum as well. We must cover some ground quickly, as if that pigskin held tightly to our chest is the most important thing in our life! (Well, most folks will get that.)

Yet we also have to remember, we are admittedly a little different than most people walking around. Perhaps a few examples would be helpful.

I know, in the deepest part of my heart that there will be people who know me who are just cracking up when they read that subheading above. (Thanks a lot!) Clutching our Guidebook, I regularly ask God to assist me in my daily walk, how I conduct myself amongst men (and women). Yet no matter how hard I grasp that wondrous Work, no matter how humble and steadfast or how long I find myself in prayer, I later find that I have forgotten every whispered prayer, every promised word. I have forgotten all those things that I've asked God to change in me, to assist me as I make this walk.

Sometimes, I believe I approach this, too, wrongly. Soon I am stiff-necked and arm tired and hearing myself spouting off words to my Lucy, words that should have remained 'forever locked away, or someplace else', anywhere but where I'd used them. Notice I did not recommend stuffing them, or keeping them within. Sometimes we just need to walk out underneath God's vast canopy and spout off, if the neighbor's windows are closed.

It seems as if the more I struggle with being decent to my wife, or others, the more difficult this focus becomes. And right now, dear God, I'm trying not to blame the deterioration of my mind on my own weaknesses. And sometimes I even find myself trying to recall that Your strength is sufficient, as our Guidebook proclaims. *Yes, I do believe it.*

This, reader friend, is quality of life? This is me, living and loving the best I can for family and friends, and my Lucy. Part of me knows that I should forget the past and press on toward the goal. Brother Paul so well knew what territory existed ever in front of him. Friend, tell me you have not heard God's voice. Tell me you are unable to discern what is right or wrong. And yes, it's true, some folks it seems, no longer can. (And here's the down part of that statement: Some folks are not going to buy it! Trust me.) Try to save one, just one, you'll be glad you did.

Believe it or not, some doctors that write about AD have discovered that there are a multitude of reasons why the patient wanders. But guess what? Not all the wandering has been labeled bad. So long as we return home and do not become road fodder, or completely lost, it is one of the okay ways to exercise. For those of us who figuratively die in the hot sunlight, nighttime strolling is important!

Yet I would never feel completely at ease recommending to anyone or being one who encourages even one patient to wander, not today. I do it because I wear a bright orange and yellow vest, wear a GPS bracelet and my *Safe Return* bracelet. Or I am wrapped within my bright purple and white Alzheimer's Association banner that was given to me upon our trip to Washington, D.C. Yet, unfortunately, with our rate of violence continuing its statistical rise, I DO NOT recommend it. Besides, if you as a patient have been told you cannot walk alone, then you should be a good patient and listen. <u>It has been said for your own safety</u>.

We had a teen-aged kid shoot another teen a few weeks ago. He lived only a couple blocks from us and the victim is now six feet under. The world has certainly become a changed place, thanks mostly to parents who don't take time to sit with, learn and love with their children. Naturally there are many other factors. But how we raise our children (to me) dominates the climate as well as the habits of a lifetime.

As we more and more discover new findings about the disease, I sometimes feel I am less and less prepared to live it in a quality way, yet I will continue to strive to do so. And perhaps that's the best we can sometimes hope for, our striving, our dreaming. But no! It's not where I want it to end it. I am praying that you will do your best to push your way through your disease; that you will Never Give Up! That you will keep striving, hoping and dreaming, always.

—Quick Tip—

Also, my striving to honor God and to live the best possible life I can, is so that I will not send *Doll Face* away in tears, at least not as often. Try it, strive for it. We can help each other. It is my recommendation that the caregiver's side of the Alzheimer's meetinghouse and the patients' side meet together, at least for a few minutes each meeting. This enables not only time for sharing information, it also allows communication to be shared between caregiver and patient that might otherwise never be shared and/or understood. Sometimes some of us do better in public.

—Individuality—

Individuality is tied to all of this as well. It's tied-in because even as we mature as Christians, we yet struggle to be our own person. I suspect that our pressing on, our striving to be better, might necessarily have to take place one step at a time. So often, in the heat of battle between Donna and me, I've found myself too much trying to desperately hold my ground, to make my side of whatever the argument, the stronger side; the side that dictates, the side that wins. I am not sure God wants it that way.

Are we all not somewhat like this? Do you not find yourself sometimes being so stubborn that you later whisper to yourself: *That was not smart,* or perhaps ask yourself: *What were we discussing?*

Pondering whether or not to concern myself with winning or losing a battle, I realize as so many before me: *Man, I may have won a battle, but I think I just lost the whole war!* Fortunately, Lucy and I have learned when to back down, and little by little we are learning the six-lettered word that is most vital to any good relationship, especially marriage.

L I S T E N is that magic word. Unfortunately, some of us never learn to listen. There seems to be one point we just can't seem to get beyond. And what a shame that is. What a selfish, stubborn shame. So many lives surely have been changed by that one simple inability, the strong-headed stubbornness, being unable to bend. It's not all about us. (I have also made an attempt in this short life to recall, God gave us 2 ears and only one mouth, there must have been a reason.)

When we begin to believe it's all about us, the story of life, it may well be time to find that quiet, private spot I spoke of earlier. A time and place where we can contemplate what it is that causes us to continue to place ourselves first. Or as I am sometimes advised, "It's not all about you, Wayne!" I realize that. But sometimes it's a real stretch for me. I have an ego, too. And sometimes it is as with others, way too big!

I also realize that my neurologist's carefully chosen and insightful words, delivered to me this morning at one of our meetings, were very important. He had asked me a question about a particular arm of the government—you know… the one I never quite name. And when I replied: *It's still standing,* he had a quick reply as well. It was about being accountable. I understand, believe in and cherish Dr. John's words and insight. Thanks, Doc. I have talked to God about it.

Back to Lucy's words: that it's not all about me. I agree. But getting from that agreeing area to doing something about it is a stretch for some more distant than God's grand earth-warming sun. As far as that goes, are we not to be *warming up* as we TOGETHER work to agree? Or at the very least, as we work toward a compromise of sorts? Doctor John had felt my obviously heinous response in all its non-splendor. And at that same moment it did flash before me, that I would not look good in numbers or a jumpsuit. Hatred is a very dangerous and often wasted emotion that can get most of us in trouble, and it is the sort of arena the evil one would love to see us enter.

I believe that striving for quality of living and a dash of individuality is fine, but above all else, we must (patients must) submit to striving not to drive the caregiver nuts! It is one of my prayers, friend, no matter what your connection or your interest in this topic, strive to be at peace with everyone. Maintain quiet within your soul. You will find it a much easier march, a lighter load to carry. The very best part of it all: If we are able to concern ourselves with those around us, we might just find that they may show more concern for us as well. It is not being conniving. It is being decent and fair, as God would have us be.

As for the aforementioned peace and quiet, I encourage you to read I Timothy 2:1-2. No, I'm not showing it to you; I am going to pray that you'll find it and read it for yourself. It deals with God, and quiet, and peace.

I yet strive, Lucy. I really do. I strive with my whole being, and I love you. To those of you that I may have appeared more insensitive to during my lifetime, my apologies. There are never enough years to make up for our sins, my sins. Is that not true of most of us?

TIME ZONES (Slipping away…)
Wayne Glenn TERRY

Chapter 12

—Humor Or Horror?—

Time for a great example of how a writer makes it doubly difficult to find a publisher. What I am about to show you drives most editors nuts. Never preface a chapter or sub-chapter with totally different stuff. No, I'll take that back slightly as I see that this segment is on looking back and looking ahead; it is akin to changes. As of the smoothing of this chapter, this time at least, I'll call it the smooth, and as we approached Memorial Day, 2007 (back then), I got that *Ugh*! feeling in the pit of my stomach: mixed emotions. As we prepared to remember fallen heroes, I realized that another one of my nephews was headed for Iraq that very week. Having already lost one nephew in December of 2005, this nephew, Samuel Dewey's, scheduled departure put me on my knees in thanks and in fear at the same time. (So, government agency whose name I do not mention, ask me again, why this old Vietnam vet suffers chronic PTSD.)

Brothers and Sisters-in-Arms, whose heroism and passing we honor this weekend, my regimen to *Never Give Up*! is nothing short of a tribute to you (that I had written at that particular time). How you have blessed this Republic with your personal sacrifices. His eternal blessings upon each one of you, your families and friends; there are no words to cover my respect and admiration for you and yours. Thanks so much.

—Looking Back And Ahead—

When Lucy had first asked me in the quietness of a day's dawn about a change in my demeanor, I responded, "Yes, I have noted that, too." I had become more docile, and had explained how I felt much of it had been due to my work (this labor of love).

Inwardly I also thought how relieved I'd felt as Congressman Forbes had begun talking with a government agency concerning my (at that time) eight-month-old application for assistance. (You will no doubt note various time differences as these segments were not necessarily placed in order of their original creation, and now it has been way beyond a year and a half since I had first contacted that particular agency I never name.) In fact it has now been well over two full years. Their progress and speed is under-whelming.

Also within me was a very strong desire to turn it all over, for I had found that I could no longer go it alone; that I felt I could possibly do something very stupid if I kept carrying that burden. Thus entered God's gracious hand and the many prayers of friends and family in all these happenings. All served to cause certain change within.

I had at last begun to think differently. Maybe, just maybe, it was best that I not only think of myself as diseased, but that I might begin to think of myself as if I were normal, healthy and filled with God's love and grace. Okay, maybe one would perceive it as some form of denial; I'll take it!

One reason I state this treatise is because I had read somewhere, I'll never tell you where now, but I had read about the study of one hundred brains (at autopsy time) of people who had been suspected of having had AD. I recall that of all one hundred people killed in accidents that not one of the diseased patients' brains showed the dreaded AD, but all of them did have some type of abnormality, vascular or previous trauma, for instance. And those are also under the AD umbrella.

Yet as I read the words, I wondered if it could be possible that one might think himself into disease and not really have had it. I do not sense that is the case for me, as my symptoms too closely mirror so many atypically diseased people and fall too much in line with what I have studied and sense myself more and more becoming. Also, the PTSD factor seems to mesh quite well with many AD symptoms. There was no doubt in my mind that something was/is amiss in the old noggin.

Thinking these thoughts in the wee hours (as I stared at pictures nearby on my makeshift writing table) assisted me in pondering that maybe if I strive to be normal, whatever that is, maybe if I act as if nothing has happened to me, perhaps it might serve as a background for longevity and better quality of living also.

In the pictures I found myself at play with grandchildren, relaxing with grandchildren, hiking with them. All appeared happy and normal (as far as anyone can tell). And although I have often felt as one of the titles to another Alzheimer's work, *I Am Losing My Mind*, I began striving to revitalize my entire being.

I guess it is when the **Never Give Up!** guy started to materialize from within. And again, I apologize for any regurgitation. I admit at the time of this final rewriting that I am not as clear as I'd like to be. Sorry.

—No model—

Father has, after all, created such a complex vessel, we humans, and now I speak not simply of the brain dilemma; I speak of God's infinite glory, His power and might. He created us, and as we know not everything, nor shall we ever, I began again thinking that there may be more than one way to look at this rather morbid situation. With that thought in mind, habilitation arrived on the scene and therefore I gradually had fewer thoughts about a debilitating disease.

At the same time I was concerned and puzzled about one particular question that I had recently asked at my local Alzheimer's Association chapter meeting. I had asked the rest of the group (other patients) if any tired easily. I did not get a sense that many of them do/did. I was therefore suspecting that my chronic PTSD was affecting a tiredness that the other folks with dementia were not sensing. Later, however, I was to learn that yes, many of them suffered the same symptoms and maladies that I do, and yes, some were also suffering from PTSD. As I probably reiterated before, there's no model for the disease, yet many of our symptoms are very similar.

At the same time as I wrote those words, I listened to *I Want To See You,* a zippy little church song I so love. It has passionate words in its refrain: *Holy, Holy, Holy, I want to see You!* How appropriate I had thought. And how wonderful my siblings and friends have been to me, that I can not only create, but at the same time listen to beautiful songs.

Yet I must confess, at this same moment, the time of this final rewrite, feeling myself not as lucid and coherent as I'd like to be, I am taking a break from this writing. I am going out underneath God's glorious night sky. When I return, I will continue with what is probably some much needed rest, and then later I shall return to this tired old keyboard. Or rather, tired old me will return to the keyboard.

I have again learned how magnificent it is; how awesome it is; how tremendously mysterious and yet true it is. God can do whatever He wishes, however or whenever and wherever He pleases to! And you and I can do little to change that. If you don't agree with that, that's all right, too. Refreshed and reinvigorated, not feeling as 'cloudy' as I had, I this morning begin again. Please keep in mind, if you are one living with the stress and strain of AD, I not only prayed for you before I nodded off for the final time, but also upon awakening this morning.

—Do Not Wallow—

As I began thinking of being young-feeling again, revitalized if you will, I realized that the *Never Give Up!* attitude really falls more in line with habilitation, the fighting against what may otherwise seem inevitable. Again, it's a challenge. I mean that for YOU also! For this work is not only written for Someone more special than all of us combined; it is written for the truly wonderful people who face debilitating and cumbersome lives.

With this in mind, I now approach each new day differently. I am sensing that I might approach the entire theme of life somewhat differently.

I had started out by taking my very deepest, fullest, yoga-type breath that I could muster. Then I praised God. Next, I exercised, and then I praised our wonderful God. Finally, I read a few words of faith, and once again I praised our living Lord.

As I slowly, yet successfully began looking at my life as a new and great life, instead of wallowing in my worst fears, I actually felt somewhat better, at least in my wherever-I-was noggin I felt somewhat better. Now, why my friend, you may be asking, why hadn't I done this in the very beginning? At the time I had first received word of my diagnosis?

Partly, it is because we must walk our way through various phases, floods of emotions, the sharing of the prognosis with family, friends and a return to our God if necessary. Then and only then, after we have completed all of that and read all we can on the dreaded subject and praised God all we can (and by the way, you can't do that too much), then and only then might we come to the conclusion as did Paul. No matter what my lot in life, I find myself content. Talk about change, and a challenge!

And then I began feeling, rather mysteriously feeling, more combative. It had only taken a period of a few weeks. *What kind of disease is this?*, I had asked myself. That is indeed a lot of material to digest at any one time. However, when one feels God-led, when one scribbles thoughts in the middle of his nights, regardless of his background, one begins to realize in his own finite way, that with God, all things are possible, even when you are feeling combative.

My fingers shook as they searched for the third chapter of Ecclesiastes: "TO EVERYTHING THERE IS A SEASON. A TIME TO BE BORN, A TIME TO DIE; A TIME TO BREAK DOWN, AND A TIME TO BUILD UP; A TIME TO EMBRACE, AND A TIME TO REFRAIN FROM EMBRACING..."

—I Want The Best For You—

Why Father, why do I feel led to these words at this particular moment, this time, at two a.m., in the morning? Why in this stillness of place and time, with only music and the ever pumping, thump-thump-thumping of my oxygenator behind me; why do You, Lord, insist I look more toward rehabilitation?

And if I were one who would tell you that I had heard it from God, but alas I am not, I hope you would allow me to continue. It is as clear to me now, as it had been at that initial moment. And it is why I share this with you. I did sense, and feel it in my bones, that God had said, if I'd heard Him correctly, internally, *"You are thinking of habilitation, Wayne, because you know I want the very best for you..."* And further came, *"...as I do, for all My children."*

How awesome is that? I felt that same lump in my throat, the one I'd felt when I'd received word of my father's death, so long ago. The one you get at the birth of your children, or even at the time of picking up a tiny adopted baby from an institute in India. I sensed God's grand, mighty, scary and yet warming Presence as I realized that He had once again entered my very being, my home. Actually, He's always here. Remember that.

I am certain that God's Presence is sometimes more difficult for us to sense than someone else's, (You may know who I speak of now, and not favorably) who may well be lurking around. Pay him no heed! We are strengthened by our adversities and our God at the same time, and the sons and daughters of Christ are to fear no one!

Lucy and I and our great neighbors, Bill and Debbie, had shared much of the previous day together. And sprinkled throughout it all had been praise music and snippets of conversation about our Lord. I thought as I wrote these words: "Friends and pictures and a church family--that to me includes extended family." I thought about people from my past, about people who had come in and out of my life. As I pondered all these things and felt humbled by God's mighty Presence and His pure Holiness, I came to this understanding: not only does God want the best for me, He also wants the best for you!

In effect I had written it on my picture mirror weeks, perhaps months earlier: "God's love is inclusive. God created each one in His own likeness!" (I don't know if it's written there, if any longer those words are there, for the pictures kind of took over the mirror/memorial.)

Yet within moments, I was reading words I had uttered during our day together. They are words from Philippians, more of Paul's. In the second chapter, the words that caused me to well up were mainly about every knee bowing, every tongue confessing, yet in that same passage is something more. And it's vitally important as well. It is the second part of verse 7, chapter two: "...AND COMING IN THE LIKENESS OF MEN..." My mind's eye was drawn to previous words in the same chapter next: "LET EACH OF YOU LOOK OUT NOT ONLY FOR HIS OWN INTERESTS, BUT ALSO FOR THE INTERESTS OF OTHERS..." To me it is why the preface before this segment (just created this day) rings true.

Yet at the time of the initial draft, I had to further dress myself and get myself outside, as I did only hours ago in my fog-like personhood. I had to get out underneath the vastness of God's grand stars, for I could at this point take it in no longer.

Underneath the magnificence of Father's stars, planets He'd hurled from His fingertips, I could not shake it, I could not depart from it, nor could I depart from Him! It was a time of being filled with God's incomprehensible love, what divine elation! There is none other like it.

Were these changes, my docility, Lucy's acceptance of the new me, and then later my combativeness, had they been offered to me from a God who really cares? My soul shouted: "Yes!" and then, *Thank you, Savior...*

—Sense Of Humor—

It would be easy to say there's nothing funny about AD. Yet to me it would signal a certain admittance of defeat. And as you know from early herein, I am not ready to call it quits, not yet. Besides, I will fight to the end! Can you imagine life if we were unable to laugh at ourselves, our situations and dilemmas? Why we would never laugh.

Allow me to share a humorous moment or two that I've endured. My sweet Donna (Lucy) helped me recall some of these, only because I could not. Most of us suffering dementia deal with similar things:

One day I put an oven mitt in the microwave. I've been known to put my toothbrush in the refrigerator. Once I turned a 7-hour trip into one closer to twelve, and Grandson and I even got to see New Jersey (of course that could have been guy stuff/not asking for directions).

The being unable to ascertain what is up ahead or behind you can be a little disconcerting, that is, landmarks no longer help.

Red is becoming my favorite color (I didn't know it until I read about this one). I'd wondered why it **STOOD OUT SO BOLDLY,** it does for many of us. Hence the background color of this book's cover.

I sometimes dream about a pond in the middle of my living room. I recently punched up 204 on my microwave, attempting to tune in one of my favorite TV shows. Realizing what's behind the lovely faces pasted on my mirror is what really matters (not so funny, but comforting).

Not long ago, I walked the dog's leash halfway down the driveway. Fortunately I'd left Lucy's little dog inside the house (this time).

We had really laughed at that last one, or should I say I wasn't real ecstatic about it until Lucy guided me to seeing the humor in it a day or two later. There are many confusing, agitating happenings where it just might be easier to laugh where you can, and I am thankful for that. Oh, about the leash without the dog, we used to call that *walking the leash – oooh-oooh!*

So thankful am I for a loving partner (most of the time) who has helped me see humor in the midst of dilemma, or as Grandmother used to say, 'Now that you're in a pickle...' Without humor, life would be so very dull and bland. Especially now.

Although sweet Doll Face sees colors differently than most of us, she's enabled me to see the beauty in nature, in music, in poetry, in the faces and the antics of our children and grandchildren. I not long ago saw humor in our playing one of our first board games after I'd been diagnosed. It had been frustrating and challenging at the same time. Yet we had become better friends throughout the process. It would have been much easier for Lucy to remain angry, but she learned instead to love me all the more. I need to remember that.

Never take away one's right to their emotions, after all, would you try to cheer up a one-ton gorilla who appeared hot under her fur? (That's a joke.) Do not attempt to cheer people up when they are hurting! They need to hurt, and we need to support them in their hurting, not cheer them up. (Besides, God agrees with me.) See the book of Ecclesiastes....

Encouragement is grand, but we do not need to always be cheerleaders. Trust me. **It often lacks empathy and does not mean a thing to the person hurting.**

I've often wondered about God's sense of humor. Many times I've muttered, "He'd need a great sense of humor to allow this old world to go on today." Can you imagine how God must feel about what's taking place around the globe? It sometimes puzzles me that He has not already returned; has not wiped us all away. You've seen the stories: 3 teens beat up an old man, or worse, beat him to death. There are many of them.

Have you met the lady who lost her mate and remained angry with God until the day she died? Would it not have been easier, more delightful to everyone (including her) had she learned to recall the beautiful memories that she'd had instead of locking herself away in her madness?

I find a sense of humor almost essential, especially this morning. The original line there would have been: I find a sense of humor essential, and then I go into some other things. But it was this morning, (back then) in November 2007, I awoke somewhere between a dream and reality, not knowing where I lived or how to get to my home. This is part of the tale no one has yet read. (Nor have I shared it with anyone.) I had stepped outside of someone's house and could recognize no other homes or any landmarks. It was, without a doubt, the most traumatic recollection (or foretelling) of my entire life. But as you may have figured out by now, I have been able to get to my computer, and able to turn it on properly, and get to the task I normally begin sooner or later each day. Only today it is (was) quite different.

Now that I have realized where I am, and that I had long ago retired from the Navy, and that I no longer need a retirement order number, as I have been retired since 1984, I will continue with the page of the manuscript that I had left off with somewhere during the night, for now it is very close to the time that I will take my sweet Lucy her tiny breakfast, put out the dogs, feed the cats and so on. (By they way, those days are gone, and now it is Lucy who does the morning chores with the animals before she departs for her workday.) You see, that line, too, was *back then.*

And no one, except the next publisher that reads this will know what has happened. To me, it is as if I had departed, crossed that line I sometimes talk about, but have been able to come back. The first thing I am going to do is fix myself a cup of coffee, and attempt to get re-oriented to time and place.

—Suspicions—

I am sensing, since my spouse, my *Bug,* my Donna, had attended an all day Alzheimer's conference yesterday, that some of what she had shared with me went right to my very core, that somehow the fear and emotion she was exposed to had at least temporarily been transferred to me. I suppose that would be transference. But first, as I said, I am going to have that cup of coffee, and then I am returning to that line about humor.

Okay, so far so good. Coffee next to me, the original line read: I find a sense of humor to be essential. One of my loving daughters had presented me with a small picture book of grandsons and me. Yet there are other pictures within its pages. I had not realized what was so funny until very early one morning (as this one is), soft music playing in the background, my writing light nearby, I began to laugh at what was not such obvious humor in many of those captured scenes.

I suddenly realized that it is not so much what's in the picture; it is very often the dreaming of a grandson on a bank, fishing pole in hand, recalling how we'd spent wonderful summer days together, of his wading in the shallow water, his fishing pole (by now) fast asleep. Victor would seek out a crawdad or a shell or a rock, exploring our world, his world and God's world. It all had caused me to chuckle to myself. (But as the publisher, and now reader knows, I am not exactly in that jovial mood yet. I am, however, working on it.) Were the truth to be known, I am actually a little shaky this morning. Somewhat suspicious.

(You will learn the first reason, as I said, because you will be one of the first to read it. The second reason is because I have two more books that I would like to complete before I really DO totally and completely cross that line.) So, dear friend, now I am asking for your prayers more than ever! And continue with them, please.

For me, there is more of a strong tie to pictures now. For a change, I don't think it will take an expert to explain that. I've seen a book or two about what doctors do not tell you (us). At this point I love my pictures, I've glued many of them to my mirror (as you know). Will it one day be my way of blocking out the face of a stranger, some happy old guy? Now that's humor.

At least for now, it's humor. All right, it is humor and horror at the same time. They say there may come a time when I will not recognize myself, and I can identify with that right now. (Again, the Never Give Up guy is a little nervous this morning, sorry.)

The fun-filled scenes (I keep attempting to discuss) say so much to me. I look at one grandchild and see her standing with a tree-branch, her first fishing pole. I recall the curly-haired Rebecca when she would come running up from our tiny stream with one of her first leaf fish! She will deny it now, as she is older and more knowledgeable. But trust me, it was her first 'leaf fish', Grandpa would not tell any fibs!

I visit another picture, a child standing tall, erect. I recall the day my young woman/daughter, the day Anjuli and I nearly tumbled down a hillside getting to a secret fishing hole. Later, I WATCHED IN HORROR, A DIFFERENT KIND OF FLASHBACK NOW, AS A HUGE SNAKE SLITHERED THROUGH THE UNDERBRUSH ACROSS OUR PATH BEFORE US. Angie had heard it first, but I got to see it with my own eyes, every foot of it!

I am noting in my drafts, (and of course that would be back then I had noted in my drafts), I'm beginning more and more to find words with fewer letters therein, or the other way around, sometimes with extra ones. Yet some of them still sound much the same to the ear, thus my gradual decline I suspect. I wish I could tell you that I am not afraid, but it's frightening! If I turned that a bit… if I said this grandpa's writing has become off-kilter, could you perhaps note a sense of humor in that? I surely hope so. I pray a bit of humor for you, too, dear friend.

You see, without humor, I've sometimes pondered how very long and dreary the journey would be. I myself laugh when I hear my brother, David's, loving laughter on the other end of the line as I share with him, "You know, I've always been a little wacky."

I also laugh when my close friends and neighbors' faces light up and Bill and Debbie cannot believe what I've just said or done. As far as that goes, I see humor in my changes of behavior as well. I guess that's all part of the plan. Right, Lord? Right?

Humor IS the glue that often allows us to keep our lives intact. Humor is the spice that enables us to get a flavor for the not-so-humorous dishes that we might later be served. It is my belief that humor is from God! Humor is what must suffice when we are unable to have the drug of choice or whatever we feel we need to ensure more of our neurotransmitters stay in circulation. And naturally, I will never rule out faith. But sometimes, to one meek and shaky, as I now am, faith does not seem to be enough. Shame on me. I will pray and ask for patience, courage and diligence.

I sense humor when I hear my old sergeant friend, okay, Gunnery Sergeant Leonard, on the line from the Lone Star State, *"And this is something new for you, Squid?"* So many wonderful friends and relations, sons and daughters, Momma, so many have been joy and strength for Lucy and me. Many have helped us get through some tough times. Thanks to each one of you. You're the best! And our Lord, He is in and through it all, thorns and all.

I beg of you, never forget how helpful laughing at yourself can be. For no matter how bizarre our lives become, a sense of humor before, during, or after the crisis may well be the surfboard that thrusts you through and over troubled waters. And again, is it not all from God?

This segment was not intentionally written to be insensitive to anyone. I fully realize that we are all at different points, different stages, so perhaps some of you will not find humor in my lacking faith words earlier. I also find that we are all changing as I write these words, and I sense the various emotions and their affects upon me. We are after all, human, are we not?

Perhaps your time of humor has passed. I pray not. Whether you are patient, caregiver, or a friend of one with AD, you might wish to look at Ephesians 4:32 or Deuteronomy 7:7-8. When I read the Deuteronomy passage, about folks being brought out of bondage, it was as if God was saying, *"And you thought Wayne's words about humor were empty?"* And there's the former writing, I've often found this Ephesians passage hauntingly comforting, a real heart-starter... "AND BE KIND TO ONE ANOTHER, TENDERHEARTED, FORGIVING ONE ANOTHER, EVEN AS GOD IN CHRIST FORGAVE YOU." *Wow!* Double wow! How can anyone not sense His loving presence in those grand words?

I've called them haunting because they haunt me daily, the being tenderhearted and forgiving part. Might there be one you have failed to forgive, or perhaps even you yourself? That act (of forgiveness) can open a whole new chapter in your life. Communication is far better than any pill on the market and so very much better than 'stuffing it' as I have for too many years done with my PTSD song. What a horrible and ugly 'beat you up' game it has become to me. I wish it were a game.

Unfortunately it is a syndrome that is triggered by events and sounds and smells and places, and it is not as easily filed in the back of our minds, as some would have you believe, whether they are shrinks or good friends in the pulpit.

One last attempt at humor: There was one other time when I awoke and could not recall what country I was in. That's not a grand feeling the first time, yet I have laughed often since that experience took place. I realized it was God's way of enabling me to travel without leaving home! I don't believe we should challenge God on His decisions as to what happens to whom and when. I know I'd be scared to challenge God on anything. But I know this, too. Sometimes I do.

†

Thank You, Awesome One, Savior, Friend, for Your sensitive ways and words, Your loving care to us. It is a wonder how You've promised to always be with us, go with us, even unto the end. What a comfort You are! Thanks, Jehovah, for giving us a sense of humor, a way that we might escape our seemingly difficult times and traumas. Your way is always one that brings us back to peace and joy and resolution. Might Your Holy name be forever praised!

—Variances And Selfless Love—

Having attended many meetings (again) with other diseased folks, meetings on both caregiver and patient sides of the house, I have noted many different personalities and adaptations. These differences (our brain compared to normal-brained folks) I am convinced you may never fully recognize. It is difficult enough for my neurologist friend and myself to recognize them. I did, however, sit with my Diplomat of Neurology this very morning (at the original time of this writing), and he had verified many of the sensations/realizations that I continue to have about myself. He also helped me understand that the *fried brain*

- 247 -

theory and the brain stem swelling stuff I have talked about are more likely to be that I simply have limited reserves, and that the brain-swelling thing is 99% more likely to be the bone spurs located near my C5 and C6, earlier reported to so many, who never seemed to care one way or the other.

But back to the theme at hand. You may not know you have it until you've experienced it first-hand and then are gone. And I'm not convinced that we'll learn of it then. I mean, how will we hear of it? Will anyone?

What I'm again sharing is: do not buy into the possibility that you have AD, for you may have lived for years and years, as I have some already, with your zombie-like walk at night, finding yourself often tired to the bone, only to learn that you never really had it. Or it may be you DID have it, that no one ever figured it out, perhaps even family and friends, yet it's a moot point once you're gone, is it not? (I also apologize if this is territory I already covered, or I have repeated myself. For to me it all seems somewhat repetitive. It is one of the problems with rewrites and lapses of memory as well.)

You have no doubt often heard my tale about my broken tooth. I realize that post-traumatic stress has been a horrible burden. I began to wonder if my *brain thing* really is or is not a result of AD. It is a very uplifting realization, when you get right down to it, that we still, as alluded to earlier, control very little, whether the diagnosis is right on or totally off! Then again, there are many different forms of dementia. It doesn't even have to be called Alzheimer's. Often I just wish it would all go away.

That is, what you and/or loved ones may have believed to be AD all those years may well have been a vascular disease or some other indistinct problem that remained hidden until your skull is one day opened and the obscure is made clear. I apologize if I once again repeated myself, such is the disease. Such is the life of one often tired.

How I wish I were some great brain-honed professor of this school of thought, but I'm just an average guy with a casual writing ability. *Sorry, Lord, I am thankful for and realize any gifts are from You.*

When you get right down to it, do you really believe it matters what exactly the situation is or what name it is given? My neurologist friend advised me that getting out into sunlight and its ultraviolet rays would have a really grand affect upon me. That's a free one. It has something to do with the 'feel good' chemicals our body makes/releases. For me, it ended up that the hot sun just made me very weak, very fast.

To me, is it not our learning what God's will is for us that matters most? And as for will, are we not bound in our Christian walk to be humble and devoted to His decisions for us, fair or seemingly unfair? Why yes, of course we are.

These variances, these differences, begin who knows when or where. My desire to examine this topic more fully is that you might come to this end: No matter what you or your care partner are now enduring, no matter what the trial, or how long the journey, or what name it is given: there is help promised to you and yours! It is a line worth repeating, and so I shall. There is help promised to you and yours!

I do apologize for any waning faith, but I know God provides care and love, and that He goes with us through these troubled times that perhaps we cannot overcome due to our lack of faith, at least, it would be more difficult without Him. His promises come from His selfless, devoted love for the ones He so wonderfully made. And as for my apparent lack of faith, men greater and much stronger in faith than I (includes women), have suffered similar atrocities in life and lost the battle. Yet isn't it true, don't you believe God was (and is) there with them all along? I do!

I once again turn to our beloved brother Paul: "AND HE SAID UNTO ME, MY GRACE IS SUFFICIENT FOR THEE: FOR MY STRENGTH IS MADE PERFECT IN WEAKNESS. MOST GLADLY THEREFORE WILL I RATHER GLORY IN MY INFIRMITIES, IN REPROACHES, IN NECESSITIES, IN PERSECUTIONS, IN DISTRESSES FOR CHRIST'S SAKE: FOR WHEN I AM WEAK, THEN AM I STRONG." —II Corinthians 12:9-10.

Those most powerful words (probably seeming crazy to most of us) are meant for edification, not the tearing down or apart of anyone. The new Paul, not the old Saul, had a way of looking on the God-filled, Spirit-filled side of things, even when they seemed godless. And certainly as he penned the *building up* words, did his mind's eye not see what he'd already endured and perhaps what was yet up ahead for him? His eye, you see, was always on the mark.

Now, turn with me to Micah 6:8 (KJV, Amplified Bible, Zondervan): "HE HAS SHOWED YOU, O MAN, WHAT IS GOOD. AND WHAT DOES THE LORD REQUIRE OF YOU BUT TO DO JUSTLY, AND TO LOVE KINDNESS AND MERCY, AND TO HUMBLE YOURSELF AND WALK HUMBLY WITH YOUR GOD?" (They are words I should wear around my distrusting, unbelieving, frustrating, conniving neck.)

Can you not, friend, identify with Paul? Can you not see that no matter what our condition, whether in the same boat or in one with an entirely different frame or destination, can you not see it simply does not matter?

A grand friend, (you've heard me mention before), Dr. Reid, put it to me a little differently within hours of this original writing. It had dealt with a totally different subject, as she looked me squarely and unwaveringly in the eye: "I want you to settle down. Do you really believe one more day is going to make a difference?" Even though the one more day had turned into one more month, I readily understood (later) the good doctor's sage advice, especially as I am not one to argue or instruct persons who are in distress. I would much rather listen to them, support them. After all, she is the doctor and I, the patient. But trust me, it was not her in distress.

Now, as I've been through all I've endured with our different institutions (?) (Amazing description). I certainly agree with the good doctor even more. There is no rush today to get any paperwork to anyone who is supposedly in the field of assisting folks in need. Trust me. And if you care to share your opinion of how they are going to handle you, or of what they will have to say, you well may only make the whole situation worse. Trust me again. No, trust God.

When I recently spent some time making out my will, I thought it again: Do you really think one more day will matter? It is a question we should delve into: our differences and we. Or what we perceive to be reality.

I met a young woman, Amy, only weeks ago. She shared, after I'd inquired about a sling-like contraption wrapped around her hand extending beyond her wrist, that she'd suffered severe pain for the past seven years!, pain from an accident that literally had torn her hand loose from her wrist!

She continued on about what was to take place the next month, that she had had no feeling in her hand, and that they, the doctors, were planning to remove her hand, take out the pins and plates and screws, and then reattach the now motionless, feeling-less appendage. After I had prayed with her, right there in the store, I later could not rid myself of her story, the journey she is 'having' to make. It is indeed a variance, a difference extraordinaire. Not only that, she is one extraordinary person! God be with you.

You need to know (a few months later), Amy is doing well now, and her post-operative recovery seems encouraging. Praise God. How gracious is He? We cannot comprehend it.

And yet, as much as Amy's story and your story and perhaps my story, as much as they all differ, we have a commonality. Some dilemmas may make us different from each other, yet we are all bound together in/by our differences. "SO THAT THEY CAUSED THE CRY OF THE POOR TO COME TO HIM; FOR HE HEARS THE CRY OF THE AFFLICTED." —Job 34:28.

Do you see how afflictions sometimes cause us not to have so much self-pity? And that is interesting. You may be attempting not to show that you are in the middle of distress and dilemma, and yet all around you, you may also be noticing that there are those who say you are acting badly, and using your disease as an excuse to behave badly. Is it any wonder at one time or another that all of us seek and run to a place where we can hide?

In our variances, God is telling us in this masterpiece of literature, Job, oppression causes God's intervention! How many weighed down, fail to turn to the Creator? On the opposite hand, how many can no longer go it alone, and finally admit it and acknowledge God's rightful sovereignty, His power, and His almighty dominion?

I just suffered another leg spasm so harsh that people in the place I was seated thought I was having a heart attack. I would guess it's something that stress brings about. Do you think I thought of Him? I certainly did. Just as no man knows when He shall come again, very few of us know of our final moments. No, I'd say none of us knows that, not unless we have chosen them, and that can be one very sad and dark decision.

I am not declaring that God necessarily causes oppression to bring us to these professions, these awakenings, yet it is true that these situations are allowed throughout our lives, are they not?

We all encounter an uphill battle of one sort or another now and again. Surely all are smitten or wounded or accidentally harmed in some way, sometimes even maimed or killed. We call it accidental, but is it? Are they?

I've heard it so often declared: If you feel far from God, you might want to check to see who has moved. (Oh yes... He moves, but as God is in and through everything, everywhere at the same time, Omnipresent, He is also with you). Or as Joshua declared, "FOR THE LORD YOUR GOD IS WITH YOU WHEREVER YOU GO." —Joshua 1:9. Pretty much self-explanatory. The book of Joshua enables us to see God's working in human situations, God's divine interceding. Does it not reconcile us to Him? I believe it does, and it always will! *There are no accidents!*

Variances? Yes and no. Different situations? Some. Different choices? Certainly. I surely feel deep within the very fiber of my being, if we remain God-centered instead of believing all of life revolves around us, what a difference there can be in our daily lives. For that matter, for the entirety of our lives! You may wish to read that one again.

Yet there are times when it takes practically an entire lifetime to get that *stuff* into one's noggin. Sometimes it takes the allowing of certain albatrosses hung around our tender necks, does it not? I believe it has with me.

And then there are times I recently learned, no matter how much a diseased person attempts to behave, it isn't necessarily going to happen. *NEWSFLASH:* This is the portion you may want to share with your caregiver, because it is indeed a tough, not-full-of-happiness time that tests your love to its limits! That is, I had been having a great time on a recent cruise, but learned not too long into it, my mate was about to throw me over the side. You heard it before. And even though my neurologist had said he felt the experience would be good for me, it ended up that I had to listen not only to those near me that I love, but also the one who is supposedly closest to me--my beloved partner. I soon found out, my wandering eyes and my desire to dance with anyone and everyone onboard was not an occasion that everyone was finding part of the fun cruise. Trust me.

†

...ʺBUT GOD DEMONSTRATES HIS OWN LOVE TOWARD US, IN THAT WHILE WE WERE YET SINNERS, CHRIST DIED FOR US.ʺ —Romans 5:8.

Can you imagine it? Comprehend it? Compare it to any earthly thing? I see a soldier spread prone atop another in battle, his sole purpose to take the rounds and shrapnel for a friend, or perhaps one he does not even know; I picture another entering a fiery building to pull out a total stranger; and always there are those pictures of brave people entering our nation's World Trade Center on that fateful and devastating day in 2001: Selfless love shown by so many, after the dastardly atrocity.

Variances? I believe God waivers not. You see, He is constant, always here, there, everywhere! Guess what I am about to do? Thanks to my early morning meeting with my neurologist friend, I am going to take a meritorious morning off from this effort. I am going out into God's brilliant ultraviolet rays and see what becomes of me. What a blessing it often is, talking to another; after all, did He not mean us to have communion one with another? Thanks, Doc. Thanks again. *And thank You, Heavenly Father.*

†

Holy One, thank You for the depth and beauty of Your constant and selfless love for us; Thank You for the beauty with which You daily surround us. Even if we are without sight, can we not yet sense and hear and touch Your beauty? For You, our shield and protector, have been so wonderful to each one of us, even when we would find ourselves daily suffering. Suffering from/in all these variances of life. Help us, Creator, to realize that Your constant, awesome, selfless love for us is not something that just happens, that You had long ago planned

*these things even before our first thought, our first awareness.
Assist us in understanding the depth of,* "RETURN TO YOUR
REST, O MY SOUL, FOR THE LORD HAS DEALT BOUNTIFULLY
WITH YOU." —Psalm 116:7.

—Still Here—

Praise God! I'm still here. I so love life. Although my
reserves may be limited, when you've had a rich and full life,
you enjoy each and every day, commune with Master more and
more, your attitude usually changes for the better. If one's
attitude is right or as someone once penned, *If the man is right,
his world will be right.* Simply put, I know and am convinced
attitude affects much of life and leads to a happier, longer life,
even for those of us diseased; even for those of us who cannot
seem to change enough, and may never be able to LIVE as we'd
like to profess we live.

I do admit the 0100 and 0200 rising is tiring, but on the plus
side: I am still here, still working, reading and writing. There is
however, one portion of my life I wish I had by now rid myself
of, and that is the looking over my shoulder and feeling
someone is watching me. It hasn't served me well. Suspecting,
suspicion, always looking around, being on guard, it's a big part
of PTSD 'stuff', stuff they were talking about once again not
that long ago when the deplorable conditions at Walter Reed
Hospital in Washington, D.C., (March 2007) hit the street.

Washington did another one of their band-aid approaches
and moved quickly on. PTSD is a small item to some, it seems.
After all I've shared with you, can you believe it? That part of
the story is not yet over. And in October, a full seven months
later (during a rewrite run-through, now even further out) I
noted headlines of one Florida paper and others that read how
on the rise was wartime trauma and situations associated with
PTSD. This story will continue on and on, and for some: it will
never end.

Though I'm yet here, the early rising is most likely caused
by dementia, as well as combat memories (and again I regret
any repetition). When one has that inevitable 'mare, there is no
mistaking it. I yet ask Creator God to rid me of these
albatrosses. It is not over on the PTSD. On 4/24/07, I notified a

particular agency, as well as others, that I had just completed letters to two more senators and four additional congressmen, it sounds akin to Chapter Six, does it not?

It was shameful: the response I received! I have heard that short of dying or being destitute, there is absolutely nothing you can do to expedite your claim. So if you're one fortunate to have a claim pending, friend, try to hang in. No one seems to want to go up against Uncle or any other outfit that SHOULD be monitoring the progress of these matters, partly because everyone knows these departments have enough other situations to manage at present, partly because they believe we will go away, or fade away, or die.

It is a shame that this, too, has become a handy excuse for their inaction. Today, in the midst of this re-typing and re-reading of this chapter, as I ready to be nearer to printing it out, I will write yet another letter to a Virginia Congressman, from the 11th District. Cross your fingers and toes. (That was quite some time ago, and you can well imagine what the return was from it: *nada, zilch, zippo!*)

Longing to report these atrocities vanished, my friend, is an understatement. Regardless, my regimen is going quite well. I remain fit. I eat properly and have actually ceased smoking! Thankfully I maintain a strong accounting for daily exercise. These have become hallmarks essential to a world I attempt to maintain, as you'll read in chapter 13.

I wish I could somehow realize a breakthrough on why I do not sleep much, (or at least understand it more clearly) and/or learn how to sleep (And that is improperly worded because I know WHY I don't sleep, it's just that it may never change). I guess in the long run, it will simply mean finding time to *remain at rest* when I am not actually getting that big two to three hours of sleep. All right, sometimes only one or two. Then again, I get another segment, or so.

Some of this, again, is caused from wartime memories and current happenings. There is nothing as much as war to help recall old friends. Lots has happened since the sixties and then the early nineties to refresh and revitalize a veteran's memories and emotions, especially those of long ago. I guess this malaise which literally thousands of other veterans besides myself face will be considered less important than the energy problem, now that they have screwed that all up.

†

I looked this morning with fondness at pictures of my niece, Autumn's new son, and one of my brothers son's new set of twins as well. They reminded me of an older niece's sons. Her name is Michelle, another former uniform-clad warrior of yesteryear. As I looked at all the babies and ones not so much babies any longer, I also reveled in the recent birth of my son's first son, Daniel Wayne.

At that same time I thought of baby's sweet mother, Debbie, my son Chuck's wife. Next, I recalled another daughter by marriage, lovely Jessica. Jessie's baby was to follow when I had first typed these words, yet now little Abigail is with us! *Wow!* is what I'd conjured up at that moment. Jessica belongs to Lucy's side. But to me there will never be any sides, for we are ALL God's, just as He has offered himself to all of us! Just as God leads us through life's dance!

The grand arrival of these new little ones has already offered us richer fuller lives. Lives granted these earthen vessels only through God's abundant, never-ending grace. You see how wonderful is our God? Can you sense His wonder and awe, God's infinite love?

†

So how is it with you, friend? Are you seated in a wheelchair, as is my good friend, Mr. Nelson? Are you closeted away in a world that you're not allowed to yet depart? Can you even read these words? I pray these words find you well this day or evening. *Really.*

I long ago learned to be in prayer for the entire world. Praying only for those close at hand is a sad reminder that we should not forget the rest of humankind, even as diverse, divided and often bruised as it seems and sometimes is. I know and understand that our God's love is inclusive; that is one reason I offer up prayers for whoever might take this book in hand.

No matter what your lot; no matter where you may be; I have prayed and am praying for you. I mean that. Though I may never meet you, I love you. For you, dear friend, were created by the same Almighty who created and loves me. We are all of a piece; part of God's gloriously awesome creation that stretches so far that we will never fully understand its length or depth, it's infinite height! Why, we're even learning that what we had once called a planet is really (at least one of them) a moon, and that there are stars out beyond that. We are just now beginning to get a glimpse of/at a portion of God's wondrous, abundant and infinite creation. (What do you suppose will happen once they tweak our 18-year-old Hubble telescope?)

Is it not by God's majestic grace alone that you and I have been afforded so many grand sights and sounds; so many exciting years? Even if you only feel those well-defined marks beneath your fingertips, created for those without sight, do you not feel blessed by Him as well? Blessed by a God a writer once penned: *to Whom a thousand ages seem as an evening gone?*

These words were typed only hours after I had once again *dumped* the entire two hundred and seventy-plus pages of manuscript that I had already typed for the umpteenth time! And I had spent an evening and the better part a morning moping about, and asking myself whether God really wanted these words to ever appear in print. Yet it was not long until He once again took me by the hand, reminding me of my value and of how much He loves each and every one of us, even in our feeble attempts to describe His wonderfully marvelous attributes for the rest of the world.

It was during that glimpse, that tiny fraction of time, when He once again told me: *Keep on. Be of good cheer and faith.* He always astounds me! And it was not long thereafter that my beloved brother, David, presented me with a brand new laptop computer as he said, "See if this one will hold all those superlatives." My brothers and sisters all have been so wonderfully gracious to me during this time of need and transition. Mother, too. And again, children and grandchildren, how wonderfully blessed I have been. I'll say it again. You have made my life wonderful. Really. Each and every relation and friend and many strangers have showed me so much compassion. I am very thankful indeed.

When I think of and thank God that I am yet here, I also thank Him that you, too, are here; that God is granting you the courage and strength to enjoy even more moments, more days. I'm learning to take it one day at a time, as our Guidebook tells us, even those days when I have accidentally *dumped* all my precious words that God may well laugh at. Yet I don't believe He does. I believe our gracious God hears each of our longings, prayers and praises. I believe He seeks to hear them, and that He savors them as well.

The Sunday school song of long ago rings true today: *Yes, Jesus Loves Me.* It is so worth repeating for all mankind. And yes, Jesus loves you! And He will love you forever. Trust Him, reach out to Him, and praise God forevermore!

†

Prince of Peace, Wonderful Counselor, Teacher and Friend – thank You for loving my reader friend, and for loving me. Thank You that we are allowed yet to be. How You love each and every one; how you forget not one. It is all so very amazing to me. God, You are the balm upon our slightest wound, even those hurts that no one else knows or cares about. Thank You, Father, for the real possibility of healing – for the very real possibility that there yet may be a miracle for so many. For I have watched and been a part of so very many miracles. Your gracious love is beyond compare. You are Lord forever and ever. Might You more and more lead us to disease cures? But more than this, make us brave warriors when we must live with disease, with hardships that some will never know, let alone imagine. How we love You, Father. And how we look forward to living with You for eternity, where we will sing and dance, pray and praise!

"YOU DID NOT CHOOSE ME, BUT I CHOSE YOU AND APPOINTED YOU THAT YOU SHOULD GO AND BEAR FRUIT, AND THAT YOUR FRUIT SHOULD REMAIN, THAT WHATEVER YOU ASK THE FATHER IN MY NAME HE MAY GIVE YOU." —Job 15:16.

Chapter 13

Memorial Day, as you might imagine, has always been a tough time for veterans of many wars. In remembrance of fallen heroes, we yet continue on. Word search puzzles are becoming increasingly easier for me, that is one of the benefits of continuing to work the mind, of pushing through that which you do not feel you can push through.

What I am reporting to you, dear friend, is that the challenging of the diseased, of our mental, physical and spiritual selves aids us as we become more and more attune to the spokes of the wheel-paradigm presented herein. You need to know the Hebrew name for Ezekiel is Yehezke'l, and that it means *God strengthens*. I am hopeful this regimen will be nothing short of remarkable for you. I encourage you to attack a routine, what your senses tell you will work for you, and then stick to it with all your might. *And never, ever give up!*

—Socializing – Ezekiel's Wheel Vision—

Socializing often means a great deal in any progress-making mode. Since AD often causes folks (such as me) to *shut down* (that is their normal routines and functions not only quickly change and become diminished), but they (referring to a patient) wish to be alone at times. A lot. I have nevertheless prayed over and studied, and as I wrote this work have been led to this paradigm for assisting dementia-affected folks in order that they (You) may maintain quality of life for as long as possible.

Unfortunately, as earlier stated elsewhere herein, I have found socializing to be the most difficult portion of this regimen. It is also another item that is customized, indeed, it is different for each one, how they (we) cope or do not cope when engaged in socialization. The paradigm (model) below, with arms (spokes) radiating with God the center, our Creator and Father and Friend, are addressed herein. Perhaps this is a good place to gather all these rascals together.

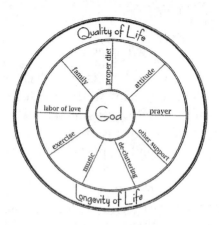

The wheel diagram contains the following labels: Quality of Life (top), proper diet, family, attitude, labor of love, God (center), prayer, exercise, other support, music, de-cluttering, Longevity of Life (bottom).

Graphic Art by Susan Ash, *www.completepicture.net* Phone: (804) 598-6969

Each spoke as you can see, is an area that requires dedicated attention, where possible, always with God at the center of the circle's very core. For God, the Creator of life is also the very center of life. Without Him is death. He is in and through everything. He gave and continues to give us life, and He allows us to drink from those everlasting waters that sustain us throughout this life and the life yet to come. *That is the Christian's great hope.*

—Spokes—

Attitude. A good attitude is the acceptance of what we believe to be factual; it is a presumption that longevity and quality of life are more than possible. It, for a moment, dismisses the notion that AD is not only very stressful and emotion-filled living, but also that it has devastating results upon our daily lives. But with God as our center, and His leading us to the best possible attitude, I believe we can achieve and maintain an optimal daily regimen regardless of the situation or dilemma. God has a way of making the rough roads smooth, the weak strong, those in fear quite unshakable. Indeed God is able to remove stressors that would normally hasten a more speedy demise. He enables those seemingly powerless to become advocates for others who are broken. He heals! This attitude of utmost confidence must be believed and lived to its fullest in order for the patient to become successful. I do not feel it is a total denial of our individual dilemmas, but that it gives us hope as we look to Him. After all, God is our greatest and only hope that enables us to not worry so much about the things of this world. *He can change gray skies to blue, and make the best become of you!*

Labor of Love. Another important area: If there is only one hobby, one interest, one affection that attracts the diseased individual, their being enabled to pursue that *one love* can for them bring about great change! Patients need to be allowed and/or enabled to feel in control of their lives, as far as possible. They need to feel useful, and should not be argued with or told what to do, again, as far as possible. This non-threatening environment should be broken only for issues of safety. A *labor of love* enables them (us) to focus. It keeps them more active; indeed at times it will rejuvenate their very being. Remember, many people do not lose their ability when it comes to skills that they've earlier learned. Some who cannot now talk, still play piano, for instance. One of my AD-friends used to be a dancer; she loves to dance. It is that 'allowing' that assists people in feeling useful, something many outside the circle fail to understand. Folks outside the circle have a tendency to baby or be overly protective and/or cautious. Yet sometimes that, too, is necessary.

Unfortunately, some close to the patient become bossy, and that is not what is needed for anyone's regimentation. Frustration is detrimental for everyone, but more so for diseased folks. Again, reading and puzzle-working are great! One reason I love writing, my labor of love, is because it activates my hippocampus and cortex, keeping frontal brain lobes in the best possible shape!

Music. Remember those deep-seated emotions, that part of us not easily erased? How easy it is to invite and/or enable patients to sing along? Remember in an earlier segment how their eyes shone, how they rocked back and forth? AD does not mean an end to participation in life, not by a long shot. And shame on the facility that allows their charges to sit asleep through much of the day, slack-jawed in front of soaps or other garbage on television, 'stuff' seemingly more important to their tenders than what workers should be focusing upon. Notice I did not use *caregiver* then. (Those who allow patients to miss out on opportunity that might assist them or in someway enable patients, those workers in my estimation are NOT caregivers.) Aides (and others) who allow patients to be treated as if they are being 'baby sat' contribute little or nothing to a habilitative process. God forgive us! (And if you're an early onset patient who could have helped this situation, God forgive you as well.) Admittedly, it is more difficult for those diagnosed, and/or in later stages to assist in any alleviation of the difficulties of living with the disease. Music though, is a balm to our bruised souls. And the baby-sitting remark is not always aimed at the ones watching the AD folks; indeed it more often falls squarely upon the shoulders of the supposed leadership of the facility, for they are ultimately responsible for this remarkable (unplanned?) atrophy of the human spirit and existence.

"De-cluttering." Sometimes I get caught up in the order of things, and perhaps this is one of those times. Remember how relieved I'd felt as I 'de-cluttered' my living area, especially my room? There is the possibility that de-cluttering may of necessity be one of the first things an AD person should accomplish. De-cluttering gives the patient great potential that he/she might otherwise have never sensed. It lessons confusion and often assists patients in feeling more in charge. Here again, however, is a caution, for some, stripped of too much too soon, may feel more quickly abandoned, and this happening may therefore cause a reaction we need to be concerned about. The reactions are what cause concern, or should. This unnecessary defoliating of their personal garden can be akin to your first flight in the F-22, the hundred and thirty-million dollar jet fighter that will show you what eight to ten Gs cans do to your body. It can cause sudden barren devastation to the patient with no good end. Therefore, some de-cluttering may have to be done slowly, carefully, nothing at all like the speeds of the F-22.

I have found it particularly easy for me, de-cluttering, (as I desired to have some say about what keepsakes and personal treasures went where and to whom). Here again, it would depend upon what stage the patient is in as how it will affect her/him. Regardless, allow the AD person freedom to be involved in these decisions if they are able to. (One of the single most unfair mistakes people close to AD patients make is in not allowing the patient to be a part of certain decisions, again, where possible.) There are times of course when patients cannot be part of the decision-making process.

I hear my beloved, *I Surrender All,* playing softly in the background. To me it is music from God. De-cluttering in a sense is surrendering as well. Now, this works differently upon the moving of a patient, for one uprooted and moved, if it indeed must be accomplished, may well require that certain mementos and/or pictures accompany them, so they may retain a sense of *home* when at all possible. At the very least, these items, if the patient can connect with them, can be of great comfort to them. (Some other good information: seven out of ten patients are able to live where they've always lived, at home.) And if it's possible, so should it be!

If an AD patient can no longer live at home, at least be sensitive about your manner and the way in which the patient is moved. It is an agonizing time for everyone, even under the best of circumstances. Be gentle, kind and considerate. Listen as much as you are able. This is a special time for teamwork. It is also a time to continue in prayer with Creator God.

Exercise. This spoke of Ezekiel's Wheel cannot be over emphasized. It is 'breathing', 'moving it', an aliveness that is essential, (again, where possible and/or under a doctor's watchful eye). The portion alone which addresses deep breathing is essential, and can be a great releaser of stress. That alone is worth striving for.

The moving of muscles and appendages. I have before diagnosis and after, been upset by the lack of concern for the moving about of patients in some facilities, that is, they are often kept sedentary for too much of their day. Frankly, it sometimes may end up that the home front, and/or visiting caregiver(s) must take charge here, and/or gently, slowly, attempt to enable not only the getting up and moving around the facility of the loved one, but also the physical movement of the person's appendages, whether it is in the form of stretching, light aerobics or simply walking about. It is also necessary to add: patients should not on the other hand be forced against their will to participate where it may cause a bad reaction. AD patients should not be argued with and/or cajoled in any way. Yet once they are 'on the move' it can be a rewarding continuum for the patient and caregiver alike.

Unfortunately, medical workers and other attendees (aides) assigned to some facilities seem to take pleasure in having fun with patients at the patient's expense. It is not slander friend, it is fact. I'm sure you've worked somewhere and realized how it is 'on paper' and how it really is, that the two are, simply put, different animals. God forgive us. You see, without God at the center of this wheel, much of this regimen will not work. We need honesty and compassion and clarity in our living, especially when it comes to those debilitated. Many patients cannot, after all, fend for or defend themselves. And I know too much sometimes takes place behind closed doors. This is not a figment or imagination of some old minister's mind.

Finally, I can honestly say that exercise and its benefits are more important than we will ever realize to persons who are diseased. Not only does it set you apart from the average diseased person, it will go a long way to enabling you to live longer and healthier (and happier) than many parts (other spokes) in this wheel regimen. (See the NEWSFLASH, earlier in this work—words from a famous Chicago doctor and national panel.)

Proper Dieting. Diet is an essential element to every living being, and to every good regimen on the face of planet Earth! Having been on more than one occasion 'called in' over this medical reading and/or that test, I have learned that one is often able to assist in 'righting' those numbers that had indicated further testing might be needed; Often it was accomplished by changing a habit, or ensuring that I simply started to intake whatever had been lacking in my diet. When people refuse to go to doctors, or are not followed by a caring family physician, they are more liable to have problems that could have been successfully avoided. Good dieting not only assists us in 'running' at our optimum level, it can certainly affect our daily feelings and attitude. (Just the lack of fiber alone from our daily diet is one example of how bodily functions can be affected in a negative way.) Thankfully, some facilities/institutions can be 'messed up' in other areas and yet be good about providing a proper diet, but as you know, any and/or all spokes of our wheel can easily be modified, their intent changed or altogether ignored. (That's not paranoia, which does exist with patients, it is just plain factual!) I am hopeful that enough has been said in this, one of the most important spokes of this paradigm. Often it is true: we really are what we eat. One more thing: The importance of patients remaining hydrated, is often overlooked or underestimated. This fact alone, that we are made up of over sixty-six percent water, should be more than enough to be a good guide. I also fear that this particular thing, hydration, may often be overlooked by personnel who are more concerned about not having to change a soiled person more than one time during their precious daily duties, instead of seeing to it that fluids are regularly offered. Sometimes patients need assistance in getting hydrated. This is more than humane, it is life-affecting, and can as well mean a great deal to so many of our bodily processes and functions, without even mentioning the better dissemination of medicine (s).

Family. It is one of my prayers that you will recall my sureness concerning family, as addressed in *Family Is Everything*. I can never give this small segment the benefit that family deserves. As I slowly built my memory mirror for the cover of this work, I realized how important (to me) were the sweet faces, the memories behind each one thereon. As you know, I had invited family as well as a few close friends to mail pictures my way. Family, too, includes your care partner. And the care partner requires and deserves lots of love and appreciation! This is a very tough and exhausting life for them. Family plays an important role in keeping stress levels down. What a great benefit it can be, simply enabling AD folks to live more peacefully when and where possible. And again, dementia in Alzheimer's terms means the brain's gradual deterioration. It is not at all pretty. I strongly recommend that you spend as much time as possible with family, (and I'm talking to the patient now, and/or the person who cares for a patient). Ensure where possible that the patient is able to love, laugh, and to reflect upon the good times they've shared, as long as is humanly and physically and psychologically possible. Even in this devastation, reflect upon God's wonderful mercy. Somewhat paraphrased, but here it is. *Thou changeth not, Thy compassions they fail not, great is Thy faithfulness.* All of this serves to remind me of family and of how very great is God's faithfulness. Always thank Him for being with you (us) through the storms of life! *After all God is the Creator of Family.*

Indeed, family is another one of those segments (spokes) that will be somewhat different for each individual, as for me, I would be *dead in the water* were it not for the love, the exchange, the embrace that I have felt from family in so very many ways. Indeed family is what much of life is about. Is it not simply a reflection of what God wishes for each of us? A special and safe place for us to stay? After all, will we not be with family when we are before Him, in praise and adoration, forever? You bet we will! (If perchance you don't have one, or haven't had one, now is the time to make one. Find a church that will treat you as family does. It should be able to provide a lot of love. That my friend is what it (and we) were created for, that, and to lead you Home.

Father God, Creator-Redeemer, allow me a few moments to languish in my personal tears as I reflect upon the love and work of sons and daughters, sons-in-laws and daughters-in-laws that Lucy and I count also as sons and daughters. Without their able assistance only a week before completing this final rewrite, many came from the north and west of us, to assist as we prepared these grounds and home and pool for a grand church baptism. Let me not wipe away these tears of joy, which so remind me of Your constant and tender love. That incomprehensible love that none of us deserves. And Father, we are so very thankful for that great and Glorious Love.

Prayer. Prayer is a necessity for daily, constant communication. It enables us to maintain the God-centeredness of this paradigm, a regimen, and our lives. Without prayer much of this program's success would be greatly diminished. (And that is, I'm certain, an understatement.) Not only are prayers what assist us in our daily dialogue with God, they are also a great 'embosom-ment' of our hope, our praise, our eternal all.

He seeks our prayers, longs for and listens for our prayers, no matter when (day or night). He loves the heartfelt sincerity of our every murmuring. It is another way that God teaches us how binding and strengthening prayer is to the greater Body, His church, the greater Family.

If you have ever stood with or been exposed to folks in need, you soon learn how vital prayer can be. Sometimes even the first-time-exposed person yields fully to their first-ever prayer. That is, they are able to readily enter the world of prayer and later on become faithful prayer warriors. Prayer changes lives! Prayer heals! Prayer brings us to the foot of God's throne. It is here that you will experience euphoria like none other.

†

God has many ways to contact each and every one. I cannot help but recall an old wartime saying I've many times heard. It came about long before me: *There are no atheists in foxholes.* These areas: prisons, combat zones, and hospitals are good examples of areas where people seem more easily drawn to prayer. They are areas of trashed lives, forlorn lives, scarred and burned-out lives, lives of the lost and lonely. Those afraid. There are many paths that lead us to this grand communication, this, the greatest of all conduits of love in action.

†

Allow me for a moment to reflect upon a time when my son's son was born with a hole in his young heart; of how quickly that burden was shared and turned over to God's people; of how great was the peace with which God flooded my soul. Not only is He mighty, His servants' prayers are also mighty and powerful. He graciously and powerfully heals! *Let not your lack of prayer be the slightest hindrance to your entrance into God's forever kingdom!* And of course, it is all by grace! And please, never believe it was your lack of faith that prevented a miracle. Our loving God is not that way.

Other Support. An Alzheimer's Association support group and other caring people, for example a loving church group, are priceless for the strengthening and proper functioning of the wheel as a whole. I cannot proclaim it too heartily. The numbers of beautiful people yet to be met will astound you. The other support spoke is vital to the patient's socialization possibilities. Socialization works hand-in-hand with family. It assists us in our striving to obtain longevity of life. Other support is different from 'Family,' and yet it is much akin. Yet ties inherent to family are in place when it comes to the support of other groups as well.

†

Just as family should not argue with the patient, support folks need to understand how to work with diseased members. Endure me a while longer? I realize this is a big piece. My brainstem, or perhaps my heart, feels it, too. Out of family and other support often comes the result of our being bound together. *Miracles!* What else would I list as a priority for supportive folks? That would be ***learning to listen***. Be able, as far as possible to go with the one hurting. Attempt not to be too opinionated, for it means little to the patient what your opinion is, especially as they (patients) struggle to merely survive daily living, but also since their days and way of life may well be much different from yours. IS DIFFERENT. And again: strive not to be bossy around traumatized folks. Often they are doing the best they can. Trust me. Really.

This so reminds me of the fact that approximately 1% of our Republic's people (warriors) strive to keep the other 99% of us free. There are 1,300,000 men and women serving on active duty for our entire country, and when you add in reserves and others, the total goes a smidge over two million. All right, so maybe it's not quite one percent. These warriors, though, are similar to AD patients, in that warriors need supported, too. They need your opinion very little (which in all likelihood today may do nothing more than bring them down.) You see, 'Family' means going with someone and understanding them, not criticizing them. Now there's something the troops could use: YOUR SUPPORT! YOUR PRAYERS, YOUR SINCERE, LOVING, UNBLEMISHED PRAYERS! I am on my knees here.

God's ways are often so different from our ways. Do we not become, however, more properly aligned with God as we gather to serve Him and seek Him? Therefore, support groups should always be aware of this: *God can do anything, anywhere, anytime. He cannot and will not be contained.* Our God of wonder and love, through His victory over the cross has shown us the way to His very heart of hearts. From our Sovereign God comes escape from death. So let us, friend, together climb that historic and beloved hill of Calvary! Let's climb it with Him!

†

Thank You, God, for leading me to this paradigm, this regimen for disease-afflicted persons. Your answers to prayer humble me and lead me more in the direction that You would have me go. Surely, Lord, there are no mistakes with You. Father, I so look forward to becoming a star in Your great canopy, for we know You have named each one of them. If not, perhaps I could be a simple flower in one of Your gardens. Your Spirit renews the entire face of the earth, and You revive my very soul. Your name is ever-praised great God and Friend!

A parting reminder: Find the regimen that works for you or your patient, and stick with it! I'll be praying for you! And yes, I would not turn down a prayer from you. Thanks.

—Yes, There Is Guilt – Yet There's Also God—

When one returns home from war, there is always that wondering why it is that you were allowed to return at all. Feeling good about it is sometimes simply not possible, for years. The guilt with the dementia-laden world is somewhat different in that we as patients feel that we are deserting our spouse, deserting our family and deserting our friends as well. It scares me, yet I know it's better to get out into the ultraviolet rays of God's glorious sunlight. I pray you do not close yourself in! (And although I wish I could affirm what my neurologist said, about the feel-good stuff created by ultraviolet rays, although it may be helpful, I didn't quite sense it. In fact, I learned the sun beats me up (or down) so quickly that I suddenly became Mr. Shade Tree or Mr. Inside. I have no idea why the sun now seems so powerful and drains me so quickly. But it surely does.) I am also certain it may be because of the many warning signs on some of my meds, and that I served so often in sun-drenched lands around the globe.

Not only do I feel as if I am robbing those I care about; robbing them of this relationship, these relationships, I also feel that I myself am being robbed. Robbed of the rest of my life, robbed of/from what could have been. Shame on me, for God has given me so much. And when I think about it, I've had more precious years than I'd ever suspected or ever deserved. And I remember this as well that at least my life was not cut even much shorter than this. After all, I could have been 'taken' long ago in the far away land of rice patties, humid jungle, and waterways with endless adventure. And perhaps you might want to think about this, friend. Most of us have had many more than a mere thirty-three years that our Special One endured as He showed us the Way.

There's also guilt that's a little more farfetched even for the wee hours, that my grand attitude about the natural habilitative approach to the disease could have 'put a dent' in the disease, yet it may not. It may do nothing. My fighter's approach for the early onset folks, that it might merely be a matter of exercise, support systems, attitude, diet, prayer and so on, working the noggin. That's all good. The not only reaching for the miracle, but that blessed assurance, that's all good, too. Yet through it all I yet feel guilty. *Are you there?* (Then again, nothing ventured, nothing gained. **So push ahead with me toward victory!**)

Perhaps I have entered my child's guilt. My Dad, Glenn G., had died at forty-three years of age. He never got to see me marry; never followed my adventures around the world, never even got to see me get commissioned. Dad never saw the ministering or rearing of three great kids. There are times when I feel guilty about having been away from home after he'd died. I never returned home when the funeral was completed, with all those little ones left behind, that included Glenn G., Jr., my fishing buddy, and Dave, my other pal, and the rest of them. (No, that one's not guilt that I can really hang on myself.)

I had called Momma, and she'd given me her blessing to move ahead, to remain in uniform should I feel called to do that. Never a thought for herself. How I revered that, revered her. *How I still do!*

But fortunate am I as I look back over it all, for I realize that I'd do it all the same again. Yes, I'd even relive the mistakes I'd made all over again. Don't you believe the hard times, the low times, the struggles, the often tough lessons of life assist in molding us to become who we are meant to become? Do they not either cause us to become fighters, or spoiled folks who had so much handed to us? And right, there are plenty of variances between those two extremes.

Yes, there is guilt. Yet I seek to keep it in the healthy-guilt arena. Anyone can think himself or herself into some kind of guilt, worthwhile for a moment, or never worth wasting time and emotion on. For me, the fighter, my tack is to realize that if my life is to be shortened, that I've already lived a rich full life, and how very blessed it has been! You have been privy to much of it within these pages. To me, the one thing that always beats guilt down, hands down, is God's amazing love for each and every one of us, no matter what He has allowed to occur to and around us in our lifetime here upon this blue marble.

Think of that lovely, unforgettable picture that you cannot get out of your head; that one place or person, landscape or scene, the love you have for that unforgettable object or background, or better yet Something or Someone not visible. Well, most of it simply pales in comparison to God's grand and incomprehensible love for You. Pales in comparison except for that Someone that you may have attempted to envision Who is invisible, thus far.

So although there's some guilt, for me it's usually short-lived guilt. There we were, and are, grand times, people, and places, experiences that most people would have loved to have lived. The scenes, the conversations, Momma's look deeply into my loved self and soul, the love of a wonderful woman or two along the way. It is all part of the colorful blanket of life woven by experiences, laughter, and love as well as God's steady, abiding, loving hand, and His infinite Omnipresence.

Then there's having been able and allowed to watch your children and grandchildren, each finding his/her own way. Making mistakes as they seek their own loves and fortunes. How privileged we are to watch, often from afar, the choices they will make, roads they will take. How often we pray that their choices will be for God, or with Him in mind, that they will be decent to their fellow citizens, unlike some of us, sometimes, that they will learn of patience and kindness, compassion, and most of all, the love of God.

How proud I am of each and every one of these kids. There is no guilt whatsoever here. There is love and laughter, the unfolding of each little flower that blooms either into a rose, a daisy, or forsythia! Not a dried-up old cactus in the bunch. (Yet even the cactus, God often causes to bloom, does He not?)

†

The grandchildren. The hybrids. I grow dizzy pondering what the lives of the youngest might be, what they are yet to see. I place it all in hands larger than any tender capable grandpa's hands, those hands of course being God's tender hands. Father is The One who keeps guilt away, even as He can drive darkness from a room or a life! For there is God. Thankfully, He was and is and always shall be!

†

Lover of my soul, Creator of each soul, thanks for this planet which You have packed full of vibrance and wonder, abundant resources, worlds yet untapped. Thanks for this grand gift of life! Whether we travel to Your deepest depths or the great beyond, space, we find You everywhere. In a blazing home, in an overturned vehicle, in the devastation of war or a disease, in all these places we find You. Yet sometimes we also find guilt. Thank You, Father, that there is also a rising from guilt, a rinsing-away of all that 'stuff' that we sometimes fear and feel. Thankful are we God that Your Ascension is our ascending, too. Thank You for awaking certain wisdoms within us, and thank You for the wonderful sacrificial cleansing of Your Holy blood. It was Your walking here below that allowed us to be forever aware of Your tender care. Thank You for doctors as well as other helpers who share, it is only our reserves that are limited. And Yes, even reserves can be changed by You; all things are possible with You.

†

I love and feel prompted to share Daniel's words with you, friend. "Daniel answered and said: 'BLESSED BE THE NAME OF GOD FOREVER AND EVER, FOR WISDOM AND MIGHT ARE HIS.

AND HE CHANGES THE TIMES AND THE SEASONS; HE
REMOVES KINGS AND RAISES UP KINGS; HE GIVES WISDOM TO
THE WISE AND KNOWLEDGE TO THOSE WHO HAVE
UNDERSTANDING. HE REVEALS DEEP AND SECRET THINGS;
HE KNOWS WHAT IS IN THE DARKNESS, AND LIGHT DWELLS
WITH HIM. 'I THANK YOU AND PRAISE YOU, O GOD OF MY
FATHERS; YOU HAVE GIVEN ME WISDOM AND MIGHT, AND
HAVE NOW MADE KNOWN TO ME WHAT WE ASKED OF YOU.
FOR YOU HAVE MADE KNOWN TO US THE KING'S DEMAND.'"
—Daniel 2:20-23.

How I love the fact that another Daniel, Daniel W., is my
newest grandson. O how God loves you and me!

—Camaraderie Among The Diseased—

Camaraderie, or the desire to have and maintain good
fellowship, is not unique to those of us with AD. I have shared
that intimate 'closeness' with brothers and sisters-in-arms, in
church bodies, and in various fraternal organizations throughout
my lifetime. I used to believe that those of us with various
forms of dementia are more docile than folks at a veteran's
meeting, but I have backed down on that somewhat. That is
because sadness, sensitivity, caring, indeed a host of emotions
are found within all circles. These emotions are part of the
human existence.

Yet in a veterans' meeting you're more likely to hear one of
us become inflamed more quickly than you might at a meeting
for folks suffering AD. I know there's a book or two written on
group dynamics. It seems to me that folks with one or another
form of dementia are probably more docile across the board, but
I may be all wet! Would you rather get this from a neophyte
Alzheimer-diseased layman or from one who studies
psychoneuroimmunology? Well, pardon me for expressing this,
but you'll get more out of me unless the good doctor decides
that he/she has a week of free time to give you.

While I'm on that aforementioned ten-dollar word:
psychoneuroimmunology, try to say that ten times real fast, I'd
like to quote from an article in the May, 2007 issue of *Best Life*
magazine, page 104. "People who have poor social ties are at
greater risk of sickness and premature death than those who
have good social ties," one such study begins. "Indeed,
friendship can, among other things, reduce coronary-related

morbidity and mortality; it can protect against the onset of AD; it can help you bounce back from illness quickly; it can decrease employee absenteeism; it can extend your life."

Is that not amazing or at least impressive stuff? It is one of those studies, unlike so many others I believe will not change. Think about it. We are all privy to the fact that enjoying, living with great company DOES affect us in a positive way. It just makes good common sense.

I've also pondered, some, about the bond formed by folks of the various Uniformed Services, that this is indeed a world unto itself. But now that I seem rather ambivalent concerning this area, and completely out of any personal expertise, I simply repeat, camaraderie of one degree or another appears in both different and similar organizations. Being in the same boat after all is 'being in the same boat' period.

You might find that you encounter more frequent 'flare-ups' at a veterans' group meeting than you would on the AD front, as I began above. Part of that I believe is because combat vets are different in that our flashbacks afford us more spontaneity when we are *triggered* by certain stimuli. We often end up shouting, stomping our feet, and/or cussing.

It seems to me that I am seated with more docile types when attending my Alzheimer's circle of friends, folks suffering a different form of head trouble. It'd be a rather sketchy oversimplification if I omitted that one can and does encounter flare-ups and combativeness amongst dementia-laden folks, too. I've seen it in action.

And who is to say: it may well be that AD patients, too, encounter certain 'triggers' that cause and/or enable us to take on a certain behavior or the being dismayed that sometimes accompanies us to meetings. What assists me in becoming even more confused, amidst my already confused state, is that somewhere, my worlds of PTSD and dementia merge (as I've bored you with time and again). Hey, a little recall coming into play, that's not a bad thing!

That is, these worlds have become enmeshed or are just plain not that far divided one from the other. I believe I have noted more 'gazing' in the world of dementia, particularly as we progress to more advanced stages of becoming entangled. Yet whether we're part of a group continuing to relive wartime experiences, or one continuing more and more to live in a different kind of past life, all (of us) are involved nevertheless in camaraderie, a bonding that evolves more easily, more quickly simply because of our sameness, our commonality, our sharing, everyone being in the same boat.

You hear it more readily expressed in post-traumatic groups, "This is your family. This is family here!" Then again, in the quieter dementia-laden setting I've never heard it expressed much, yet it does (even though more nonverbal) exist here, too. There is a strong sense of family, a wordless sense of 'welcome-ness' to all who enter. Normally. Veterans (to me) seem a little more skeptical about who has entered the room, at least for a time. I'd say more warm-up time is necessary for veterans.

But back to the gaze. And again it is a time I do not wish to appear insensitive; however there is a look about us, as we progress to and through various stages of our disease: AD. That is, our countenance does change. I spot it quite easily. This, too, is not unique to the demented. It is possible to have persons with various debilitations and a look about them, present in any and all groups. Enough. I will not pretend to know it all (as I am sometimes accused of). Far from it; most of what I am doing is purely reporting, observing, the going through of it as I live it and endure it. And yes, I am thankful I usually can.

In each world of camaraderie I've noted a *Never Give Up!* attitude. I've noticed folks ignited by another's words and/or example. In fact, I have at times ignited them, I believe. Yet, not quite so much with AD, for we sometimes seem less concerned or cannot always express our affectations (our unnatural speech or conduct). Yet that is not totally accurate either.

I am certain I am not the only one with the *Never give up!* words imprinted upon my brain, dementia-affected or otherwise. Who cannot help but love that fiery declaration, no matter where your camaraderie finds you? *Never give up!*

Let the long ago young writer's famous words be kept alive for some: "Approach thy grave like one who wraps the drapery of his couch about him and lies down to pleasant dreams." *Baloney*! I'm not going out that way. Yet I did want to share it with you. There are indeed times that that line comforts me, at other times it does not. It does remind me of what I'd more than once shared from the pulpit: Many of us think we're going out with a bang, when in reality most of us go out with a whimper.

Me? I've whimpered early, and much. And contrary to what some might say or believe, I *DO* realize that it's not all about me. (How sadly quick we are to point out the flaws of our fellow man, even within our own families.) Then again, maybe it's simply a case of being straight-forward and honest, who knows? I'll give that one away.

This day I talked with a son and two of my daughters. (Again, recall that I consider the extended family sons and daughters, too. It can be confusing at times.) Amy, in her somewhat mundane yet *grand work* assisting the elderly and disabled; Angie in her studies and plans for a complete dental rework, and then a special challenge: nuclear medicine: *Ugh!* And Chuck, at that particular time happened to be awaiting the arrival of his firstborn (who I earlier reported as already being here, again, the difficulty with the rewriting of stuff, later on). This arrival though, of a baby, is something he had awaited for twenty-plus years. Twenty years after being married, that is. (Again these writings are simply not always in chronological order, so don't try to figure it out.)

This same day I got incredibly lucky and talked to a brother also, concerning the current Middle East mess. I don't know why I say 'current' though, that is, it's been a disturbed mess for a very long time, long before this Republic became involved or was even in existence. But when I think about where our Republic has been headed of late, one might call it a toss-up, eh? I mean, sometimes we seem in as much turmoil as the Middle East. Yet if we turn to God, once again, we can be more proud, more honest, far more loving. *Indeed I fear for our young America.*

Every person I'd talked to that day (that day that had been 'this day') easily shared their life with me, each one striving for the common good, ever looking forward and upward. It was unique and welcomed, indeed a blessed day for me. They are all blessed though, are they not? Yes, that includes you and me.

I will always be convinced that within a group, or without, that nothing is by accident. He alone is Holy and worthy, "O praise Him!" Outside again, the chilled yet sun-filled air had cleared my head, somewhat. As my neighbors departed for a visit to the West Coast, I awaited the return of my Lucy from a conference. Momma had at that time sold her Tennessee chalet, so her remaining days would not be as tightly controlled by the dollar, thank goodness. Those who turn to God normally find it all works out. Do you believe that, too? Actually, it works out with the dollar in the picture or without it. The money-part just doesn't matter that much in the grand scheme of things. Why we keep chasing after it is a constant source of amazement and amusement to me. It is also an area that causes men to become older much before their time.

Donna (otherwise known as *Lucy*), had been having some sleepless nights, but continued smiling, her huge heart filled with tenderness, most of the time. She, too, was and is another comrade, a consistent fighter! Nothing by accident, dear friend, nothing. And yes, we always belong to some group. Let's pray and strive, and so live that it is part of His Holy Family.

Thank You, living and loving Lord, for camaraderie, for a sense of family. Thanks for people, well or debilitated, who easily share their lives, their love. In so doing they live Your love, Your selfless, compassionate, pure and eternal grace. 'THANK YOU, LORD, FOR YOUR GREAT AND WONDROUS CREATION, YOUR WONDERS WITHOUT NUMBER.' —Job 9:10.

So thankful am I that You bind the realization that even our camaraderie rings as this: "FOR BY HIM ALL THINGS WERE CREATED THAT ARE IN HEAVEN AND THAT ARE ON EARTH, VISIBLE AND INVISIBLE, WHETHER THRONES OR DOMINIONS OR PRINCIPALITIES OR POWERS. ALL THINGS WERE CREATED THROUGH HIM AND FOR HIM. AND HE IS BEFORE ALL THINGS, AND IN HIM ALL THINGS CONSIST. AND HE IS THE HEAD OF THE BODY, THE CHURCH, WHO IS THE BEGINNING, THE FIRSTBORN FROM THE DEAD, THAT IN ALL THINGS HE MAY HAVE THE PREEMINENCE." —Colossians 1:16-18.

TIME ZONES (Slipping away…)
Wayne Glenn TERRY

Chapter 14

Just Feelings

—I Didn't Want To Know—

AD happens to be one of those diseases that affects many of us in many different ways, especially as we enter our later years. (That is, the latter years for us in the disease, not necessarily the later years in life.) As we become more set in our ways, perhaps the plaque inside of us hardens more quickly and we more easily begin to isolate, therefore, often we can become our own worst enemy. It has taken me literally months, as well as a few friends, to eventually get much attention regarding an application for help from a governmental agency. You've too often heard it. I do apologize. But I am not going to regurgitate here what has already been stated in another work that is more wholly devoted to that particular subject. Whether I will work it to its final conclusion, I remain uncertain as well as unsure.

Yet I must, here and now thank the Department of Health and Human Services. *Really*. I think I earlier advised you that I am finally a MEDICARE cardholder.

During this time of additional stress, due to that arm of government I never mention, I began to ponder whether stress had caused me to more and more forget immediate happenings, locations and names, just as epileptic episodes are brought about by stress, and or a clouding of the consciousness. I therefore sometimes wonder in my own layman's mind whether these two worlds are not somehow related, even though they are also different. (That stuff's for the more well schooled in those particular areas.)

Something positive. I realize that it is something scary, yet I *DO* have something positive to report. I caught a show (on the evening of the 14th of August, 2008, CNN) concerning returning Iraq War vets. I was delighted to see that an outfit or two had contributed portions of money to outfit a van for some of the men (and women) who have their legs blown off in wartime. So some of them have been enabled to drive utilizing hand controls only. But admittedly, you will not hear me saying a lot of positive stuff about what has happened for wartime returnees; the other side of the coin is a total atrocity.

I just didn't want to think about what I already knew to be taking place within myself. I did not want to face the scary but real possibility that I *had it,* AD. To me, even admitting that I'd gone to a psychologist or two would have been vastly easier to share with folks. You see, one or the other happens when you tell someone you have AD. Either folks enjoy what they think is your little joke, that is they laugh and say how they, too, have it all the time (*ha, ha*), or they seem to be thinking that you're just such a *nut case* that they either reply 'interesting' or 'I'm sorry', and/or they totally shut down, unsure of what next to say. Thankfully that last one probably covers most of us.

I need to review all of that from time to time, especially when someone in my own family is having difficulty accepting the fact that I am a patient. Some never get it. (And while I'm on that, I would attempt to explain, *do not allow that to trouble you too much,* it simply seems that many folk who love us, especially ones close, do not wish to think about us being debilitated in any way.) That's natural.

†

More Paranoia. I returned a call an Alzheimer's support coordinator had originated. She had simply wanted to relay information about a TV taping of a documentary on AD. I hadn't been able to get Lucy as she was away at a job conference. (One place it would be a taboo for me to contact her.) As I later talked with someone about the interview on AD, I was advised that a lady would later still, contact me. I scribbled a couple questions onto a piece of paper. I had wanted to know who the caller was, what outfit she represented, and when the airing of the show would take place and so forth. Next week, I had surmised to myself, would be good, as my Lucy would then be back home and she could assist me with all of this. I had also begun to get a little concerned about my driving ability, or the lack thereof.

All the while my mind continued to play the fact that this (the initial true knowledge about Alzheimer's disease for me) had all begun almost a year before, and that due to their (a government agency's) bureaucratic attitude that seemed much lacking in empathy, I had documented it with the local Field Office Manager, that there was little warmth felt by this applicant, in fact, it appeared that at almost every checkpoint I had encountered comments such as, 'I just think your timing is poor' from a nurse or doctor, or this one from an initial screener: 'Oh, I see you were just here, and you're back for more' (*ha, ha, ha*), flipping of the hair and so on.

(And if we've already been through this part, I apologize. I am well aware that this work contains quite a lot that might be considered *paranoia*.) I recalled having talked to a lady **four months later** (I'd kept notes on all of that) whose reply had been, "They're working on it." I never did learn whether they'd received my initial application. **A full nine or ten months after that had taken place,** Lucy drove me to the local government office where we learned (from yet another screener): 'Why there's nothing in your file about any medical evidence, Mr. Terry.' (Laugh, laugh – hair flip, innocent look.) That was when Lucy pulled out the doctor's diagnosis/prognosis letter, which by the way the particular government agency tells you doesn't matter, because they (the government agency) hasn't said you *have it* yet. That is, *you are not diseased until we tell you you are diseased.* Now ask me again about *paranoia*.

Part of this mess was because we had been talking about all of this in late April of 2007, and the diagnosis letter written by my neurologist was dated 12-12-06! In **January**, before we had received a letter from a third party in which the local government office (their letter of 1/26/07) had stated in part, paragraph two: "Mr. Terry requested we expedite his case because he was in dire need of support in order to meet his bills/responsibilities."

Later I of course learned that you have to either be dying or declare bankruptcy to get anywhere whatsoever. Down a little further in the letter: *"Our records indicate that Mr. Terry's reconsideration was received on October 27, 2006. As of the close of business on January 25, 2007, we have expedited his case to the* _____ _____ (blanks intentional), with an 'Expedite' flag attached." (My turn: *Interesting.*) I must admit I love the banner on their (90-day time-lagged letterhead): ***"Committed to Quality and Creativity in Public Service."*** I thanked God for this portion of Psalm 37:7: "REST IN THE LORD, AND WAIT PATIENTLY FOR HIM;" Can you imagine, all of this BEFORE our meeting with their office in April, when we were informed: *'there is nothing in your record...'* God bless the senior citizens of this *above board* Republic. Can you imagine being in my shell, living with AD, PTSD, and on panic pills as well, in order to even go out in society. Is it any wonder why people do crazy things today? (I know, Dr. John: accountability.) Lord, still my soul once again.

†

The *new me* had wondered at the time, if these agencies simply enjoy this gamesmanship? Or had it just become an inherent game of conniving and frustrating and misusing people who are in need of help? (I had by this time had to promise the Alzheimer's Association chapter that I would NOT talk about government agencies during the TV documentary taping, can you imagine that? Yes, I can, too, as I look back on what parts of it I can or care to remember.) And this small portion of reporting and/or *paranoia,* call it what you wish, well, just imagine the thousands upon thousands of tired, older, more debilitated folks who simply have given up.

Imagine that this example is a very minute portion of what one soldier/citizen has endured during this past year. *Imagine.* Imagine that now (at this final writing), it has been well over two years since I began setting forth what I had suspected two years prior to that! Imagine how many others simply walk out the door? Can you blame them?

So here I am, the good writer that usually holds something back, now seated in the library, waiting, my cell phone turned on. (I'm not too far from a sign that talks about the penalties for doing same.) I hate to turn the heat down now, especially when it's just getting interesting. No, let me check one more thing, I say to myself.

The next day, at 5 a.m. on the morning of April 27th I checked my voicemail. Sure enough a call from a media services person who relays that they are indeed doing a program on Alzheimer's disease, that she is from Henrico County. She further states that she'd attempt to contact me again on Friday. Finally I decide that it really is a medical documentary and not governmental agency folks jerking me around… *(Paranoia.)*

Back to my *I Didn't Want To Know* segment, and the President's impending veto of a bill that had just been passed calling for a troop withdrawal from Iraq. Do you think that kind of topic might affect an old veteran in any way? What a mess our *'me first'* representatives have made of things, I think one more time.

Part of what initially had smacked me squarely between the eyes is much the same as what caregivers think when they finally understand that their loved one *has it.* For me, the worst part is what had been written in earlier pages of this work, that the fear of not being able to recognize someone close to you and/or to no longer be able to verbally communicate is nothing short of a panic-striking death-hammer-blow, we just plainly speaking, do not want to know! We especially don't want to know where we'll be when we arrive at stage six or seven, or the later on part, that part that no one knows about, not really. Not totally. (If someone reading this *does* know, would you kindly notify me before I arrive there?)

As I begin to close in on the latter part of this travel fantasy, I confess that we do not yet know if there are other ways to communicate. Yes, we know there is the sense of touch of course, other's and our own. Perhaps a simple flashback will readily help me realize this as I cautiously revisit places not so fond in my military head. I recall even those in combat who'd had half their world blown away, torn away, even those either quickly realize or slowly learn new methods of conversing, and hopefully of becoming close to being mobile again. It's somewhat akin to that pregnant lady many of us learned that we had to be tenderer around. It's a totally new world. (Thanks again, CNN, for sharing a good story about returning Iraq War veterans.)

Patience and communication. Patience is a subject that I take a glimpse at now. It would have been easy, perhaps I should have written more about it, perhaps an entire chapter on patience. Actually, this work could easily have been accomplished on a much larger scale. There are so many directions that you can go with it. It is actually a difficult task for me to cut it short. But patience is not only important for the caregiver, it is also important for care receivers to remain patient with helpers, our mate, and others.

We should be especially careful as well with those around us who are making this journey with us. Patience is such a very real necessity, although often it seems illusive. Sometimes in life, as I've said before, when I figured I'd had it altogether was a time I later realized that I had been quite confused. There's a lot of that nowadays, not simply with AD people.

Patience is the leaf of understanding that forms a heart-shaped tree of love. Patience is hope and caring and trusting, understanding and sharing. Patience is vital to anyone suffering with/from dementia. Yet often it is something that doesn't come to one with AD, not even the most lucid of patients. Some of the processes you might expect to be in automatic just are not that way. Sometimes instead, there is rambling, confusion and frustration.

†

I've visited many healthcare facilities where I've seen either from afar or close-up that workers, too, do not always get the idea of patience. They just do not share its essence. But to be fair; each facility usually has an angel or two. Thank God.

One of the reasons I never wanted to know I have dementia is because of the desert of life one quickly becomes secluded in or can. One can quickly become stranded. It is unfair, unrelenting, and very uncomfortable to say the least. It is the mind's personal Sahara.

As a young man ministering to others, I've watched from afar families making the grave mistake of pretending to take the patient (the diseased one) on an outing or a picnic. Not long thereafter, when all the loved ones have disappeared from the 'picnic', and the patient finds herself alone in this new, strange, usually frightening environment, it had almost caused me to become physically ill. Sometimes we can be so very undisciplined and uncaring, even when we believe we are doing the best we can for our loved one. (It puts me in mind of folks who attempt to counsel others, when in fact they hardly have their very own life under control, and have no idea whatsoever about counseling/listening, and are very opinionated about someone they know little about.)

As I recall just how horrific is that moment as it unfolds: that *dropping off* of a loved one at a retirement home, what has (in the name of love) been thrust upon the patient, it makes me want to go back and get right in the middle of all of it. But as you know, sometimes it's none of our business, not our place, is it? *Well, it needs to be our place.* Too many of us have learned to be content about not saying anything, not writing to anyone, not attempting to right the wrongs of our society. Too many of us have become insensitive and indecisive, concerned only it seems about the 'piling up' of money. Money we will never take with us.

One valuable motion that I have learned to carry out, and therefore I gladly pass it on to you, dear friend: I have learned to dial 1-866-272-6622. It is the switchboard phone number for the White House. I recently wrote an essay about it, and I am hopeful that if there's anything you ponder that might be changed or assisted or righted by your call, that you'll use it. And use it as often as you'd like to. (Note: it's a free call.) On December 11th, 2008, just before this work went to press, I heard our *leaders,* shut down the White House lines. Interesting, huh? (I'd love to know who made that decision...)

But let me return to travesty. Another possible travesty of the wondrous 21st century: watching the motions of care and love some families initially show when committing their loved one to a residence, only to see them (the family) go away and hardly ever again return. "*Buh-bye* now. It's been real." The patient is gradually reduced to little more than part of the building, no longer visited, no longer thought much of or about. Then again, remember, sometimes we cannot see it all, do not know it all. I base my reporting on what I've observed and know to be true. (There are other family members of course, who can barely stand to leave their loved one's side, and some do not, hardly for any great length of time.) I'll admit it though, those are the ones I admire most; the ones who share God's continuous, wonderfully amazing, unconditional love.

The inaction or uncaring attitude of a few of today's healthcare workers is a scary subject that many folks do not want to hear about, let alone face head on. It is one of my prayers, one day the healthcare system will either be able to properly monitor itself simply because of pride, dignity and the conscientiousness of its workers, or that it might more properly be monitored by a new system that truly displays care and love for people. (I do not suggest anything dealing with government.)

I so tire of the *fighting fires* attitude many retirement communities/nursing homes cannot yet seem to get beyond, the video-game-like type of existence that is now lived out; the putting in of time, as opposed to genuine concern and professional assistance.

(And while I'm on this topic, make no mistake, I am addressing 'leaders' and 'owners' of such establishments. If anyone is feeling 'froggy', as if you are willing to leap without thinking, remember that I retain the names and addresses of MANY folks who had loved ones in your 'caring' facility. That is a fact. It is not said as a challenge, or to place a burr under anyone's saddle. It is said out of love for those ones who seem to be forgotten so very often; that is as softly as that idea will ever be administered by this author.)

†

I sometimes wonder if surveillance cameras and listening devices are going to be standard fare in retirement homes of our grandchildren. I mean, we have cameras out in the open at our traffic signals where people daily fail to stop. Please tell me things don't go on inside (where workers don't think they're being seen). Tell me again. We had a local report not many days ago of sixty-plus traffic tickets issued for red-light runners at one intersection, and it wasn't the entire day's total! What has happened? How is it our confused lives follow us to our vehicles? (Oh yeah, we already covered that.)

Yet we still seem to retain exceptional people in all walks of life. I remember long before joining the ranks of those with dementia, a young woman coming home late one night, telling her dad (as she finally stood with her baby in her loving, tired arms) about her night of work. Okay, she told *me* of changing each person on a 50-person floor, single-handedly, and through tired tears relayed how when she'd finally completed rounds for the lot of them, it was time to begin all over again. That, dear friend, is simply said: sadly unsatisfactory and demeaning and antiquated. Yet indeed we have arrived at the 21st century.

What admiration I have for people who care for our elderly population, especially when they have love in their hearts. It is her simple, pure, love and devotion that keeps my sweet *baby girl* going. She is a college graduate who could teach any grade level, and yet she finds great joy in working with seniors. Thank you, Amy. You are indeed unique and special. God indeed has a place for you.

†

Simply put we have not seemed to make great strides in our care to seniors. I have worked in some fine facilities, where patients are attended to rather nicely, but I noted they were also very top-of-the-line, expensive places. Unfortunately many of our facilities are yet understaffed, personnel underpaid, and sometimes there persists a general malaise concerning what the whole process is about. Some so lack in dignity and caring and a general knowledge of how to be a good caregiver.

Unfortunately much of this is because although it is all about very specialized personal care, it has also become reduced to nothing more than a business. It becomes more about numbers, more about callousness it seems, more about dollars and cents, and less and less about caring and service.

A friend of mine recently advised me how the 'in service' training at nursing and retirement facilities tells workers how they are to be/provide service, then he gave me the *newsflash,* that it just isn't happening the way it's supposed to happen. Is it true that things can happen differently in real life than the way they read in our internal instructions and directives? That's a rhetorical question.

I thank God for volunteers, especially ones genuinely concerned about people. Folks that can listen, pray, and let others know there is someone who really cares about them. These are some of those angels I've mentioned: folks who daily go and care and do for others, over and again, day after weary day. Some do it rather lethargically, others with grace, charm and vivaciousness. God bless 'em.

I'll not continue much more. Yet I must say it is evident that the remainder of the staff today, working within these residents/homes, surely reads the attitude of management, and soon (if the attitude remains as it is: often not good), the task at hand, no matter how miniscule or great, is reduced to little more than a babysitting service.

When it comes to the care of the elderly and/or debilitated, it takes much more than just a handful of sitters. If there is no love, no respect for personhood, then life becomes so debased and meaningless that it is as though we're in different *time zones* already. Is this what we wish for our children and children's children?

Most of us must feel the same way in our hearts. Who wants to live a full life that has overflowed with great memories and friendships, only to watch it gradually become reduced to a room not much larger than the size of a state-run prison cell? Speaking of which, isn't that the way many of us feel about leaving our homes, never able to return? Incarcerated, I've heard it said, first-hand, and those people were not at all in good humor.

While I'm talking about personhood, I want to share a couple more gems with you before I get too close to capping off this work. I have noted during this process, and as I've grown and changed (for the better) I believe; I have also learned that it is not necessarily a good thing for us (and now I'm speaking of and to patients) to rely too much upon the caregiver. What I am saying I am certain my neurologist would agree with.

It seems the more we allow others to do for us, whether we are or feel disabled, the more it is that we are allowing ourselves to become disabled, capable of doing less and less. That is a warning and a gem of wisdom for you (and myself). It is not *tough love* or *suck it up,* or any other statement that might seem rather loveless. What I am saying is: do as much for yourself as you possibly can, you will be better off for it in the long run, at least for as long as you possibly can.

I also learned, and this has nothing much to do with AD, but I learned a 'Sam-ism' as I was painting our fence around our pool (getting read for that grand baptism). Towards the end of this unpleasant and rather hot and steamy project (which I had thought I could not do), I learned not only that I could do it, but also that the paint roller would actually fit between some of the slots in between the slats of the fence, thus making the job a whole lot less complicated and even quicker. I hope you remember *Samism's* from a previous chapter.

Yes, I surprised myself as well. I am thankful that I can yet break a sweat and do a little light work. I would pray this great insight for you as well. That is, *I do!*

I've sat bedside, where the patient's strongest desire, their one remaining hope, was to be allowed to die in peace at home. To them it was dying with dignity and dying where they'd laughed, lived and loved. And it has been my hope as well. Dying in the palm of God's loving hand, for our homes, as God's hands are, are that place where we lock the rest of the world out. Our homes are our sanctuary. And if our homes have been designed with God in their midst, then they are a natural progression, a divine progression; a place from which we march forward into Forever.

But while we're yet here, let's each work for good change! Let's strive once again to cause life to be filled with love and care and dignity and professionalism, as far as possible.

Would you ever have thought a PTSD-ridden, Alzheimer-diseased person who suffers panics could write a helpful guidebook for you? No. Neither did I.

†

On the evening of August 15th, 2008, again on a CSPAN network, I watched with great interest and listened intently to words of Governor Mike Huckabee and others, as well as Lou Engel, founder of *The Call*. I liked what I'd heard as they spoke of spiritual renewal, of pro-life activism and words about the spiritual deficit in today's Republic. Although wherever they were sequestered sounded as if there were only 20 people in the room, their comments and thought processes are worthy of our attention. I reveled in the words about a clear voice, and then I cringed at the realization of the horrific tragedy of the abortion of some 40 million (and then later heard 50 million little beings). ***Shame on us for our years and years of silence.*** (For a more complete picture of how abortion destroys not only lives, but how it has lead to the collapse of our economy and culture, read Ron Bourque's book, *DISTURBING QUESTIONS: Has God Stopped Blessing America?*, ISBN: 978-0-9795394-0-4)

†

I know a God who cares about each and every one: about our being loved. He even speaks about the mansion He has planned for you.

Thank You, God. Words fail me when it comes to Your wondrous Omnipotence. Oh that each one of Your creatures could treat others as You have treated us. Your abundant rewarding love remains unsurpassed. Father, it is here that I need to back up, to do some patching-up work. For in a previous section and this one, too, as I talked of healthcare workers, I later realized that we must be careful not to sit in judgment. For I know words from the first book of the New Testament, chapter 6: 14 and 15, "FOR IF YOU FORGIVE MEN THEIR TRESPASSES, YOUR HEAVENLY FATHER WILL ALSO FORGIVE YOU. BUT IF YOU DO NOT FORGIVE MEN THEIR TRESPASSES, NEITHER WILL YOUR FATHER FORGIVE YOUR TRESPASSES." Father, give us the grace to forgive, for daily; we, too, cause You to be saddened. All glory be to the Father, the Son and the Holy Spirit. "As in water face reflects face, so a man's heart reveals the man." —Proverbs 27:19.

—Be Honest Or Hide Your Feelings?—

Yours truly, has attempted to be as honest as possible about this writing, indeed I have not tried to sell you anything that I would not myself attempt. I am not sure why I have added that caveat at this particular time, perhaps it is because the aforementioned heading has something about *honesty* therein. Without it (honesty), our writing and words are worth nothing.

Never did the question appear so personally important until I heard another man's words about seeing the light. I've thought since then, how much there is to be said for honesty. Honesty should be the base which we work from, the position we draw our strength from. It should be our foundation and emanate from our very core.

Too often I've heard it said, "You need to quit thinking about that. Do not revisit those things that trouble you, those situations that haunt you." Well, when we allow ourselves to continue to ignore our dilemmas, or to mask them, sooner or later they must be dealt with, so it is my opinion that reliving your hurts with a reason in mind can be very important as well as cathartic. And, you are entitled to your emotions! You, yourself, will have to be the one to decide when it has been long enough that a wound you would now wish to heal, or have healed can indeed become healed.

I have also learned that it is best to be honest with your doctor, in fact, to be honest with everyone. This information after all will lead to better living for you and perhaps longer life as well. When I realized that those dimly flashing and often fading light-plays were part of my disease, it enraged me. First of all it angered me because it only served to further verify my disease, the one I did not want to believe I had. Secondly, I was angry that no one had shared the 'light thing' words with me. I had had to learn it on my own, through Lucy, who'd read the words. I love honesty. Most of the time.

On the other hand, I must also fear it because I had never shared my light story with anyone. Not ever. I do not encourage you to do as I: to keep things hidden away inside yourself. So in a sense, I guess I don't love honesty as much as I sometimes declare. Confusing?

Doctors, plainly said, do not have the time or the opportunity to sit down with each one of us and download all they have learned or are aware of; it's just not practical let alone possible. Not yet. Thankfully there are some who will spend more time with you, doctors who are willing to share, and even make time for you. Some, unfortunately, just can't afford to do that. Mine, thankfully, my neurologist, has been an exception. The problem? I was just with him today and forgot all about asking him about the *light shows*. I did however have the opportunity and remembered to discuss difficulty socializing, and learned that this is fairly normal with AD folks.

This is not territory drastically new or innovative, but I wanted to share it with you. Often, it seems, we just do not know how to go about helping ourselves. With that being said, I regret that I have mostly seemed as one who is a shrink basher, when indeed my heart realizes that there are times they can help us through some thinking and conclusions that we could not come to on our own, at least not in the midst of our tiredness, anxiety and confusion. I do believe, however, that short-term counseling is the best. I have never bought into the fact, as some of them would rather enjoy us to, that counseling needs to be drawn out and long term.

To me it seems: if you are so entirely 'messed up' that you are in need of years and years of therapy, then I would hope that you are in the slammer so that someone else is picking up the tab on so many wasted sessions. Keep in mind, however, this is testimony from a layman, not one schooled for many years in great mind and heart matters. Would you rather have a layman perform brain surgery, or a real surgeon-type surgeon? (Yet still, I will remain with my statement about short-term counseling being the best.)

†

In an unseasonably warm winter morning of a year, I sat with the administrator of a facility, having only a couple days before shared with his new admissions person my knowledge of their escaping residents as well as other matters. No sooner had I sat down (later on) with the administrator did I hear: "We, er – we want you to cease your… er— services for a while."

Let's just say I was ticked! And actually, as one of my grandchildren might say, actually, I was mad for having been honest with any of them. When honesty no longer allows that warm, fuzzy feeling, or you are unable to do your duty, or what you consider your duty, you know you are being threatened. I just felt turned upon, bitten, and somewhat wounded, all of that and more. For a moment I died inside. I no longer wanted to be honest.

Not only had there been conniving and maltreatment within that facility, but I also was aware that certain workers and/or management persons would lie about anything they felt they needed to lie about in order to achieve their goals, their total dominance over people. One good example: leaving a patient's pills with the patient and saying, "Here, Dear, take them whenever you're ready." Those words are not only taboo in most states for the nurse or an aide dispensing medication, they are illegal. (And if I have shared this with you prior, again, I apologize.)

The person handing out medicines is supposed to remain in the patient's presence until the medications are swallowed! Doesn't that make sense?

I had not died inside. Yet part of me had died for ones who would no longer smile, pleased to see me again. Honesty had not caused the administrator's "...Let's just say, I've had complaints" allegation. I knew after all the months that I'd served this facility that his insertion of the go-for-the-jugular-vein words of "complaints from the residents," had been a crock. It smacked heavily of words fabricated prior to my arrival for a corporation's immediate resolution concerning someone who knew too much, someone who had been honest, someone who had attempted to share with them. Sometimes we easily sense it: it seems better to hide honesty. Yet I'll stick with honesty, regardless of the outcome. At least I attempt to, don't you?

Any desire to hide honesty is not a godly trait. It doesn't take a person of the cloth or a commentary writer to tell you that one. Paul's valuable words in Romans 13:12 and a portion of verse 13 following, inspired me the night I had written those words. By now you know it was during the wee hours, much closer to dawn: "THE NIGHT IS FAR SPENT, THE DAY IS AT HAND: LET US THEREFORE CAST OFF THE WORKS OF DARKNESS, AND LET US PUT ON THE ARMOR OF LIGHT. LET US WALK HONESTLY..." Or as most Bible commentators explain, *'Let us walk as those who belong to the kingdom of light.'* *The One Volume Bible Commentary*, Reverend Dummelow, Queen's College, Cambridge.

Think also upon this for a moment. "...JUST AS HE CHOSE US IN HIM BEFORE THE FOUNDATION OF THE WORLD, THAT WE

SHOULD BE HOLY AND WITHOUT BLAME BEFORE HIM IN LOVE." —Ephesians 1:4.

This speaks of man's love to God and his fellows. Again, this from The *One Volume Bible Commentary*, cited above.

Question: Had I been wrong in pointing out a facility's deficiencies and now their obvious attempts to hide them? No, I had not. I had offered useful ideas for people with AD, ideas that would aid them in not becoming lost and/or injured. I had gone on to share about a man who had sat without eyeglasses for months at a time, perhaps they'd thought he was just another patient, I did not. To me the direct and honest statements could have proved fruitful, especially as that particular man had every right to see clearly. (But in all fairness, sometimes these very lost ones are eventually forced to go without seeing clearly.) I still don't think it's right. I believe it only assists in causing the acceleration of dementia and its obvious deterioration.

You see his inability to see clearly is not habilitating in any way. Instead, it enables him to give up more easily. I'm certain there are those who will say that that patient's just letting go. Well, that's your opinion. I call it folks being uncaring and/or unwilling to work at securing and maintaining a person's dignity. And if he could not retain his eyeglasses, they could have worked to help that, too. They could have provided a necklace or eyeglasses chain. If it were placed upon him in the a.m., and then retrieved daily before he retired, he would have been able to keep them and keep seeing properly. I simply tire of their excuses for neglect, their unwillingness to consider doing good because it's the right thing to do. Their proclamations, *I don't have time for that.* If there is not time for the residents/patients, then another line of work needs to be considered for folks who don't have time.

And so it goes: the man who I understand is by now somewhere else, that man if yet alive, will be awakened and once again seated daily at a breakfast table; a table where in the bareness and dimness of it all and the poorness of his vision, he will yet sit, unattended, forgotten, until the next meal is served. That is, as I said, if he is even yet alive. How I ache for him. Ache for a brother. I indeed ache for anyone in this obvious aloneness that does not have to be alone. This is archaic and unfair, as well as uncaring.

I also ache for the fraternal organization that my sister and I had attempted to contact on several opportunities about getting him eyeglasses. I surely hope it was simply a case of someone on vacation, or that we had the wrong phone number. But it is doubtful. Doubtful and sad. It seems that it is getting to be more and more difficult to assist persons in need nowadays.

In the wee hours I sit, once again scribbling words that will one day be read, I am convinced by Father, so that somewhere someone will read what he or she already knows is honesty. Maybe it's what they already realize, and if we are fortunate, something or Someone will enable folks to take action for those like my old friend, seated at a table all day. Seated alone, unattended, just there, as if he were another piece of furniture; this old friend that I am no longer allowed to visit. (I may yet, trust me.) He became not only someone vision impaired, he also became the man who would no longer hear my voice, and as I could no longer hear his and see his smile and catch that gentle chuckle, I would continue to be haunted by his *Why do I remain lost?* look. Are you familiar with that look? That sense of fear?

It will always be with me. Sometimes I wonder how long it will be until I join the ranks of folks such as this one. It is a natural thing. We all wonder about our own finality.

†

There was another. It hurts me to tell you the story. He had *gotten out* and was fortunately escorted back to his unit. His Parkinson's shake so bad that he could never dress himself, never put his own undershirt on over his sweat-covered body. Most of the time his tortured body was covered in sweat as if he were still back in a steamy Vietnam jungle. It is a place where one can actually see steam rising from the ground, that's how unbearably hot and humid it is! A place filled with leeches and crawling at times with the little man from the north that we called Charlie.

When it was time for Steve's shirt to go back on, I'd often ask him why he didn't ask an aide to help him with it. Then one day I witnessed the answer firsthand: "I don't have all day to put your shirt back on!" a worker screamed at him from across the room. It would be only weeks later, I would learn that God had called this one *Home*. Yes, another one who had gotten out of the facility and fallen down. I often wondered where one of God's angels had been that day. One had not appeared at that place, or Father had decided to take the man *Home*. Either way, it made me sad and mad. The fact that my brother, Steve, is in a better place, just doesn't cut it! *(And yes, Dr. John, this is accountability!)* And it feels good.

There are not injustices solely in the healthcare system. This friend, another one, years ago discovered a crack in a new missile; he would not allow his company to ship it out to the troops. (Thanks, Glenn. I've always been proud of you!) You would not have believed how he explained what he had been up against over that little bit of honesty, that honesty that in all likelihood could have saved several of our troops. What has happened to honesty and pride in workmanship? Our caring and resolve for safety?

Be honest or hide your feelings? Strange and wondrous, how God directs our thoughts. How he continues to guide my hands even with this knotted entanglement of a brain that I must surely possess by now, as I wear this GPS bracelet, as this shrinking mass that causes me to sense that I am ensconced by a cloud or cobweb. Sometimes I get so tired that I call it being fried. It makes for many short nights. I tire more easily, more frequently now. My neurologist friend tells me the feelings are all caused by low reserves, that I just won't be able to do things at full capacity any longer. (I'm sorry, I think we may already have shared that. Perhaps I have too often been through this particular work.)

It reminds me of my family doctor's words (the being honest), to my Doll Face, "Roll with it, Baby." They were well said and filled with great meaning, and clarity.

I feel his leading as I share how God gave us superior brains for wonderful work. Read it in Psalm 8:5-9. The words there tell of our being made a little lower than the angels, to be placed over all other living things. Those words end with some of my favorites: "O LORD, OUR LORD, HOW EXCELLENT IS THY NAME IN ALL THE EARTH!" Now to a commentator's wise words: "…a little less than divine. Man, the only creature made in God's image, stands nearest to Him in the ranks of the universe."

A little lower than the angels? What does it tell us about honesty, and about our wondrous position in life? You can obviously discern that it's not a mere suggestion. I'll tell you what my low reserves tell me. God has created us to do our very best; not only with all the birds and beasts, He has also positioned us to watch out for one another. Just as the wandering lady, yes, another assisted living resident years ago had asked me, (when I found her searching and confused nearly a half a mile from her facility), "How do you know my name?"

I know He calls us each by name and I knew it that day as well. God even cares about our quiet 'whimpering', those senses that we may not be able to express or totally feel perhaps. Maybe we have even been able to mask those feelings for years on end.

"Honesty or hiding?" Bring light to something or hide it away? Sweep it under the old carpet? Ship it out to the troops? How do you sense it all, and what, my friend, what do you choose to do about it? Merely exist for yourself alone, or reach out in an attempt to right a wrong?

Are you aware of the *Veterans of Foreign Wars* magazine article of May 2007, that speaks of a 6 to 800,000 backlog of claims for veterans in need of assistance? *That 100,000 claims are wrongly decided every year?* Are you aware of GAO's Daniel Bertoni's words in that same article: … "after more than a decade of research, we have determined that federal disaster programs are in urgent need of attention and transformation"? A Harvard professor, Linda Bilmes, said, on the average an appeal claim is resolved in 657 days! And that's just on the appeals portion, folks. Is that incredible or what?

†

But let me get back to other healthcare issues, other inequities and injustices, not just robbing the veteran. Another facility? Yes, I've visited many. I recall this one vividly: how when the middle-aged woman 'got out', they later found her lifeless body in a stone quarry. I will not share the grizzly details. Is that what we want for our elderly brothers and sisters, whether we know them or not? Do you really think that ending had been planned for her? That's a topic for a completely different book. Perhaps I'd call it, *The Reformation of the Nursing Home System in America*. How I wish I had the heart and stomach and clear-headedness to author it.

Sometimes honesty can be misinterpreted. I again reflect upon a time not long ago. My nephew, an Air Force veteran, had been killed in an operation supporting the global terrorism demon that will be with us from now on.

I sped to my niece's side and stayed with her a while, her and her two small boys. As young warriors with row upon rows of ribbons appeared kaleidoscopic before my field of vision, I was flung back in time to my rows of ribbons, my combat remembrances. Later, unable to bring myself to attend Luis' funeral, I yet carry a burden about it and have often wondered if my silent honesty was ever understood.

†

My heart has been warmed some, however, as I have seen welcoming committees for returning young veterans in various locations throughout our nation. That has been a grand and worthwhile effort. Congratulations to anyone participating thusly. And THANKS A BUNCH!

Speak the truth or hide your feelings? I will stick with the truth in every situation. Skeptics will come and go. Some of our intellectual types may try to explain why we wander from truth, whether it's to defend a position or to keep some sense of balance within. As for me, I count it my duty as one aligned with God, to walk in the light of His truth, our truth. (It is my fervent prayer that you have not sensed much deterioration of my writing ability or quality throughout this work thus far.)

There is one more item I wish to include while I speak upon honesty. It is a topic many shy away from, for various reasons. Or they do as I have done, and keep it for last. That topic is *intimacy*. I firmly believe that intimacy plays a huge role in the maintenance of those who are living with AD. I am also aware that I do not believe it should necessarily be up to the AD-affected party to be the one who has to always initiate *intimacy*.

Please share that with someone going through this traumatizing unawareness called AD.

Perhaps all I wish to say about this at this time is that I believe this connection is more vital than we have given it credit, or that this is territory that I have read little to nothing about. If you as a caregiver have noted that your patient-partner is no longer capable of, or unsure of what to do about intimacy, I encourage you to talk to your family doctor about it as soon as possible.

It is my belief that this powerful, and deeply hidden showing of tenderness and love is a vital connection for each of us, patient or caregiver. Further, it is my belief that a patient will have longevity if he or she is able to maintain this intimacy for as long as is physically, mentally and psychologically possible. So I am speaking to caregivers specifically now: It may be up to you to carry the burden of this one, and even as easy as it might be for some to dismiss the entire topic, I believe both partners will be better off for having attempted and/or succeeded in maintaining this vital tenet of their relationship. *(That one's free)*.

All-knowing and powerful Master, continue to steer us toward Your light and truth. Enable us to have no turmoil concerning whether to live or not live with honesty. For as we live purely and honestly, do we not do as You'd have us? Do we not care and perhaps assist in causing protection for ones lost and/or possibly abused? Thank You, God, for the best advice of all, that we are to walk in Your light, as You are The Light! You are our lighthouse near so many stony outcrops of certain destruction. You save us during our storms of life; You light the way for us. You lift us up and maintain us! "THE LORD IS GOOD, A STRONGHOLD IN THE DAY OF TROUBLE; AND HE KNOWS THOSE WHO TRUST HIM."—Nahum 1:7. *Help us Father, to be tender to one another for as long as it remains possible.*

—Breathe, Praise, And Big Admission—

God and life itself never cease to amaze me. On the first day of May as I worked on a rewrite of this segment, we had two praise items right off. The first was when a media services lady came to our home to do an initial interview about a taping for

HCTV (Henrico County Training Division). It would be a media services program on AD persons recently diagnosed, myself and others who could yet discuss the disease. I talked about it earlier in my paranoia section.

It hadn't taken me too long to discover that the lady doing the shoot was and is Roberta Fountain, a cousin of one retired Rear Admiral Robert R. Fountain, who was also mentioned in my acknowledgements. Admiral Bob, had been one of my first 'bosses' when I reported to the tiny island of Guam, in the Western Pacific, 1979. It had also been the year I was commissioned. It so made the meeting and the ordeal that I had not looked forward to much more pleasant. Small world. Wonderful world.

The second neat surprise, and one we had long awaited, was noting that the amount deposited to my bank account had become a little larger than usual, thanks to an agency that at long last contributed to my dementia infirmity. What a blessing it would be for us. Perhaps we could slow down some of the phone calls from various agencies seeking their money.

Thank you, Father! Thank you, slow-moving, antiquated (unnamed) system.

This segment then, had been written initially with a twofold thought in mind. As you know, writing causes me to spend concentrated blocks of time reading, studying, relaxing, and exercising my mind and body, routine. One of the worlds I've over the years always had an interest in is the study of yoga. Even though I had never dabbled in it much, I had known a little about yoga from an earlier association with India, having lived in that Asian country (that at one time, believe it or not, had been part of Africa).

I must share that in a yoga work, I had learned of the beautiful new world of proper breathing. I hate to share with you a sad song before I get into breathing, but it is as follows:

Breathe! Just breathe. Yet somewhere, something seems buried so very deeply within me. It's the conscious and/or perhaps subconscious, 'I don't want to learn to breathe, don't want to know about it. I don't wish to feel anything positive associated with this disease.' Unfortunately, all though we (you and I) are allowed that kind of thinking, it is not the thinking I desire for you.

Sometimes indeed, I lean more and more toward becoming somewhat of a recluse. Not good. I encourage AD folks to fight that strange urge. *Fight it!* And I mean fight it with everything within you! And I'll admit that I have not always been successful at this. But then again, everyone needs space at one time or another as well. And perhaps, now and again a little break.

Do you not sometimes feel that we are often our own worst enemy? Once we've been introduced to the inevitable, the bad news, some of us seem to naturally curl up into a comfortable position from long ago: fetal. *(It is a word to me that closely resembles f a t a l.)* It so disables us when and if our attitude remains poor; that is why I spoke earlier of a little break.

Comfortable or scary, or more comfortable being scared. Perhaps we set ourselves up for certain inaction by failing to do anything other than the wallowing in the news or the pews.

We feel fragile and frail, and in a sense we are. Instead of praying to God, we seem to ask to be prayed for. By the way, that's all right, too. Yet we should focus on others more. I firmly believe that, and have been successful at it. I have found, too, that worshiping and seeking God's Face is without a doubt the most exhilarating experience (celebration) that one can have in this visible lifetime of ours! Nothing compares with God. *Absolutely nothing.*

†

I once had met a lady who later died. She had died from the loss of a toe to diabetes. A toe, mind you! Now, I don't want this to sound as if I'm making light of her loss, that I am insensitive to this dilemma, and a rather drastic thing really had occurred, especially when it is an event happening to you. It's easier for me to take in with that kind of thinking.

This lady's particular curse, her maybe longed-for-all-along fate I believe, was that she had simply given up on life. Some would not give up and die from the loss of a toe, or a leg, or even the entire waist-down-portion of himself/herself. The toe, according to physicians, had not been her only enemy. Indeed, she had shown that her attitude had so much degraded her not-so-positive attitude that she had allowed her wounded self to become defeated by it. Yes, I realize that's simplistic and a broad generalization of sorts, yet it's honest and accurate reporting.

On the other hand, as I continue to strive for honesty in all I do, I must confess that if we 'stuff' (hide) our feelings as I heretofore have reported, those emotions will convulse and eventually come out with such force that they will haunt us for a very long while to come, sometimes until death.

Sometimes, and I know this goes against the grain of a few modern-day thinkers, but sometimes rehabilitation is, simply put, not possible. Not only is rehabilitation impossible, this is where *my big admission* takes place. Although what some have believed in and prayed over, and hope to one-day find somewhat true, there is no guarantee that my regimen and/or paradigm will work. Indeed, it is akin to a well-trained shrink grasping for a straw, that tiny thread of relevance or glimpse of the past that will enable the doctor to guide the patient to becoming enabled once again. Off the bench and back in the game, if you will.

Yet please do not hastily cast aside this work, for there is a silver lining and it's worth thinking about; for anything worth having *is* worth working for, waiting for.

That off my soul and mind, I'll get back to breathing, and normal thinking, whatever they are. Breathing is a choice; especially proper breathing. You may have thought it's an automatic process, and in one sense it is, yet if you have ever been caught without breath, or as some asthmatic folks might share with you, realized that you are just a breath away from death, then you more fully understand this premise.

Sometimes a choice is not involved. Then again sometimes we simply cannot do without. Perhaps what I should have more properly said is proper breathing, i.e., yoga-type breathing, is one of the most important bodily functions/happenings. Therefore, we **do** have a choice about the way we breathe. It seems we start out forgetting how to properly breathe, especially if we're never taught, and/or as we grow older.

Perhaps we stifle our own lives, scuttle the ship, therefore speeding up the inevitable. Do we? Yes, sometimes we do. I've been there. Did you know that focusing upon your breathing can increase the intensity of your love-making efforts? (I know, too much information.) That little tidbit is however, quite true.

Creator God has led me to many blessings during these long days and sometimes-longer nights. His benevolence and grace as we suffer in silence are a crescendo of love showered down upon us. Yet again, this disease is a roller-coaster ride, and my car is slowly moving to *out of control*, or at least running low on fuel. But who is not these days?

"CALL TO ME AND I WILL ANSWER YOU, AND SHOW YOU GREAT AND MIGHTY THINGS, WHICH YOU DO NOT KNOW."
—Jeremiah 33:3.

Through God's generous grace and guiding, I, too, have learned at long last how to breathe more properly. I want to share what I've previously hinted at, about breathing.

To more properly breathe, one needs to fully fill one's lungs to capacity and therefore aid relaxation and assist other physiological processes (the working of an organ's processes). I share the layman's version. First, fill the abdomen deeply, then move on up to the thoracic area, now with a huge breath, finally finish the last of this gigantic breath. Fill the top part of the lungs until your shoulders rise. Now slowly release this deep breath through your mouth, that way allowing the toxic 'stuff' to escape. Now try it again; slowly at first. (I have found that I particularly enjoy that process, that more complete breathing technique as I make the rise of a gentle climb when I am walking.) Try it some time. It is refreshing.

Once this breathing technique is mastered, you will be using a greater amount of your lung capacity, be breathing more efficiently and will have learned one of the great secrets, again, of relaxation. I have also noted various great body positions for stretching and relaxation (in yoga). You may wish to consult a yoga book or two about stretching and relaxation. Remember however, I am in no way an expert. I caution you to consult your physician. (It would not be good to have someone find you all tangled up someplace in the midst of a lotus position, unable to free yourself.) I can hear the call now: *I'm stuck in the lotus position, and I can't get up.*

And while we are here, do not forget what we shared about tai chi, earlier. I am more than fascinated by this ages-old technique (or art form) out of China. I wish you well as you continue to make your personal selections. But please, *make a few.*

Back to breathing, a technique I encourage you to adopt if you're ever in the midst of a dilemma, a poor situation, and/or disease. As addressed in a preceding segment, there is a great deal of inhospitality alive and well within our culture(s) today.

One example of inhospitality is how patients/residents of various facilities, nursing homes, and retirement homes, whatever you wish to call them, are sometimes treated. And this is an observation from one who has observed it when *outsiders* are not around to note what is taking place. It happens when they (residents) are encapsulated with the staff, alone, so to speak. And many times that translates into relentless, complete, and sometimes dispassionate control. I am not going to beat this until it becomes a dead horse, yet I have been known to make a call or drop a line to someone in authority (about unhealthy facilities).

I must share with you that it is vital that care partners and care receivers must know that care outside of your personal home is not always up to par. In fact, it can be quite dismal. Once again, as I near the tail end of this work, I encourage you, dear reader, to *just breathe.*

If possible, fix not your eyes upon the negative too long, as I sometimes have. No, I suppose it could also be considered being realistic, knowing what is taking place. Discernment.

Attempt though, to learn as St. Paul did. In his writings he often addresses it one way or another. And the really great part of it is that Paul lived his words as well. Attempt to be at peace, no matter what your lot or condition, was one of those beliefs. It is another way of relinquishing, of letting go. *It is also without a doubt, a position of power.*

I will never let go of this, my longed-for epitaph: *Never give up!* Do not allow yourself to be convinced that you are at the end of your rope, dangling there, totally alone. I realize that sounds somewhat 'preachy' and may not be great counseling. *I simply want you to contemplate that you are never, ever, really alone.*

Speaking of dangling, swinging with ease, breathing is much the same. It is of course a natural, free-flowing gift. Breathing is not only intoxicating; it is part of what keeps us alive and invigorated. There are studies that show as we age, our breathing capacity lessons. Is there some correlation between proper breathing, oxygen, blood and all that? I would suspect so. Persons much sharper, more active, much more fit than me have indeed received the same Alzheimer's diagnosis. Many have already departed. I pray that they first discovered God. (It is noted, for your information; I also live with oxygen during periods of rest; I had heretofore been oxygen deprived.) So is one of my sisters.

This breathing portion is not written simply with the diagnosed person in mind. To me it is meant as much for a caregiver, a close friend, anyone concerned about the person suffering this devastating disease, (and/or the person who loudly snores). Remember this, too, it is the caregiver who unfortunately *holds their breath* the most, in most instances.

That is easily understood. After all, when that hammer-blow comes down, when the news is disseminated, is it not as though the caregiver's whole world has like some kind of Jericho wall come crashing down around them, upon them? The care receiver goes in one direction; the caregiver almost immediately senses a devastation that makes him or her want to head quickly in another. Any direction! Sometimes they do, too.

Does it ever get any better? It is painful for me to report: yes and no. On a recent Saturday afternoon, my wife advised me how she needed my help weeding, since she works and exercises and does this and that, that she could not do it all alone. All I could offer rather meekly was: "I'll help you as I can." Honest, direct, matter of fact. But I tire more easily, more quickly now. Be prepared. Sometimes your very own loved ones forget your plight. Then again, in fairness, perhaps Lucy was assisting me in *pushing through.* And it has worked, somewhat.

What I have learned during this research and the living of this thorn in my side is that although folks attending to you may be doing it out of their love for you, if I have not said it before, I encourage you to accomplish as much as possible for yourself. In so doing, you will be able to go further, to last longer, to be stronger. Who knows, you might even be around for the miracle drug? Or you may be one who God chooses to do a miracle on!

I had written it down some time ago, back when I was yet a licensed driver, wondering where it might one day fit; words I wrote during some hours before the rooster's first sound. He now leads me to share them. Half asleep one morning, my loving wife connected with me somewhere in the house, you may have read it before. We bumped into each other in a darkened living room, or was it that place that I have set up and affectionately call my workplace? Either way, at my side half frantic, "Honey!" she had begun, "I thought you were gone! I heard the car start up!"

All too often our natural conscious or subconscious visits places because of how we have lived our daily lives. *Much has to do with our environment.* I over and over, normally once a week, realize that my mind is incessantly visiting family and friends. And that is not all bad. I'm still here, right? Many of them are all still here. And God? God will always be here, there, everywhere.

—Younger Ones—

The young ones sense dementia's depth somewhat differently than the way Lucy and I sense it, feel it. You can't hide much from kids. They are ones who continue breathing, but you are unsure what they are wondering. Shards of Grandpa's disaster have cut them as well, as it does everyone around me, near me. You cannot live with this deterioration and not affect those near you. It is shown and/or felt, and I'm not convinced it'd be too good to attempt to cover it up. I have done that enough. And I did it for far too long.

†

We've had our share of teenage suicide in this country. Nowadays we seem to be watching even crazier times; kids shooting other kids, naked college parties, fighting children (wanting to film the fights)!

What do you think it is, reader, eroding everything about us? Part of it is because we do not take time for one another, i.e., some families never make time to sit down together for a meal. Many of us forget to be thankful, and we whine about that we do not have. The happiest people I've ever known are ones who daily remember to say *thanks*. Thank You, God, we can walk and breathe and talk and sing. Thank You, Lord, for whatever it is that we are yet able to do.

Senseless actions are not reserved for the young. Look at today's non-breathing men and women caught as childlike prisoners, yet again I'm entering territory above my learning curve. I ask you to forgive my flailing about as I attempt to simply tell you that we need to b r e a t h e. "THEY SHALL UTTER THE MEMORY OF YOUR GREAT GOODNESS, AND SHALL SING OF YOUR RIGHTEOUSNESS." —Psalm 145:7.

The thought and memory of a loving God helps to heal my hurting, and I hope it helps heal you, too. I know it assists my breathing, my having as much quality of living as I am yet able to have.

A recent Memory Walk (for Alzheimer's awareness), with hundreds of people in attendance; a walk to cause and represent a **VOICE** for this disease that pervades our society, was a sweet event. Lucy and I walked three miles, and we were happy to be a part of it; happy to be among those affected by this disease, happy to be part and parcel of this loving family.

†

A picture of one of my grandsons, Victor (by name) and I doing one of our favorite pastimes, fishing, is often brought out. What a time of breathing that is! I always recall that it had been allowing our spirits the freedom to enjoy life more abundantly. It is the unleashing of all those tiny elements that hurt us inside, as we not only make an attempt, but also *do,* fully enjoy breathing our way through this sweet life.

The picture (to me) is a memory of God's goodness. A sweet memory of that first divine breath, His breath. Is not our breathing akin to walking in space? Is not breathing watching with love the 'care freeness' of our grandchildren as they curiously spend time frolicking in tree houses or seeking that next mud puddle that they can plop their feet into, in its deepest spot? Even my cat does it, with her spirit-like form. She's almost snow-white in color and loves splashing at her water dish instead of drinking it. Playtime for her.

Yet that was a while ago, for Snowball is gone and now Ray has taken her place. Thanks to one of my mentors and heroines, Mary Ann. Ray had been found outside prostrate in the grass, rain beating down upon her, therefore my shortened version of rain became Ray.

†

Dad used to say that we would hear him in the wind. Was it his way of saying, *Breathe, I'll never be that far away from you?* (Somewhere I have read words of the wind being God's messengers.) I can't pull all of that out of the old noggin just now.

What a grand morning! I wrote about sun downing, this morning (that morning). As I walked along, hearing the rooster's cacophony, I felt a light breeze kissing my face and sensed that my dad was there, and to me, very real, another Father was there with us. Your Father, and my Father; the Father of the entire universe. It was and is a humbling experience.

†

Take time for yourself caregiver… patient… sibling… and angel at a facility, reader friend. Take time to get away, to rest, to revitalize, to get a view from another vantage point. Take that deep cleansing breath and simply breathe. How calming is God's balm.

For unbelievers: I'm praying that you will one day seek God out, if you really feel that you have not, and are truly a nonbeliever. I have great difficulty convincing myself that there can be any such being in God's universe. It is because I know God can be your fortress and strength, as He is mine. He desires to be your constant Friend and Guide.

Take time, and breathe. Learn of God's enjoyable, enveloping comforting Presence. I pray that you have not felt self-made, or that you have come all this way believing you are on your own. For surely one day you will reach out for a Power above you. I only pray that it is before you are crumpled-up upon your deathbed. And even if you are fortunate enough to 'go out' in the midst of your peaceful sleep, I always remember that sooner or later every knee shall bow… every tongue confess… those words I recall from our magnificent Guidebook. "… TO GIVE LIGHT TO THOSE WHO SIT IN DARKNESS AND THE SHADOW OF DEATH. TO GUIDE OUR FEET INTO THE WAY OF PEACE." —Luke 1:79.

What comfort I find in those divine words; not simply earthly peace, but peace from God. Eternal peace.

Then there is this: "THUS SAYS THE LORD GOD TO THESE BONES: SURELY I WILL CAUSE BREATH TO ENTER YOU, AND YOU SHALL LIVE. I WILL PUT SINEWS UPON YOU AND BRING FLESH UPON YOU, COVER YOU WITH SKIN AND PUT BREATH IN YOU; AND YOU SHALL LIVE. THEN YOU SHALL KNOW THAT I AM THE LORD…" —Ezekiel 37:5-6.

What power and splendor and grace and love God gives each one!

Just breathe, as God first did for you, into you, when He allowed your very existence to begin, and that was long before you encountered your first dilemma, your first joy. This then should count for each of us, but especially for those suffering from a form of dementia. Never think the worst, and *never give up*! I know it is repetitious, but no matter what the odds against you, *Never give up!* **God didn't…. for God will not.**

†

Father God, eternal One who first breathed life into each one of us, we have little hold upon or control over our lives, let alone any control over You. Thank You for breathing life into us. Thank You for sustaining us; but above all, thank You, Almighty, for coming to a stilled place that had been devoid of life, to show us Your wonderful ways. Thank You for leaving Your eternal Home to come here. Breathe on us again. Restore us, and show us Your divine way, Your everlasting peace. Remind us that the clouds are surely traces of Your mighty footsteps. Continue with each of us as we approach our final ending. But let us keep in mind that that final ending is only for an instant. We so look forward to Your coming again. Perhaps Father, perhaps You could guide us in the offered paradigm in chapter twelve, the positive spokes of disease. "*FOR GOD DID NOT APPOINT US TO WRATH, BUT TO OBTAIN SALVATION THROUGH OUR LORD JESUS CHRIST, WHO DIED FOR US, THAT WHETHER WE WAKE OR SLEEP, WE SHOULD LIVE TOGETHER WITH HIM.*" —I Thessalonians 5:9-10.

What a blessed, glorious and eternally awesome thought. A love-thought draped in joy!

TIME ZONES (Slipping away…)
Wayne Glenn TERRY

Chapter 15

—Capstone: Four Wayne's, Fame, Shame and Pride—

(A fast-paced walk was my intention before writing the capstone chapter. I had begun underneath bright clear shards of crystal cast upon God's vast black and beautiful canopy. Soon I commenced a slower stroll, something that comes quickly when you're awake too soon and are an AD patient too long. When I began to awaken more and to walk more confidently, smelling the sweet air of an unseasonably warm May morning in Virginia, (way back then), it had been a good start, for I'd had no combat nightmare, nor a weird dream brought about by my AD medicine.)

The cock's crowing and the fading of God's stars seemed almost simultaneous. Having come full circle from dawn to dawn, I mulled over the previous day's bounty that had obviously spilled over into a new dawn. As day began to come alive I no longer felt as one who had given up on anything, no longer felt combative in any way. I felt hopeful, thankful, renewed; my mind and heart more attune to God's.

It was then I whispered age-old words: *"More of Thee; less of me…"* The caring, sharing, love and prayers that I have sensed throughout the beginning of my transition from where I was to somewhere else, this *slipping away*, this time, has pointed me to the most remarkable event of this world traveler's entire life. It flashed before me in a rather obscure manner. Yet whether I had encountered my hairnet fog-like feeling or a sense of simple listlessness, it had for me been a wondrous, blessed privilege, realizing how many tired eyes God would one day allow to read this work. Dare I say He might direct to read or listen to it?

I was and am in hope that their lives might be somewhat better for it. And it would all be through His remarkable grace alone. There was and is another blessing, friend, one I would know until my knowing is no more: that God can accomplish whatever, wherever and whenever He desires. I will continue, thorns in my side, to walk with Father in the light. Should the darkness become more abundant, I'll call upon Him to allow and enable me to recall that He not only goes with us, but also allows us to be strong and filled with great courage and strength, even unafraid.

After all, it is God who is my Collaborator, as well as my Savior, Redeemer and Friend. It is God who strengthens me and lightens my heaviest burdens. And He will do the same for you.

This Awesome Collaborator has also shown me, the small collaborator, these comforting words, "FOR I CONSIDER THAT THE SUFFERINGS OF THIS PRESENT TIME ARE NOT WORTHY TO BE COMPARED WITH THE GLORY WHICH SHALL BE REVEALED IN US. FOR THE EARNEST EXPECTATION OF THE CREATION EAGERLY WAITS FOR THE REVEALING OF THE SONS OF GOD. FOR THE CREATION WAS SUBJECTED TO FUTILITY, NOT WILLINGLY, BUT BECAUSE OF HIM WHO SUBJECTED IT IN HOPE, BECAUSE THE CREATION ITSELF ALSO WILL BE DELIVERED FROM THE BONDAGE OF CORRUPTION INTO THE GLORIOUS LIBERTY OF THE CHILDREN OF GOD. FOR WE KNOW THAT THE WHOLE CREATION GROANS AND LABORS WITH BIRTH PANGS TOGETHER UNTIL NOW. NOT ONLY THAT, BUT WE ALSO WHO HAVE THE FIRST-FRUITS OF THE SPIRIT, EVEN WE OURSELVES GROAN WITHIN OURSELVES, EAGERLY WAITING FOR THE ADOPTION, THE REDEMPTION OF OUR BODY. FOR WE WERE SAVED IN THIS HOPE, BUT HOPE THAT IS SEEN IS NOT HOPE; FOR WHY DOES ONE STILL HOPE FOR WHAT HE DOES NOT SEE? BUT IF WE HOPE FOR THAT WE DO NOT SEE, WE EAGERLY WAIT FOR IT WITH PERSEVERANCE. LIKEWISE, THE SPIRIT ALSO HELPS IN OUR WEAKNESSES. FOR WE DO NOT KNOW WHAT WE SHOULD PRAY FOR AS WE OUGHT, BUT THE SPIRIT HIMSELF MAKES INTERCESSION FOR US WITH GROANINGS WHICH CANNOT BE UTTERED. NOW HE WHO SEARCHES THE HEARTS KNOWS WHAT THE MIND OF THE SPIRIT IS, BECAUSE HE MAKES INTERCESSION FOR THE SAINTS 'ACCORDING TO THE WILL OF GOD. AND WE KNOW THAT ALL THINGS WORK TOGETHER FOR GOOD TO THOSE WHO LOVE GOD, TO THOSE WHO ARE THE CALLED ACCORDING TO HIS PURPOSE.'" —Romans 8:18-28.

At the time of this first writing (way back for me) and now this final rewrite, it was at that moment (back then), my twenty-four-day-old grandson was being wheeled into heart surgery, and I then was writing and reading of my love for another Daniel: "HE REVEALS DEEP AND SECRET THINGS; HE KNOWS WHAT IS IN THE DARKNESS, AND LIGHT DWELLS WITH HIM." —Daniel 2:22. *Might Your light once again remain with Daniel, Daniel Wayne, loving God, I had then written. That had been some 18 months ago.*

Know you why I refer to myself as a collaborator? It should not take much for it to penetrate. It is because I know God is the Author of Life! So lest there be any doubt whatsoever, I have counted it the greatest honor having had our Lord God, the Prince of Peace, guiding many of my thoughts, every word, each moment I spent awake at this keyboard. So much was taking place when I wrote these words with His able assistance, and my mind not always clear. Actually, I was the assistant, was I not?

God had guided the doctors' hands with Daniel. My great representative and his wonderful staff had been working my paperwork for a government agency regarding my compensation request. At the same time as Grandson Daniel Wayne was in heart surgery, Grandpa Wayne was on his way to the oral surgeon. That dentist was and is Charles Wayne Martin, and Daniel Wayne's daddy is Charles Wayne Terry! *The four Wayne's*! How about that?

You see, our loving God was in the midst of all of that, even as He comforted my family and friends and so many other believers at the very same moment! Is there any wonder why God is often called Awesome God? And yet He calls us by name! Who can understand that? And one more thing, God has finally granted me a psychologist (at the time of this writing, back then), appointed by another agency, who finally stated: "If they deny you this time, Mr. Terry, for dementia, you need to try again." Of course, as you now know, that was some time ago, and things are into an entirely different segment by now, an entirely different *time zone*, if you will.

Never give up! friend. Not ever. Our loving God can fight all these battles for you at the same time. He can prevail throughout all of them, too. He wins battles daily for believers around this world, and who knows, perhaps others as well. And so it is, this life and story is all about Him. About Creator God and His great love for *you,* for us! Even as I had all those years often wished I could have died in war, instead of learning of, as well as knowing of the death of so many friends, I am now learning that God can even forgive us when we are grieving in vain. But I don't necessarily believe that either. That is, some grief is quite necessary, and is not in vain.

He even forgives us as we fight to be assisted by a government that appears not to care, a government's *leaders(?)* who seem incapable of listening. Today's Republic. That should be difficult to say! Yet I feel bound to share this. It is simply that the processes for veterans and non-veterans alike take too long, they are too cumbersome, too antiquated. Too many people die before they are awarded assistance, and that, simply put, is not right!

My heart has all too often ached when I heard the stories: too little, too late, or for some widows and widowers, not at all. I have a personal friend who was a door gunner on a chopper during the Vietnam War. His primary care physician recently proclaimed (at the time of this final rewrite) that *none* of his 'stuff' is connected to PTSD, so today's Republic's stellar representatives **denied** my friend's request. You might have some idea how this writer feels about that. That, my friend is part of the *shame.*

Lord, be it known now as I paraphrase it, I pour contempt on any pride. I ask You Father to bless our troops, and this work. That it might be as a shining star in the hands of all who need it; all those who might read it. Might their feet be set to dancing, always, always, always. Thank You, God, for that special dream, chapters ago; that dream where I smiled deeply into each tiny face and each head that nodded up at me as I spoke of fishing and flying kites and going for ice cream. Thank You, Jesus, for special good-bye times. Thanks for each and every good-bye.

*Thanks for special visits, and those who never gave up on my Lucy and me. Might we live each day as if it were our last farewell. Thank You Lord, for Your torturous wonderful way, how You so humbly trod the treacherous path to the cross. That, dear Lord, was and is the **fame**. Thank You for that amazingly wondrous rising after death! Thank You for loving us before we were ever formed. Omnipotent Creator, I see Paul's words once again:* "EYE HAS NOT SEEN NOR EAR HEARD, NOR HAVE ENTERED INTO THE HEART OF MAN THE THINGS WHICH GOD HAS PREPARED FOR THOSE WHO LOVE HIM."

†

My grandson, Daniel, the new one, had arrived home on the 28th of March of that year. How ironic that it had also been the very day the entire world and Lucy and I would watch with our collective breaths held as we listened to a (female) British sailor's monologue (no doubt prepared for her).

You may recall that I had discussed <u>Delta Force</u> earlier, its early formation and a little about Colonel Charlie Beckwith (back in chapter three). Now, as we listened to the young British hostage sailor's supposed light-hearted words, I could not help but wonder what might be going through Colonel Beckwith's head.

Whatever his thoughts and emotions, and mine; regardless of the outcome of this additional saber rattling, I realized again that it had been just another point in history, another time we would need to be in special prayer for this fading world. Being a resident of Virginia (a commonwealth for lovers), I must mention another sad happening that seemed devoid of love that day. For on April 16, 2007, (way back then), a crazed gunman took many lives at the Virginia Tech campus. If I could say anything good about it, it would be about so many stories of college heroes, students and a few professors, stories worthy of another type of *fame*, folks that had reached out and taken selfless action to save others.

The drama that unfolded that day is akin to my disease, it singled out no one in particular, a vast cross-section of cultures was affected that day. And that, too, is a ***shame.***

As this work nears completion for press, I cannot help but think of the many memories this Virginia disaster must have triggered for others, not solely for me. It has only assisted me in the reverberation of a very sad song. How can anyone not understand our personal grief? How can they deny us closure? It must be for God alone to shore us up; at times I believe that's the case. God, and you alone; God and myself alone.

These are strange and challenging times, my friend, times of hearts hidden and hands outstretched, of closed minds, (that sometimes includes mine, too). In early May it was becoming evident that my world was growing ever larger. I just didn't realize how much larger until HCTV, a media services outfit out of Henrico County, Virginia, taped Lucy and I (and others) for a documentary on Alzheimer's disease. (I must here insert that Roberta Fountain and her co-worker won an Emmy for that presentation! My *kudos*!) (I also think this is something mentioned earlier on, so my apology to editors, readers and all of you who can remember better than I.)

The world got bigger still, as the next day I began packing to depart the house. It had been another experience that I wish I had shared with the producer of my taping, sweet Roberta Fountain. Lucy and I were not three miles down the road when I thought, *Wow*! Roberta should have heard about this! I must have been in a state of denial, or I'd simply never had this particular sensation strike me quite this way before. I was leaving everything I knew behind. That included my safe haven. My shaking caused me to take a panic pill as we rolled along and I held on for dear life!

Suddenly I felt, as I'd earlier hinted, yet never so strongly that I was becoming as one grandson, Nathan, had said. Nathan is the one who calls me "that grandpa that lives far far away." Not only was I on my way to feeling far away, but I also felt more childlike, less and less in control; the world that I'd had control over farther behind me with each spin of the wheels.

Bound for another niece's wedding, Amber, I was excited for the young couple and myself, it would be a mini-reunion; only one sibling missing, the illusive Gale (Dancing Waters). Hopefully it would not be the last real look into Momma's eyes for me.

The striking setting atop Afton Mountain, Virginia, was not only breathtaking, it was God-filled. I had always felt as though I was in His mighty palm when amidst the mountains. This time was no exception.

In the tiny, pre-World War I chapel, nestled within a valley, surrounded by gravestones, some of which were washed so smoothly by time and elements that they were unreadable, the early evening vows had momentarily removed the world's stress from me, at least my personal worldly stress.

Some time later I gathered more precious pictures of other nieces and nephews, their children, and one I particularly favored of my brothers, this old boy and two other Navy guys. We stood with a Malaysian-like abundance of greenery in the background. When you have that many Navy men together, that's a lot of firepower. It was and is also a lot of love.

I learned one last very valuable lesson at that wedding/reunion/retreat. The heart's true value is **L O V E.** *There is no possession or desire greater than love.* I could not help but recall my neurologist's quiet words to me only a week before (back then). "Make the most of it. Live, love and laugh as much as you can." He had been spot on once again.

The next day Lucy's daughter, Jessica, capped it off with the birth of Abigail! I trust they used the Scriptural spelling. Poor Lucy I thought as I typed those words, always on the go.

A letter went out on the 10th day of May, one to a myriad of creditors and helpers. It once again addressed my PTSD request. Some of it addressed today's apathy within our Republic, or my waning excitement perhaps concerning a country I so love. A place I had been so proud of back in the sixties, when I had reenlisted to go to war.

The letter had been my last volley at those supposedly in positions of leadership, well, at least somehow appointed or voted-in, aren't they? I advised them that though I was not pending death, not yet, or even bankruptcy, that I did feel AD is very similar to dying. You know what helped me more than the mailing of those fourteen little envelopes? It was something I'd read many times before. "THE LORD IS RIGHTEOUS IN ALL HIS WAYS, GRACIOUS IN ALL HIS WORKS. THE LORD IS NEAR TO ALL WHO CALL UPON HIM, TO ALL WHO CALL UPON HIM IN TRUTH. HE WILL FULFILL THE DESIRE OF THOSE WHO FEAR HIM: HE ALSO WILL HEAR THEIR CRY AND SAVE THEM." — Psalm 145:17-19.

And then, suddenly, just days before this final rewrite I was so filled with pride as one named Tiffany, stood beside her mother in the front of our wonderful congregation. I was as proud as I had been (way back when). You see, Tiffany, is on her way to Iraq soon, to do what many of us can no longer do for this great country. We laughed and silently cried, shared and prayed for her, for them, for all of us. August, 2008.

Later, in October, (sounds funny now, as it was way back again), at the time of rewrite number umpteen, I was in Heaven as brothers, sisters and Momma, and the good Lord only knows who else, arranged for Lucy and I to join them all on an ocean cruise. I had felt so buoyant and blessed as I greeted and held each one as if it might be the last time. You see, some of my dreamland stuff, when I do dream, is now so outlandish, sometimes so devoid of any warmth whatsoever, so strange that I am often afraid to lie down again. It is quite possibly one of the reasons I sleep for such short periods of time.

Remember this, dear friend, in this brief summation, this *capstone*. The story is not about you, not about the tiny baby Daniel, not about the latest hostages. It's not about Virginia Tech's campus carnage, and it's not about the four Wayne's, or even this one Wayne.

It's not about institutions or government arms that are sometimes forgetful of their own. It's not even about processes or psychologists and psychiatrists. It's not about the thousands upon thousands of veterans who have completed applications and yet await replies. And it's not about all the thousands who died before they ever received assistance. That has to be one of the greatest shames I can think of in the history of our country.

It's not about my fear of leaving my safe haven, or the birth of Jessica's sweet new baby girl, Abigail, who by the way takes nothing away from *revved-up* Rebecca. And it's not about my last cruise. That last slice of Heaven attended by sweet Lucy, Momma, and all my siblings and other relatives that I so hold dear, respect and love.

There is so much more I could have said about an old sailor's visit to the ocean once again. Any ocean. The feeling of sun and salt-sea air on your face again is much akin to going home (for a sailor). And then to be surrounded by so much love, so much you love period. It's not even about all these crazies that we keep calling candidates, who mostly run around resting on their laurels and hardly ever say anything new or even impressive. Yet I know it's not in the talk, don't you? Even the golden-sounding notes seem tarnished to the ears of us tired of sensing that *"We the people",* just doesn't seem to be the case anymore. (Then again, I did sense some good things when Pastor Rick Warren, who'd written *A PURPOSE DRIVEN LIFE*, questioned the final two candidates on the sixteenth of August, 2008. Thanks, Rick.)

The story is not even about a previous publisher who had the gull to ask for my manuscript, one who then returned it to me after 7 months! Talk about a sweet house and staff! Yet now you know the actual outcome, and that another house has come to bring the work home, and to your doorstep as well.

No... you see, this story is about our God, the King! It is He who is to be exalted on high! It is not about what we have obtained or believe we've earned in life, for all belongs to God, and you and I are merely passing through these *time zones.* As for Father, He who was and is and always shall be, God is the one who shares, gives, and out-loves each of us! That's just the way it is.

"FOR THE LORD SHALL DESCEND FROM HEAVEN WITH A SHOUT, WITH THE VOICE OF THE ARCHANGEL, AND WITH THE TRUMP OF GOD: AND THE DEAD IN CHRIST SHALL RISE FIRST; THEN WE SHALL BE CAUGHT UP TOGETHER WITH THEM IN THE CLOUDS, TO MEET THE LORD IN THE AIR: AND SO SHALL WE FOREVER BE WITH THE LORD." —I Thessalonians 4:16-17.

✝

Father, I praise and thank You for two good women: Jean, who was at Daniel Wayne's heart surgery when I was far-off and could not be there, and my sweet Lucy, the Lucy who stood with tears in her eyes on Easter Sunday as I attempted <u>He's Alive</u>! to Your honor, in Your church. That same Lucy whose flannel pajamas that I bump into from time to time in the night's midst. Gracious Lord and Ascender unto God, I so tire of crying about assistance due to older veterans and myself, when I have been so showered with Your tenderness, abundance and love, all that really matters. I turn my face towards Yours.

I cannot help but picture a young lad in poverty-stricken India, some thirty years ago. He had knocked upon the side window of our shiny vehicle with his stumpless limb, his nose half eaten away. He had no shoes at his young age, perhaps ten or twelve. (It is difficult to tell one's age when a body is raised with malnutrition and/or only enough to daily get by.) There had been no childlike gleam in his tired, bloodshot eyes. My then 12-year-old son had responded to my quip, my words: "All the beggars do that" with, *No, Dad. He's really hungry.* His words hit hard, once again reminding me that you cannot hide much from children, especially children. As Chuck continued to stare through the back window of our air-conditioned carriage (they would call it in that land) he stared long and hard, as if he were somewhere lost.

†

Prince of Peace, forgive us for dwelling on any lack of luxury when in fact we have utilized far more than we ever deserved. Not only do we daily consume far too much, we often turn our collective backs on Your hungry ones around the world. And then again, in all fairness: this nation is still filled with many wonderful people who give much and often. Amen? Oh Holy God, let us not lose sight of the faceless street urchin who is one of Yours as much or perhaps even more than we. I have set the teeth on edge enough about my particular thorns, and what I have felt are abuses to others and myself. And sometimes I wonder, are we yet a Godly nation? Father forgive us, forgive me, as You have promised. I have said more than enough, and too often have forgotten my wonderful travels to lands where masses yet struggle daily simply to survive. Please God, forgive us, forgive the Wayne's, and forgive me for wanting to die in war when You in fact allowed me to survive. How I wish every shame could be erased. Shame on a country that has often forgotten its veterans; shame is sometimes what I have so often felt for myself, but more often it was for the orphaned beggar who worries not about rating boards or battles of years gone by. As You know, Lord, his battles—the estranged beggar's battles are daily, and they are about survival! Forgive us one and all. All praise and glory to You, Father Friend.

<u>To my AD friends and loved ones</u>: It is my prayer that you never even think about giving up! But if and when you do, only give up for God. Fully have your heart and soul and mind focused on Him: For He is the Light; and you will be guided to and by His Light. And in that you will bask. Think about that for a moment: You will bask in God's Light that outshines all other lights,... *forever!*

What wondrous love is this? And almost lastly, thanks for giving me ***pride*** once again, as I said farewell to Tiffany, one of

New Hope Fellowship's wonderful and godly young representatives. She is such a shining example displaying hope and strength and love for something above herself. Indeed she is giving back.

†

In an attempt to explain the fervor and fury for this work, what for me may be one of my last, I have striven to say as much as I could about this condition that I am now living, my day-to-day existence. I am hopeful that anyone with dementia might take this next portion of the work and make a copy of it, and feel free to place it upon your refrigerator or the wall where you rest.

They are words from the heart, and they are words that I am hopeful you might be able to adopt for yourself. For in this sonnet's words I reveal my love, and though not said, my continued prayers for you and yours. I pray you might have seen a glimpse of God on several occasions throughout this work. And that you will be strengthened by the words and by God.

Thorns Allowed

Lord of the Universe Your love is awesome.
Lord of my soul You are pure compassion.
Sweet Lord, epitome of passion,
Your life is filled with sacred action.
Forgive our feeble ways of living this life,
How beautiful Lord, I have loved this life!
With scattered dreams I approach Your holiness,
Heart overflowing I marvel at Your tenderness.
Thank You for guiding this work for those diseased.
If nothing more, might it make You, God pleased.
I sense Dear God, Your grace and how I've been freed,
Remember friend, we cannot God out give
It is this, it is for God, you and I live!

The thorns allowed, are our privilege.

By the way, did I forget to tell you, debilitated or healthy, never give up; God will never give up on you. He looks forward to your grand Homecoming! It is what you were created for.

Reader friends may contact the author at retcwo@yahoo.com. He looks forward to hearing from those living daily (and in the night) with various debilitating diseases and affectations as well as those caregivers and family members associated with the care receiver. He also cannot forget the proud and faithful warriors of this nation whether they served in combat or non-combatant roles. Be leery though, replies may be slow or at least as time permits. If you do not hear from him, you will, at the very least be in his daily prayers.

In March, 2009, the author will make himself available for a limited number of speaking engagements and/or signings for this calendar year. Please be so kind as to contact Mary Smith at stillbrook@comcast.net for scheduling and availability dates of the author. Although this is your event, please also recall that the author tires rather easily at times, and does not always go at the pace of other forward-looking folks who may be in better health and/or in an earlier onset-stage of their diagnosis.

Indeed, there may be times when the author will need to be accompanied by a caregiver, especially if it is a lengthy journey which might require his oxygen and or an overnight stay. And when an escort is necessary there would of course be additional funding needed to be made on/from the requestor's end of the phone. Especially since this is a work of philanthropy: that is, monies from this endeavor are distributed to Alzheimer's associations and to research and development. (Mary's note): It would also be appreciated if you could give me an approximate number of books your group will require, as the author utilizes his work for a reference when speaking and would be more than happy to entertain the notion of a signing sometime during your meeting/occasion/celebration. Any books left over are your responsibility, not the author's.

So then, this labor of love, ministry, or whatever you wish to refer to it as, is accomplished at no expense to the author, and as well, he retains none of the monies garnered from it. One reason for that is because there may be arms of the government who believe that this veteran who fought so diligently to eventually achieve compensation for his disabilities may appear to be suddenly intact and fully capable of functioning, when in fact it is simply that he is pushing-through and doing the best he can with his diseases and affectations in order to carry on this labor of love in behalf of others who may not be able to push through. Therefore, there will be times that the author is not that 'shining star' or beacon of hope you might wish would be in your midst. Yet, as always, with Father's assistance, he will do his best and NEVER GIVE UP!

Every writer should contemplate 'holding something back.' I believe for me it is the following: The author really feels no need to warn anyone who might attempt to challenge his compensation that they will encounter resistance, but because he has become aware of the 'games' our leadership often plays, (as anyone alive in today's environment can understand), he allows the caveat to stand. *'These words were not crafted in despair, but as I looked to that Light, and you should, once having read the contents of this work, realize what Light I speak of...'* (Author's words.) He also knows the thoughts and hearts of other agencies and the veterans of a land who have fought diligently and have sometimes died for this great nation. God bless and preserve America. Let us be now renewed, and together look forward to that re-emergence (with God at our side). Let us never be allowed to be oppressed by any culture or nation or even a small arm or governing body of a nation..., for we yearn to breathe free, just as so many other members of our citizenry, who have been blessed to arrive at this great melting pot of freedom!

'As this work is closer and closer to going to press, part of me is hopeful that you did NOT read the November 2008 article in the magazine published by and called the Veterans of Foreign Wars, specifically pages 24 through 28. No... I will back down slightly': The article addresses the sad and almost rampant suicide of returning war veterans, as well as those who have been around a while. Thankfully, towards its end there is a box entitled: 'Sources of Help' and therein the number for the 24-hour suicide hot line as well as new and growing organizations and/or campaigns to be of benefit to the devastating affectations of wartime trauma to our beloved uniform-clad heroes, past and present. (That number is IMPORTANT, and is: 1-800-273 TALK.) The article is by a free-lance writer, Janice

Arenofsky (Thanks for your marvelous work, Janice. God bless you.)

Author: Yet be not too hung up on my words or words of anyone else other than the One. Here is something needed to be heard: *'Come unto Me....'* This is the core of the Savior's sacred and wonderfully beautiful message. For when we come unto God, and become dead to the things of this world, it is then that we learn about maturing in Christ, accepting His gifts and walking in His Light and love. And although this is only a portion of His gift, recall that God will also sustain you in that new place you most assuredly will enter: and in that place of love and peace and joy and so much more you will learn that those things are because of what He has done, NOT what you or I could ever do. And please… please never forget that we are to pray and to praise Him always. Amen.